WHAT OTHERS ARE SAYING ABOUT THIS BOOK. . .

"Trzeciak and Mazzarelli have aggregated a definitive look into how health care workers and patients alike can produce better outcomes and feel happier through adversity—all through implementing compassionate behavior. *Compassionomics* shows that by focusing the lens through which the brain perceives reality, lives can be changed for the better. This is a must-read for health care leaders looking to implement lasting cultural change, health care employees wanting to change patient's lives, and consumers who need to take charge of their health care experiences."

— Shawn Achor, *New York Times* bestselling author of *Big Potential* and *The Happiness Advantage*

"Health care must evolve from treating diseases to caring for people and their families. This is much more than a semantic difference. In the Health Transformation Alliance, our experience with more than 4 million people clearly validates what Dr. Trzeciak and Dr. Mazzarelli so eloquently argue—compassion and empathy are essential to better health care. Caregivers who practice these principles encourage people to take ownership of their health care—a result that fosters better health outcomes. I hope this book catalyzes a compassionate revolution in our health care system."

— Robert E. Andrews, CEO of the Health Transformation Alliance

"In *Compassionomics*, Drs. Trzeciak and Mazzarelli conclusively demonstrate that the power of compassion in medicine is undeniable. Well-researched and comprehensive, the book will be a valuable tool for anyone with a desire to reestablish the primacy of compassion in health care."

— Rana Awdish, MD, FCCP, author of *In Shock: My Journey from Death to Recovery and the Redemptive Power of Hope*

"The health care professionals of today are constantly challenged by moral choices, whether from organizational pressure, societal expectations, or their own personal code. Under all of the mounting pressure, one constant guiding principle—to "do no harm"—drives us to do whatever we can for the benefit of the patient. *Compassionomics* provides the evidence that one simple tool, compassion, can affect not only the outcomes for our patients, but also the financial health of our organizations and the well-being of our providers."

— Donald M. Berwick, MD, MPP, president emeritus and senior fellow of the Institute for Healthcare Improvement and former administrator of the Centers for Medicare and Medicaid Services

"It is easy for hospitals—and thereby physicians—to believe that focusing on volume, rather than quality, will drive results. No one, however, comes into healthcare with this idea in mind; it is a byproduct of an age where systems are stretched thin on time, talent, and resources. Physicians want—and need—to practice in environments that emphasize focus on outcomes and experience. They want—and need—to know that their work makes a difference. With meticulous research, *Compassionomics* blends these ideas—that physicians can feel proud about their work and produce high-quality outcomes for patients. By focusing on compassionate care, Drs. Trzeciak and Mazzarelli provide a simple, but effective, roadmap toward positively affecting both physician burnout and patient engagement. *Compassionomics* can help restore the hope for everyone in health care that they can have a positive, meaningful career that is driven by human connection, not numbers."

— Robert Bessler, MD, founder, chairman and CEO of Sound Physicians

"Today, in these challenging times, we often bear the burden of the pace of change and complexity of care. This book offers so many ways to think about compassion: for patients and families, for your team and colleagues, and for yourself. I can't think of a more important path than compassion to get to the Institute for Healthcare Improvement's Triple Aim—better health, better and safer care, and lower costs. This is the best book I've read in years."

— Maureen Bisognano, president emerita and senior fellow of the Institute for Healthcare Improvement

"The foundation for providing sustainable, quality care is simple: compassion. If we want to keep healthy people out of hospitals, support the most vulnerable of patients or those with long-term issues, and lower health care costs, compassion must be at the heart of all these interactions. Drs. Trzeciak and Mazzarrelli's deep dive into the data that support this fact is second to none. In *Compassionomics*, they have built the thorough and inspiring case for anyone who wasn't already convinced that compassion was essential to health care and empowered those who are firm believers."

— Jeffrey Brenner, MD, senior vice president of integrated health and human services at UnitedHealthcare Community & State and MacArthur Fellow

"It goes without saying that compassion is a crucial element for healers and healing. Except that we don't have enough emphasis on compassion in today's health care system. This dearth of compassion in training and practice makes *Compassionomics* timely, important, and vital. Whether you are a clinician, administrator, or a health care patient (i.e., all of us), its message is a call to action for true change in the way we deliver and receive care."

— Arthur Caplan, PhD, Drs. William F. and Virginia Connolly Mitty professor and head of the Division of Medical Ethics at the NYU School of Medicine

"Hope is central to progress in health care. And hope is a byproduct of compassion. In *Compassionomics*, Drs. Trzeciak and Mazzarelli provide not only compelling evidence of how simple acts of compassion positively affect patient outcomes, but they also demonstrate that compassionate care improves the experience of those who work in healthcare. Instilling compassion throughout the delivery of health care will enable the health care industry to advance into the future."

— David L. Cohen, businessman, attorney, and chairman of the board of trustees of the University of Pennsylvania

"This well-researched book on such an important topic will be welcome news to all those who strive daily in the front lines of health care provision. They know well the importance of compassion and its effect on outcomes and overall well-being—not just for patients but for the providers themselves. With it we win, without it we struggle. This is also a directive to leaders to include compassion as a key criteria in recruitment and promotion. My congratulations to the authors for bringing it center stage."

— Michael J. Dowling, president and CEO of Northwell Health

"My mentor for compassionate care was my physician father, the co-founder of HCA Healthcare. As he frequently said, 'It's not bricks and mortar and equipment that make a hospital. It is the warmth and compassion and attitude of good employees that leads to quality care.' Trzeciak and Mazzarelli's findings not only provide us with data to show how compassionate care achieves measurable improvement to patient outcomes, but also shows gains in fiscal health and employee satisfaction. Those of us in health care owe it to our patients to review the facts, implement the solutions, and make the essential personal connections that can change health. This book is a vital step forward in transforming health care as we know it."

— Senator William H. Frist, MD, heart transplant surgeon and former Republican Senate majority leader

"*Compassionomics* is a very important book for everyone engaged in health care, including physicians and nurses, health care administrators, educators, and especially patients and their families. It documents the impressive and growing evidence base that supports the critical role that compassionate care plays in shaping outcomes in clinical practice. From ancient times, scholars have described both the 'art' and the 'science' of the practice of medicine. *Compassionomics* presents a wonderful distillation of the science behind the art of a healing and health-promoting doctor-patient relationship."

— Robert N. Golden, MD, dean of the School of Medicine and Public Health and vice chancellor for medical affairs at the University of Wisconsin-Madison

"We work so hard to master diagnosis and therapeutics that it's easy to forget that all patients get better faster if they receive compassionate care, as marvelously laid out by Trzeciak and Mazzarelli. However, it's as true for us physicians as it is for our patients: friends are the best medicine, and isolation kills. This isn't a 'self-improvement' book, but we should all read it, because we'll all find in this book a path to feeling better."

— Stephen Klasko, MD, president and CEO of Thomas Jefferson University and Jefferson Health

"Drs. Trzeciak and Mazzarelli's proclamation acknowledging the power of courageous caring, now rooted in quantified science, is so timely and essential in the inevitable transition to a consumer-focused healthcare system. This book is a must-read for health care providers—indeed, a blueprint for a high-performance culture."

— Calvin H. Knowlton, BSc Pharm, MDiv, PhD, chairman, CEO, and founder of Tabula Rasa Healthcare, Inc.

"A wonderful, evidence-based book that is a must-read for the health professions—if not every citizen-patient—especially, the leaders of health care. Drs. Trzeciak and Mazzarelli show, in no uncertain terms, that health systems that fail to embrace and prioritize compassion are missing out on caring fully for their patients and for their clinicians and employees. As the

Gold Foundation has championed for 30 years, compassion makes a dramatic, measurable difference in health care—and this book proves it."

— Richard I. Levin, MD, president and CEO of the Arnold P. Gold Foundation

"If you've ever been a hospital patient, you know that compassion on the part of the caregivers is perhaps the single most important factor affecting your experience. The medical profession, somehow, has failed to see this. It took Drs. Trzeciak and Mazzarelli to make this incredibly important and long overdue observation on compassion. Let's hope this book is the basis of a revolution on health care."

— Steven Levitt, *New York Times* bestselling author of *Freakonomics*

"If you or a loved one has ever been ill or worried about your health and have had the good fortune of being cared for by a compassionate health care professional, you probably don't need to be told that compassion matters…a lot. And if you are a health care professional who has been able to offer your care and compassion to those who are ill and vulnerable, you certainly don't need to be told that a sense of connection through compassion is what rewards and sustains you.

So why does compassion remain on the sidelines as 'nice,' but not absolutely essential, in the ways we train health care professionals and teams and in how we deliver care and evaluate health care organizations and systems? Drs. Trzeciak and Mazzarelli are trying to rectify this. By sharing stories about illness alongside highly readable summaries of decades of scientific research, they make a compelling case that compassion is vital to our collective health and well-being. Perhaps heightened public and professional awareness of the value and importance of compassion will enable us to raise our voices together to insist that compassion is a necessity, not a luxury, in health care."

— Beth A. Lown, MD, associate professor of medicine at Harvard Medical School and chief medical officer at the Schwartz Center for Compassionate Healthcare

"Research has long shown that the kind and caring gesture of a health care provider can have significant beneficial effects on a patient's health—yet medicine often operates like compassion doesn't matter. We now finally have a book on this fascinating topic that will empower patients to choose providers with a heart. Thank you, Drs. Trzeciak and Mazzarelli, for helping shape medicine's future for the better."

— Emma Seppälä, PhD, science director of the Center for Compassion and Altruism Research and Education at Stanford University and author of *The Happiness Track*

"At a time when precision medicine has the potential to make the 'art of medicine' obsolete, this book demonstrates that the power of healing lies not just in our genome, but also in our soul. Through their journey and scientific explorations, Trzeciak and Mazzarelli remind professionals and patients alike what is truly important and offer a formula for improving health care, one patient at a time."

— David Shulkin, MD, ninth secretary of the Department of Veterans Affairs

"Every patient welcomes the emotional comfort afforded by a health care practitioner with a good bedside manner, but now comes evidence that compassion from caregivers isn't only proper and just—it actually saves patient lives. This book is eye-opening—between the data and the stories that bring the data to life—for those that provide care as well as those that receive care, which makes it a great read for everyone."

— Michael Smerconish, author, columnist, and host of SiriusXM's *The Michael Smerconish Program* and CNN's *Smerconish*

"In the dawning of the compassion-centric paradigm of medicine with the new cutting-edge science of compassion, we have been in need of someone to evaluate the hundreds of studies we already have that demonstrate how compassion in medicine positively affects medical outcomes, patient experience, business profitability, and even the well-being of clinicians themselves. Trzeciak and Mazzarelli have done a thorough systematic review of all the studies to date that address the hypothesis that 'compassion matters.' They have given us the gift of a very insightful and concise summary of this work and related it to what we do practically every day. Clinicians will feel a validation of their call and their intuition that compassion really does matter. *Compassionomics* provides the scientific evidence that anyone who practices medicine without compassion is scientifically outdated and committing malpractice."

— Dominic O. Vachon, MDiv, PhD, director of the Ruth M. Hillebrand Center for Compassionate Care in Medicine at the University of Notre Dame

COMPASSIONOMICS

THE REVOLUTIONARY SCIENTIFIC EVIDENCE THAT CARING MAKES A DIFFERENCE

STEPHEN TRZECIAK
ANTHONY MAZZARELLI

Foreword by SENATOR CORY BOOKER

Published by:
Studer Group
350 West Cedar Street, Suite 300
Pensacola, FL 32502
Phone: 866-354-3473
Fax: 850-332-5117
www.studergroup.com

ISBN: 978-1622181063

Library of Congress Control Number: 2018968569

This book was published by Studer Group Publishing, the exclusive publisher for Studer Group. Studer Group, a Huron solution, works with healthcare organizations to help them achieve and sustain exceptional improvement in clinical outcomes and financial results.

Printed in the United States of America

This book is dedicated to all of the nurses we have ever worked with and that we continue to work with. Your compassion for patients has saved many a life and has inspired us to be better doctors.

CONTENTS

FOREWORD:

We are often led to believe that sentiments like compassion, love and kindness are expressions of weakness rather than signs of strength. And we are often all too ready to give in to the false belief that meanness somehow equates to toughness and that empathy is empty of power.

But the evidence—in our shared history as Americans and here in this book—suggests the opposite.

Our country was founded on the understanding that if we were going to make it, we would need to make an unusual commitment to one another. To be clear, our founders were imperfect people, and our founding documents are saturated with examples of bigotry and sexism, but these imperfect individuals succeeded in putting forward a more perfect ideal. When our founders wrote, *"we mutually pledge to each other, our lives, our fortunes, and our sacred honor,"* as the last line of our Declaration of Independence, they were also declaring our *interdependence.* They were declaring that our destiny as Americans would always be indivisible.

A commitment to one another, to a common purpose, and to our highest ideals—that is the powerful force that has always sustained us as a nation. We are a country that rightly values the ethics of self-reliance and rugged individualism, but we also understand the necessity of our larger communal ethic—that our greatest achievements as Americans are the result of collective struggle and sacrifice.

At the heart of that ideal is our ability in any moment, to choose to exercise compassion.

Throughout our history, it has been those seemingly small acts of kindness, decency, and compassion that have affected change. And as this book demonstrates, practicing compassion—caring for one another, and seeing the struggles of others as our own—isn't just the right thing to do, it's the smart thing to do.

In *Compassionomics: The Revolutionary Scientific Evidence that Caring Makes a Difference*, Dr. Stephen Trzeciak and Dr. Anthony Mazzarelli focus on the health care system to show us the tangible and significant ways that compassion makes a crucial difference in health care. They show that compassion isn't just a nice idea, it's a practice that when put into action improves lives.

At the heart of this book is the truth that it's precisely how little effort compassion really takes that makes it so impactful. In every moment, in every industry, we all have the power—and the time—to be kind.

—Cory A. Booker
United States Senator

PREFACE:
An Explanatory Note on the Origins of this Book

"Life's most urgent question is, 'What are you doing for others?'"

—Dr. Martin Luther King, Jr.

For researchers, a scientific awakening may come in a single watershed moment, a powerful event or observation that instantaneously changes their entire worldview and the purpose and trajectory of their research career. In other instances, a scientific awakening takes a much longer arc and is the product of a cumulative, iterative, and evolutionary understanding that is experienced over time. The genesis of this book was actually a little bit of both.

Dr. Stephen Trzeciak is a physician scientist (a self-described "research nerd") and specialist in intensive care medicine. He had been conducting clinical research on critically ill patients in the intensive care unit (ICU) for more than a decade. Trzeciak was not in the market for an awakening.

Quite the contrary. In his estimation, everything was going exactly as planned. His research program was hitting every milestone for "success." He was publishing his research in some of the most prestigious medical journals, receiving research grants from the National Institutes of Health to fund his work, and was frequently invited to speak at major scientific conferences both nationally and internationally. Life was good. There was no plan to mess with "success."

And then, an unexpected question from a 12-year-old turned everything upside down and literally made Trzeciak change the trajectory of his life's work. That 12-year-old was his son, who was in seventh grade at the time.

One evening, Trzeciak's son came into his study at home and asked for help. "Dad, I have to give a talk for my class at school," he said. "I know you give a lot of talks. Can you help me prepare mine?"

Trzeciak thought to himself, "What a great father-son bonding opportunity!" So he said, "Of course!" and asked his son to tell him more about his talk.

Then his middle schooler pulled out a piece of paper from his assignment book and laid it on Trzeciak's desk. This was the assignment:

"What is the most pressing problem of our time?"

Trzeciak was taken aback. He had never pondered the most pressing problem of a generation during his own formative years. But he was eager to engage now.

"Okay, whatcha got?" he asked.

His son jumped right in, with both feet. "Okay, I have these slides, and these images, and these references, so I'm almost there...," he explained.

But while the topic was meaningful, Trzeciak was not buying it. "Do you *really* believe that this is the most pressing problem of our time?" he asked. "Because if you do not *really* believe it, you are not going to convince anybody else in your class."

As you might expect from a 12-year-old, his son wanted to just finish what he'd started. "Look Dad, I just have to get this assignment done, okay?" he explained. "And I have everything I need to tell *this* story."

But Trzeciak advised him to stop and take some time to really *think* about it. *Take some time.* "Of course, there is no one single most pressing problem of our time," he suggested. "But you need to find the most pressing problem of our time…for *you.*"

Two nights later, after careful consideration, his son returned with what he really believed was the most pressing problem of our time. In *his* eyes. Through *his* lens of experience. The topic that he ultimately selected is not what's important. What's important is that his son actually *believed* in its importance. And he prepared a talk that not only his classmates found compelling, but he did, too.

This mentoring experience gave Trzeciak pause. As he contemplated his life's work, he realized that he was not following his own advice; he'd dedicated his hard-won skills and talents to research, but never examined whether he was applying them to the area he believed to be *the most pressing problem of our time.* Why had he never asked himself that question?

Here's why: research scientists typically develop a successful career in a particular way. It usually goes something like this: "I'm at the University of ABC, and here we are experts in XYZ, so that's what I'm going to study." Or, "At my institution, we have a one-of-a-kind research instrument; no one else can get these data, so that's what I'm going to focus on." Or, "My mentor is Dr. Jones, and he is a world-renowned expert who can open doors for me, so I am going to do what he does."

These are the usual blueprints for "success," as it is typically defined, in research scientist career development. Hopefully, someone who follows this path is actually quite interested in what they end up committing their careers to, and it's something they find intellectually stimulating and meaningful.

But, do they actually believe that what they are working on is the most pressing problem of our time? And, more importantly, what would happen if they actually *did?*

Thus began a period of great introspection for Trzeciak. He asked himself: Was his research at the time meaningful? Definitely. Was he working on what he believed to be the most pressing problem of our time? Definitely *not.*

This was going to torment him. He knew he had to find the most pressing problem of our time, for *him.* Through *his* lens of experience. And in his scope of influence as a physician scientist. But what was it?

You could say he was having an existential crisis. He felt lost.

As fate would have it, that is precisely when he bumped up against a request from someone who would ultimately lead him to his answer.

Dr. Anthony Mazzarelli is a physician executive, emergency medicine physician, lawyer, and bioethicist. At the time that Trzeciak was first beginning to consider the most pressing problem of our time, Mazzarelli was newly promoted to chief medical officer at Trzeciak's institution, Cooper University Health Care.

Mazzarelli had responsibility for leading a practice of more than six hundred physicians at a major academic health system with more than $1 billion in annual revenue. Like most C-suite physician executives, Mazzarelli was charged with the critically important goals of improving patient experience and physician engagement throughout the entire health system. But initially, it was not clear to him where to start.

He was well aware of the data that demonstrated an epidemic of burnout among health care providers. And he knew that burnout was directly linked to compassion fatigue and depersonalization—an inability to make a personal connection with patients—among caregivers.

Through his own clinical experience and intuition, he knew that this must have meaningful effects on patients and patient care. But he could not *prove* it. Not yet. He needed data, in order to compel others in his health system to make a meaningful change in how they would care for people. He needed help.

So Mazzarelli turned to an unconventional choice. He called in the institution's top physician scientist, Trzeciak, to do a systematic scientific evaluation of these topics that were traditionally considered "touchy-feely" in the domain of medicine.

Mazzarelli's thinking was this: if there were scientific data linking better human "connection" with better patient outcomes, then there was hope. The academic faculty at Cooper—who insist upon practicing evidence-based medicine (appropriately so)—would be more likely to buy into new initiatives to improve the patient experience. And, frankly, Mazzarelli needed to be convinced himself. So that's why he asked Trzeciak to get involved.

In their initial meeting, Trzeciak thought Mazzarelli was crazy. Literally *crazy*. Trzeciak actually had no interest in getting involved with what he then considered to be "soft" science. Mazzarelli and Trzeciak had been colleagues for years, practicing alongside each other.

However, now Mazzarelli was in his new role and technically Trzeciak's new boss. Not wanting to disappoint a colleague—or the new chief—Trzeciak nodded a lot and pretended to look super interested in the idea. (Maybe you've had this experience yourself?)

In that meeting, Mazzarelli laid down the charge. "Here's the question," he said. "Does treating patients with more compassion really matter? Does caring make a difference? Does it matter in *measurable* ways? Put as much scientific rigor to it as you possibly can. I need you to 'science this up!'"

Science of caring? Trzeciak used to think that science and caring were mutually exclusive. Of course, he always believed that compassion was a moral imperative and that health care providers have a duty to treat every patient with compassion. It's a cornerstone of the art of medicine. But scientific evidence? Really? However, his charge from Mazzarelli was clear.

Fortunately, Trzeciak already had training and extensive experience in synthesizing a body of evidence in the biomedical literature: a methodology called systematic review. Trzeciak figured that he would quickly search the available science—check all the boxes—to show that he applied some legitimate methodology, and then be able report back to Mazzarelli the bad news that there is no scientific rationale for caring. Then, he assumed they would be left with just the conventional rationale—that caring is the *right* thing to do.

After that, he figured he could go back to his search for his most pressing problem of our time. Or so he thought. What happened instead was nothing short of an awakening for both of them.

What they kept coming back to, over a two-year period of synthesizing all the data, was one distinct element of human connection, and that was *compassion*. The data on compassion was eye-opening indeed. Epidemiology data indicated that there is currently a *compassion crisis* in health care. Literally, a crisis.[1]

But, there was also crystal clear evidence showing that compassion could affect patients and health care in not only meaningful, but also measurable, ways. As Trzeciak dove deeper and deeper into the data he shared with Mazzarelli, a clear picture emerged for both of them.

The presence of compassion has the power to improve patient outcomes, and its absence can lead to devastating, and even fatal, consequences. Additionally, it has substantial impact on health care costs, both to patients and to the overall health care system. The insights that the data provide to both caregivers and health care leaders has the power to change both the delivery of care and the way in which health systems are managed.

It was an awakening to a body of evidence that was actually right in front of Trzeciak and Mazzarelli all along. In fact, it has been right in front of everyone in medicine all along. Decades of research, hundreds of studies… converging almost all in the same direction. It just had never been synthesized before, in aggregate, with a rigorous scientific approach. For both Trzeciak and Mazzarelli, it was a truly transformative experience. Compassion science became an obsession.[2]

And that is how you know you have found the most pressing problem of your time. You get out of bed differently in the morning. You put your feet on the floor differently, with purpose. For the first time in their lives, Trzeciak and Mazzarelli found that they did not need alarm clocks anymore.

It was time to get up and go! The most pressing problem of our time—through their lens of experience—needed them. It was a clear departure from the science Trzeciak had been working on during the course of his entire research career. (But major departures are common when one finally identifies the most pressing problem of one's time.)

For them, the most pressing problem of our time is the compassion crisis. Both in health care and, more broadly, in the world today.

That was the watershed moment of this scientific awakening, when they realized it was all about compassion. This became the "why" for this book.

The iterative part of the scientific awakening was the two-year-long journey through all of the data on the power of compassion. That is the "what" of this book.

But the end result is an awakening indeed. Once you see the pattern in the data, it is impossible to *unsee* it. It becomes impossible to ignore the effects that compassion (or an absence of compassion) may be having all around us every day.

Ultimately, this book is not about what Trzeciak and Mazzarelli think, nor is it what they believe, but rather it is what they *found*...

Compassion matters.

Now that they see it, they feel the need to share it. And not just data, but also compelling and fascinating patient stories from the front lines of medicine that bring the data to life.

And that is how this book came to be.

INTRODUCTION:

"Love and compassion are necessities, not luxuries. Without them, humanity cannot survive."

—Dalai Lama

The picture typically painted of early man is one of the rugged, self-sufficient hunter-gatherer: a mighty warrior whose equally rugged partner is tending the hearth back at the cave, training their offspring how to survive alone, if necessary, in the harsh environment.

This fits the notion of Charles Darwin's "survival of the fittest" evolutionary theory—where it is imagined that the strongest and toughest are pitted against each other so that they can pass on their robust, superior genetic material to the next generation.

Then, as the story goes, as humans became more "civilized," they looked up to the heavens, as well as down at their tools, and human reason took over. They began to develop a moral compass that led them to feel empathy for each other and to treat each other with compassion. Ultimately, this theory evolved into the modern day concepts of morality.

That's the narrative that everyone is used to hearing. However, it's not quite how it actually happened.

You might be surprised to learn that Darwin did not originate the phrase "survival of the fittest," for which he is known. It was actually Herbert Spencer, a notable British biologist and anthropologist, who coined the phrase after reading Darwin's views on evolution. Over time, this framing became misconstrued into the widely-held belief that Darwin's views were justification for aggressive, gladiator-like behavior.

What Darwin actually concluded was different and even more remarkable. According to Darwin, the communities with the greatest compassion for others would "flourish the best and rear the greatest number of offspring."[3] In short, the body of scientific evidence supports that compassion actually *protects the species.*

This makes sense: the hunter that shared his extra earnings with those in need could count on others to do the same when he needed help in the future. It was the other-focused, more compassionate humans that were the ones that survived to pass on their genes.

At a very basic level, research supports that compassion is something intrinsic to the human condition. For example, studies show that infants will resonate with the cries of others in distress and that toddlers are naturally inclined to altruistically help others.[4, 5, 6] There is a general consensus among scientists that compassion for others is, in fact, *evolutionary.*[7]

Furthermore, compassion is integral to the belief system of almost all world religions and has been a fundamental moral imperative in essentially all cultures and civilizations throughout history. This makes it much less likely that the practice of compassion for others was the product of human reason and much more likely that it is the manifestation of scientific benefit for advancing the species.

Compassion is also considered integral to the provision of health care. Compassion *is* explicitly included in the American Medical Association's (AMA) Principles of Medical Ethics, with item one stating that, "A physician shall be dedicated to providing competent medical care with compassion."[8]

In the United Kingdom, compassion is considered to be one of the core values of health care, according to the National Health Service (NHS) Constitution.[9]

But what *is* compassion exactly?

> **Compassion is defined as the emotional response to another's pain or suffering, involving an authentic desire to help.**

The etymology of the word is a derivation of the Latin words "pati" and "cum," which together mean "to suffer with." But a precise definition of compassion is necessary as a starting point for this book. Nomenclature matters in any scientific domain to ensure that comparisons are "apples to apples."

Most scientists define compassion as the emotional response to another's pain or suffering, involving an authentic desire to help.[7] It's different from empathy, which is the feeling and understanding component (i.e., detecting and mirroring another's emotions and experiencing their feelings) because compassion also involves taking *action.* Feeling empathy is a necessary precursor (or prerequisite) to motivate acts of compassion; so the terms are related, yet they are also distinct.

There are actually neuroscience underpinnings for this distinction in terminology. When people are studied with a brain imaging test called functional magnetic resonance imaging (fMRI), which can detect subtle differences in cerebral blood flow, there is higher activity in areas of the brain that are firing at any given moment.

When a person experiences empathy—the feeling component—the pain centers in the brain light up. That person is experiencing another's pain.[10] But when a person is focused on compassion—the action component of trying to alleviate another's suffering—a distinctly different area of the brain, a "reward" pathway associated with affiliation and positive emotion, lights up.[11, 12]

So neuroscience supports what is borne out through our own experience: encountering another's pain can, in fact, be painful for us, but taking action to alleviate another's suffering is a rewarding, positive experience. You can think of it like this: empathy *hurts,* but compassion *heals.* Accordingly, the key distinction here is that empathy is *feeling*; compassion is *action.*

Another critically important distinction is that compassion is not simply being kind or nice. As compassion is defined as a response to another's pain or suffering, it is implicit that human suffering is involved. Responding to that suffering is the essence of what it means to be human. If one lacks compassion, one is essentially lacking humanity.[13]

Compassion (or a lack thereof) can have a powerful effect on human beings—not just the receiver of compassion, but the giver too.

This being the case, perhaps it should be no surprise that compassion (or a lack thereof) can have a powerful effect on human beings—not just the receiver of compassion, but the giver too. Evolutionary science supports that compassion has benefited humankind collectively, but is it also possible that compassion has a meaningful and measurable effect on people *individually?* If so, how can that be examined through science?

The answer is to study the people that are the most vulnerable, those in the most need of compassion, to make them the subject of scientific inquiry. These ideal subjects would have the greatest capacity to be "responders" to compassion.

Rigorous review of the literature finds that these data already exist; they are the patients studied in the domain of medical science. In other words, health care is the optimal "laboratory" to test the effects of compassion at the individual person level.

It turns out that researchers in medicine have already been studying this for decades, through more than two hundred published medical studies that speak straight to the science of compassion. When you gather all of these studies together and look at them for the first time collectively, what you find is quite remarkable.

Traditionally, compassion has been confined to the *art* of medicine, completely distinct from the *science* of medicine. But, in this book, you will see the evidence that supports the overlap between these two areas and that there can be compelling science behind the art.

We call this emerging field of science "compassionomics." Simply stated, it's the scientific evidence that caring makes a difference. Just as genomics is the branch of molecular biology that studies the human genome and its function, compassionomics is the branch of knowledge and scientific study of the effects of compassion on health, health care, and health care providers.[14] In this book, you will see the evidence for the impact of compassion on each of these things.

People in health care have always understood that treating patients with compassion is the right thing to do as a moral imperative. Therefore, the vast majority of people in health care do not need a change of heart. They know that patients *ought* to be treated with compassion.

However, few health care providers realize the extent to which compassion matters. They do not realize how powerful their compassion can actually be. Science shows it's a game changer. Accordingly, the aim of this book is not to change people's hearts, but rather to change people's *minds*—by sharing the overwhelming scientific evidence about the effects of compassion on patient outcomes, patient safety, provider well-being, employee engagement, and organizational performance.

Once you understand the data, it changes your mind. You'll realize that your compassion can be more powerful than you have ever known. And when you come to realize the power of your compassion for others, you will want to use it every opportunity that you have.

CHAPTER 1:
The Compassion Crisis

"Our lack of compassion stems from our inability to see deeply into the nature of things."

—Surya Das

If you have ever been the good Samaritan that has stopped at the scene of a motor vehicle accident, you may have witnessed what paramedics notice all the time: the scene can be unusually quiet, despite the presence of wrecked vehicles, shattered glass, and, sometimes, a few people with injuries. There is typically a sense that the chaos is over, and while a few people may need some medical attention, fortunately, the majority of the time there is not a life-threatening injury.

This was not the case on a snowy stretch of highway outside of Uppsala, Sweden on February 27, 2007, when two commuter buses packed with passengers collided head-on. One of the bus drivers lost control in the icy, slushy conditions while trying to pass a parked truck on the side of the road.[15]

The result was devastating. One bus was completely annihilated, and one bus was sheared in half. It took several fire engines, multiple medical helicopters, and ten ambulances to respond to the accident and sift through the twisted metal for survivors.[16] The rescue circumstances of the scene, between the environmental surroundings and the incredible extent of the damage to the buses, was such a complex and time-consuming rescue operation that it later became a reference point in a disaster medicine textbook.[17]

Tragically, six people died, but miraculously 56 people were saved.

Five years later, researchers asked the question, "What do the survivors remember?" They interviewed every survivor and, using a rigorous qualitative research methodology, they found two common themes in the data.[18] The first was completely expected: many spoke of the physical pain that they experienced at the moment of impact. It is not surprising that the experience of such physical pain is seared into one's memory.

But the other theme that came to the surface in this study *was* surprising. Another aspect of the event was also cemented in the memory of the 56 survivors: a lack of *compassion* from the caregivers at the hospital. This finding is even more striking when one learns that these individuals were actually taken to multiple different hospitals. Yet, they all had the same experience. A lack of compassion is what they remembered the most *five years later*. This study is eye opening, indeed.

The Scope of the Problem

Before diving into the data on the lack of compassion in health care, perhaps the question should be asked: "Is there decreasing compassion in our society in general?" Maybe health care is just following general trends.

For example, the political divide in America is growing. As this gap widens, people are becoming less and less comfortable with those who hold views other than their own, regardless of whether they are conservative or liberal. According to data from *The Atlantic*, there has been a steady increase of both Republicans and Democrats who would be upset if their child married someone of the other political party. In 1960, it was essentially a non-issue among parents, with about five percent from each party that would be displeased if their son or daughter married someone from the other party.

Today, about *forty percent* of parents would have a negative reaction about party intermarriage![19]

This unwillingness to look outward from one's own "bubble" to those that have differing views is, ironically, one of the few things that members of both United States (U.S.) political parties share. By remaining in a bubble, it's like everyone is becoming unable to see each other's humanity. There is no way to show compassion if one cannot see another's humanity.

A recent survey study found that half of Americans believe our society in general is not compassionate and does not place a high value on compassion for others.[20] The preponderance of data indicates that people are becoming significantly more self-focused and less other-focused. Our disposition is shifting away from compassion for others, and this shift appears to be accelerating over time.

For example, a meta-analysis from the University of Michigan synthesized data for more than thirteen thousand U.S. undergraduate college students and found that students' dispositional empathy (and specifically, students' empathic concern for others) declined sharply from 1979-2009, and the decline in empathy was picking up speed over time.[21]

> Empathy is feeling; compassion is action.

Because empathy (the feeling and understanding component) is a prerequisite for compassionate behavior (the action component), this study speaks directly to the state of compassion in America. While these were studies of college students, do not be so quick to dismiss this data as simply the selfishness of youth or isolationist attitudes of a generation.

In fact, it turns out that grown-ups may be the ones actually at fault here. In a recent study from Harvard University, researchers surveyed ten thousand U.S. middle and high school students from 33 different schools and asked them what they believed their *parents* valued the most.

They found that nearly two-thirds of our youth feel that their parents do not value caring for others as much as they value achievements and accolades.[22] While parents may deny that they explicitly say this to their children, this study offers solid evidence of a generation that has internalized this message from older Americans.

Perhaps the most striking data is from a recent Pew Research Center study that found fully one-third of all Americans do not even consider compassion for others to be among their *core values.*[23]

> One-third of all Americans do not even consider compassion for others to be among their *core values.*

These recent studies on the state of compassion in the general population are important new data points, but the backdrop for the data was established decades ago in a famous study conducted by renowned Princeton University psychologists John Darley and Daniel Batson. Their classic experiment—a study of compassionate helping—found signs of a compassion crisis way back in 1973, even among people from who compassion is most expected.[24]

Darley and Batson studied students at Princeton Theological Seminary (i.e., pastors-in-training). They randomly assigned the seminarians to either an intervention arm, in which they received a talk on the biblical parable of the Good Samaritan (i.e., a message of compassionate helping for a stranger in distress), or a control arm that received a talk on an unrelated, non-helping topic.

Immediately afterward, the students were instructed to walk to another building for their next assignment. On their walk, they encountered a stranger in need: disheveled, lying on the side of the road between two buildings, moaning, obviously in distress. The man slumped over on the ground was what they call a "confederate" in psychology research. In other words, the stranger in distress was an actor who was part of the experiment.

What Darley and Batson learned from their experiment was truly striking, in three particular ways. The first was the overall rate of a compassionate response, regardless of the arm of the study to which the seminarians were randomized. Overall, only *forty percent* of the seminarians stopped to help the man in distress. Keep in mind that the other sixty percent who did not stop to help were also studying to be pastors of a church.

The second striking finding was the fact that the seminarians randomly assigned to hear the message of the Good Samaritan were no more likely to stop to help. The message did not matter.

The third striking finding was what they found to be the major determinant of compassionate helping (i.e., what was going on in the minds of those who did not stop to help). That result is truly fascinating…so much so that Chapter 8 is devoted to it. But the key point to remember now is that a majority of well-intentioned people failed to show compassion to a struggling stranger, even those with explicit instruction to do so.

So is the data from the bus crash the exception or the rule? Is health care an exception to what is happening in the rest of society? Isn't health care supposed to be different? Special? Like the seminarians who walked right past the stranger in distress—failing to be good Samaritans—do health care workers walk right past patients in distress?

The evidence in the biomedical literature is clear. The data for a lack of compassion in health care is just as striking as the data are in the general population. In fact, given the evidence of an erosion of compassion in the general population, it was likely only a matter of time before the epidemic infected health care. Make no mistake: at the present time in medicine, there is a serious compassion crisis.

Let's Go to the Data

Let's take a quick tour of the evidence on compassion in the health care domain. In one study from Harvard Medical School published in *Health Affairs*—one of the best-regarded health policy journals in the world—researchers surveyed 1,300 patients and physicians and asked the question, "Is the U.S. health care system compassionate?"[1]

> Nearly half of Americans believe that the U.S. health care system and health care providers are not compassionate.

The result: physicians and patients were both split on this. Nearly half of the people in the two groups—both patients and physicians—said the U.S. health care system was *not* compassionate. Even more interesting: when researchers asked this same group of patients and physicians if U.S. health care *providers* were compassionate, three-fourths of physicians agreed they were. Physicians gave health care providers the benefit of the doubt.

But patients? Not so much. Nearly half of patients said it's not just the system that's the problem...they said that the providers in the health care system are not compassionate. This study was quite rigorous in its methodology, so there's really no question about whether these results are valid; this is how patients feel.

In another survey study (a follow-up to the original *Health Affairs* report), the researchers found that 63 percent of health care providers say they have observed a decline in compassionate care over the past five years.[25] It's a downward trajectory.

These findings are corroborated by many other studies. Here's another: In a large-scale survey study, researchers found that 64 percent of patients in the U.S. said they've had a health care experience with a meaningful lack of compassion. And yet, in the same study, 87 percent said kind treatment by a physician is more important than other key considerations in choosing a health care provider—including wait time, travel distance, or cost.[20]

Since the U.S. has the most expensive and, in many respects, the least effective health care system in the world, it would be easy to just point to cost pressures and an unwieldy health system as the cause of all of the ills within the U.S. system, including issues surrounding compassion for patients.[26]

However, it's not just the U.S. that is experiencing a compassion crisis; it's worldwide. A public inquiry into the Mid Staffordshire National Health Service (NHS) Foundation Trust in the United Kingdom found, among many quality concerns, a widespread and striking lack of compassion from health care providers.[27] This report prompted then-Prime Minister David Cameron to call for an urgent renewed focus on compassionate patient care in the NHS.[28]

Similar data are found in Ireland. A survey study conducted in collaboration with Harvard Medical School found that for patients in Ireland, health care providers commonly fail to meet patient expectations for compassionate care.[29]

Obviously, a big part of compassion for patients is making a personal connection, because it is a key element in seeing, feeling, and understanding another's pain or suffering (i.e., empathy). As discussed earlier, feeling empathy for others is what motivates a person to respond to them with compassion.

So it stands to reason that if one has difficulty making a personal connection with another individual, then compassionate behaviors are much less likely to occur. There is actually a ton of data on this subject of the inability to make a personal connection, and it is all relevant to the compassion crisis. It's the research on the burnout syndrome among health care workers.

Research has identified three hallmarks of burnout: emotional exhaustion, a lack of personal accomplishment, and depersonalization.

Decades of rigorous research have identified three hallmarks of burnout: emotional exhaustion (being emotionally depleted or overextended), a lack of personal accomplishment (the feeling that one can't really make a difference), and depersonalization. Depersonalization is the inability to make that personal connection.

Specifically in health care, it's an inability to make a personal connection with patients. With respect to health care providers and compassion, depersonalization is the phenomenon where health care providers find it easier to think about their patients as a cluster of symptoms rather than a whole human being.

For example, thinking of the patient as "the chest pain in room six," rather than knowing the patient in room six by name and as a person with very personal fears, anxieties, and worries. This is an important hallmark of the burnout syndrome. A recent Mayo Clinic survey study of 6,880 U.S. physicians found that *35 percent* of physicians are so burned out that they are manifesting high levels of depersonalization.[30] Interestingly, that is the exact same proportion—35 percent—of physicians who were found to have a high level of depersonalization when researchers studied 1,393 family physicians in Europe.[31]

So it's not just a U.S. phenomenon. It's everywhere. When depersonalization is combined with emotional exhaustion, it culminates in compassion *fatigue*—literally running out of compassion for patients.

Burnout Starts Early

Trainees are also at risk. In one University of Pennsylvania study that followed 47 physicians in training over their intern year (i.e., the first year out of medical school), there was a sharp increase in depression; one-third of students experienced it.[32]

Depersonalization rose over time in the students studied, as did emotional exhaustion. As you might expect in light of these developments, researchers found that these students also experienced a reduction in empathy for patients over their intern year.

This study was building upon research published in the *Journal of the American Medical Association* (*JAMA*) that showed empathic concern decreased over the first year out of medical school for junior doctors.[33] And without empathic concern (the feeling component), there can be no treatment with compassion (the action component).

Unfortunately, burnout is a hot topic in medicine today because so many physicians and nurses, in every stage of their career, are struggling with burnout and its consequences. Look for more about the link between compassion and burnout in chapters to follow, but for now, just recognize that the association between the two is well documented in the medical literature.

The thing is, taking care of patients and working in health care is not just a job; it's a calling. Health care providers share in the most intimate aspects of people's lives, often in their darkest and most difficult moments.

> The compassion crisis could turn the profession of health care providers from a calling into a *job*.

The relationship that caregivers have with their patients—whether a physician, nurse, or any type of health care provider—is supposed to be grounded in both the art and the science of medicine. But the data shows quite clearly that some of the art is, in fact, disappearing.

In other words, the compassion crisis could turn the profession of health care providers from a calling into a *job*. There are 18 million health care workers in the U.S. alone, so this is a huge problem. If these clinical interactions are devoid of compassion, the relationship between caregiver and patient could become essentially no different than any other customer service relationship. That just can't be allowed to happen.

Why not? Health care *needs* to be a calling. Walking with people through the worst, most intimate moments of their lives is a sacred thing. That requires a level of personal interest and investment by health care workers. When patients' health and well-being are at stake, time, emotion, empathy, and compassion should be non-negotiable.

But multiple studies indicate that many health care providers aren't even hearing their patients' worries. So it's no wonder that many patients experience a lack of compassion. In one study published in *Annals of Internal Medicine*, researchers recorded the audio from primary care office visits and found that 77 percent of the time, physicians interrupted patients before they completed their opening statement of concerns.[34]

How long did they wait before interrupting the patient? *Seventeen seconds.*[34] The study that produced this data was published in 1984. At that time, the medical community took notice of this finding. As a result, a large number of medical schools, training programs, and continuing medical education programs added communication skills and techniques to the curriculum to address this issue.

Then a repeat study entitled "Soliciting the Patient's Agenda: Have We Improved?" was published in *JAMA* 15 years later. The new time to first interruption? Twenty-three seconds. Better, but still short of the time that the researchers found that patients actually need to state their main concern.[35]

How are we doing in the most recent look at this data? Worse. Much worse. A 2018 study from the Mayo Clinic now clocks the time to first interruption at 11 seconds![36] By the way, researchers have found patients only need, on average, 29 seconds to state their main concern.[35]

Do Health Care Providers Believe It?

Here's the funny thing...in so many studies, patients agree there is a compassion crisis in health care today. After compilation of all the scientific studies, but prior to writing this book, we were interviewed by *Philadelphia Inquirer*'s Stacey Burling who wrote a front-page article that highlighted the evidence for a compassion crisis in health care.[2]

> There is abundant data that physicians routinely fail to demonstrate compassion.

Within 24 hours, more than 30 markets picked up the story off the *Associated Press* wire. There was a widespread, intuitive, and immediate understanding of this problem based on the repeated personal experiences of people all across America—especially those who do not work in the health care industry.

The idea of a compassion crisis really resonates with most people. But health care providers are less sure of this and often don't believe there is really a problem. They seem to be in denial.

However, there is abundant data that physicians routinely fail to demonstrate compassion. In one University of Chicago study supported by a federal research grant from the Agency for Healthcare Research and Quality (AHRQ), researchers analyzed hundreds of audiotapes of surgeons' clinic visits with patients.[37]

What they found was that these consultations had a narrow biomedical focus. There was very little discussion of the emotional and psychological aspects of the problems those patients faced with their health condition. Furthermore, when rigorously measured, the researchers found that only *0.5 percent* of statements by surgeons expressed any compassion. Less than one percent!

"But the Docs *I* know Are Compassionate"

It's interesting how often people have critical opinions of others but are much less likely to have the same critical opinion of themselves (or others close to them), despite similar behaviors. Perhaps that's just human nature?

Here's one example: The polling company Gallup has found that while people may have a very low overall approval rating of Congress, they often have a much higher approval of their own representative in Congress. This number goes up even higher if they know the name of their representative.[38]

In the same way, health care providers may believe and acknowledge that other providers are not compassionate, but still believe *themselves* to be so. They may also believe that they are more compassionate than their patients actually find them to be. It is what psychology researchers would call a cognitive bias. They seem to have a "blind spot" on their ability to relate to and connect with patients. There's research to back this up.[39, 40, 41, 42, 43]

In one study, researchers studied doctors' emotional intelligence to understand the associations between emotional intelligence, patient trust, and the doctor-patient relationship. What they learned was that how the doctors self-rated on emotional intelligence didn't correlate with how their patients viewed them.[43]

> Research shows physicians routinely miss *emotional* clues from patients and actually miss 60 to 90 percent of opportunities to respond to patients with compassion.

In fact, it was nurses in the study who had a more realistic view of the doctors' emotional intelligence. As independent (i.e., third party) observers, the nurses' scoring of the physicians' emotional intelligence mirrored what patients said they experienced. In short, doctors' insight on their own ability to connect with patients just wasn't very accurate. But the nurses could see it. This may not come as a surprise to any nurse reading this book.

Research shows that physicians routinely miss emotional clues from patients and actually *miss sixty to ninety percent* of opportunities to respond to patients with compassion. This is even true in cancer care, despite the fact that cancer patients are likely to be in need of compassion.

The evidence in cancer care comes from a number of rigorous, federally funded studies from reputable, internationally recognized research institutions like Duke University and University of California San Diego and were supported by grants from the National Cancer Institute and the AHRQ.[44, 45, 46, 47]

And those findings about missed opportunities for compassion in cancer care? They're corroborated by a host of other studies in other types of medical practices. A National Institutes of Health (NIH)-funded study from University of California San Francisco found that in communicating with acutely ill patients admitted to the hospital, hospitalists (specialists in hospital medicine) miss 68 percent of opportunities to respond with compassion.[48]

Would it surprise you to know that hospitalists miss so many clues and opportunities? Perhaps not. Hospitalists are a newer medical specialty. As individuals who coordinate the hospital care of many inpatients, maybe it's harder for them to develop much of a relationship or rapport with their patients in the way you would anticipate from doctors who come to know their patients over many years.

But guess what? A University of Chicago study—that was published in *JAMA* and funded by AHRQ—found that in primary care clinic visits, primary care physicians missed 79 percent of emotional clues from patients and opportunities to respond with compassion.[49] So there goes that theory…

So Many Missed Opportunities

When a patient says, "I'm having a tough time," the hope is it might prompt some type of compassionate response from health care providers, either by using a "continuer" question or statement (instead of a "terminator" statement that stops the dialogue in its tracks) or just by offering emotional support.

But research shows that, more often than not, physicians just blow right past those opportunities for compassion. They don't acknowledge what was said or engage, listen, or connect in a meaningful way. Instead, they move on to a next area of inquiry. The preponderance of data in the medical literature shows this.

There are countless stories of patients who see multiple physicians before they finally sit with a physician that listens to every aspect of their history and then catches the smallest detail that can finally lead to the right diagnosis. Oftentimes, these second and third opinions finally help a patient receive the care they need.

But the inability to understand what a patient is really trying to say—or perhaps is not saying—can be a matter of life or death. It is now known that most people who attempt suicide have made some type of health care visit in the weeks or months before the suicide attempt—38 percent of them within the last week and 95 percent within the last year.[50]

The stakes are so high and the risks of missing warning signs so great, that some institutions have adopted screening tools, like the Columbia Suicide Severity Rating Scale, to assess all patients with depression in certain settings (e.g., the emergency department or primary care).[51] One of the main reasons why scales like this exist is that health care providers are often not detecting the emotional and other cues that could indicate someone is about to take their own life.

Part of the problem is experiential in nature; health care providers in these settings typically do not have focused expertise in evaluating suicide risk. But the other part is that the health care providers may not be emotionally attuned or attentive to what the patient is saying (or not saying). But what if they were?

In his book, *Why People Die by Suicide*, renowned psychologist and suicide expert Thomas Joiner from Florida State University quotes from one man's suicide note: "*'I'm going to walk to the bridge. If one person smiles at me on the way, I will not jump.'*"[52]

One smile is all it would have taken to change such a terrible outcome.

None of the people this man passed on the way to the bridge had any idea what kind of pain this man was carrying around...carrying it all the way to ending his own life. From their vantage point, this man may have looked like anybody else.

Yes, you never really know what kind of pain people are carrying around. What about the people that man passed on the way to the bridge? How do you think they might have responded if they knew that the man they barely noticed could have been saved by the compassionate act of a single smile?

They would probably be devastated to learn that they missed an opportunity to save a life. That is just how health care providers in emergency medicine and primary care feel when they learn the shocking news that a patient who just left their emergency department or clinic took their own life. They second-guess everything they did (or did not do). They are devastated by the missed opportunity to potentially make a lifesaving difference.

In fact, sometimes the end of that patient's life literally ends a physician's health care career. He or she never recovers. A missed opportunity for compassion can change the trajectory of ones' life—for both the patient and the provider—forever.

> **A missed opportunity for compassion can change the trajectory of one's life forever.**

And it's not just suicide where providers can save a life. Missed opportunities for compassionate care are also common for patients suffering during the most severe physical health crises. This is not opinion; these are the scientific data.

Consider this shocking example from a rigorously conducted Johns Hopkins study: Trained observers set about measuring health care providers' verbal and non-verbal communications in the intensive care unit (ICU). In fully *74 percent* of the interactions in the ICU, researchers found that the health care providers showed no compassion for patients or families (i.e., zero compassionate behaviors).[53]

Likewise, in another study from the University of Washington and supported by the NIH, researchers found that fully *one-third* of end-of-life discussions with families in the ICU had no statements of compassion by health care providers—zero—even though they also found that compassion leads to a better experience for families.[54]

Isn't that a little crazy? If there were ever a time that people need compassion, it would be at the end of life. It is important to recognize that, just as there is typically a bell curve in all aspects of human performance, there is also a bell curve in people's compassion for others. This variation has been demonstrated in health care providers as assessed by patients.[55]

This will be discussed in detail later, when considering methods to increase compassionate behaviors, but for now suffice it to say that variation in compassionate care between health care providers is a major source of the lack of compassion in health care. In addition to variation between providers is variation *within* individual providers—i.e., inconsistency in one's compassionate care.

There are bad days for every provider, of course. But some individuals manage to find compassion anyways. Even on bad days.

Dr. Phil Koren, a cardiologist and head of the heart institute at Cooper University Health Care, for instance once explained that he recognizes patients must often wait weeks to see him. So even if he's having a challenging day, he consciously works to set aside those feelings to muster all the compassion he can.

He recognizes that he's "on"—just like a performer on stage—when he sees a patient and that each patient deserves his compassion. Incidentally, he also finds that the extra investment of compassion and the patient interactions that flow from that actually fuel his passion for medicine and increase his fulfillment with his career. (This link between compassion and resilience will be reviewed in-depth in a later chapter).

> There is an expectation for emotional labor in all service industries. Health care is no exception.

This isn't to suggest that health care providers "fake it," but rather that they recognize there is an expectation for some emotional labor in all service industries, and that health care is no exception.[56]

Of course, there are exemplary health care providers who are truly experts at compassionate care and consistently show compassion for every single patient, every day. However, consistency is lacking with many providers, and the preponderance of evidence shows that what patients are experiencing is falling short.

Could Lack of Compassion Be a Learned Behavior?

As discussed earlier, physicians-in-training struggle with burnout just as their more seasoned peers do. This leads to compassion fatigue. In fact, compassion tends to decline over time throughout medical school. The phenomenon has been well studied so there is a lot of supporting evidence.

But there is also another dynamic at play here. In a systematic review of 18 studies of empathy in medical trainees, 17 of 18 studies identified that empathy declined during training.[57] However, they also found that a major reason was the "hidden" curriculum.

The core curriculum is, of course, the outline of the substantive knowledge to learn on a particular topic. The hidden curriculum is "that which the school teaches without intending or being aware that it is being taught."[58]

Let's pause for a moment and identify the players in medical education. Medical students, who are also known as "student doctors" or "physicians-in-training," are students enrolled post-college in a school of medicine. Resident physicians, who are sometimes known as "house staff" physicians, are recent graduates of medical school who are training in a particular field of medicine but have not yet begun to practice completely unsupervised. Finally, attending physicians have finished training in their particular field of medicine or surgery and are the supervisors and teachers of medical students and resident physicians in teaching hospitals and academic medical centers.

The hidden curriculum is what medical students learn from resident physicians and attending physicians during all of the hours they spend together during clinical rotations in medical school that is not part of the actual "core" curriculum. It's considered to be a side effect of a formal education…lessons learned—perhaps unintended—through the transmission of norms, values, and beliefs conveyed in the social interactions of the people in the educational environment.

For instance, on a medical student's obstetrics and gynecology (ob-gyn) rotation, the core curriculum may consist of learning about various types of surgeries that gynecologists perform: the indications for those surgeries, the anatomy involved in the surgery, and the steps that will take place in the operating room. It may include the complications that could arise and how to assess the patient both pre-operatively and post-operatively.

Imagine for a moment: A medical student is called to the emergency department to see a patient with suspected ectopic pregnancy (sometimes called a "tubal" pregnancy – where a pregnancy grows outside the main cavity of the uterus). Within the core curriculum, the student might be expected to know the indications for taking the patient to the operating room for surgery.

However, when the medical student is with the ob-gyn resident physician that gets the page from the emergency department about that patient, he will also learn a whole host of other things, such as how the resident speaks to the emergency department physician that calls for assistance.

Is she annoyed by the call? Is she respectful? Does she answer the page right away or ignore the page and say, "If the emergency department really wants me, they will page me again"? Does she always treat the patient with courtesy and respect and listen intently? Does she really do all the things that are taught in the classroom?

This is where the hidden curriculum comes in. While medicine abandoned a pure apprenticeship model years ago, learning the hidden curriculum—essentially learning by example—is still very much a part of how physicians are trained (or indoctrinated). The problem is that if mentors role model a lack of compassion in their day-to-day work with patients, new physicians will learn to do the same. That's how they find out "how things work around here," for better or worse.

> If mentors role model a lack of compassion in their day-to-day work with patients, new physicians will learn to do the same.

There may be no better illustration of the hidden curriculum than in the pages of the infamous book, *House of God*, a best-selling satire with a cult following of medical students and physicians since it was first published in 1978.[59] It has been described by many as "hilarious," "troubling," and a "scandalous" insider look into the hidden curriculum of medical school. In *House of God*, characters learn all the unwritten rules of how to practice medicine from a supervising senior resident they call "the Fat Man."

He teaches them all about GOMERS. That's an acronym for "Get Out of My Emergency Room." This awful term was used to describe older patients suffering from dementia who are not communicative and are repeatedly admitted to the hospital. The Fat Man teaches these trainees how to "turf" GOMERS: that is, how to find a way to transfer the care of these patients to other physicians so they can wash their hands of them.

In short, it's a heart-breaking look at the worst examples of depersonalization and passing these behaviors on to the next generation of doctors. It's the polar opposite of what you will see in the pages to follow. The lessons from compassion science will teach us what it really takes to be successful in medicine.

So remember: the hidden curriculum can have either a negative or positive effect on the training of compassion practices. It's up to individual physicians, nurses, and other health care workers and administrators to decide what they want to role model. Their choices will have a lasting impact that echoes through trainees, mentees, and those that are less senior to them, all across the organization.

Medical Progress?

The introduction of the electronic medical record (EMR) into routine clinical practice represents an important advance for patient care quality and safety. However, it likely has not helped the human connection between health care providers and their patients.

Since EMRs have been inserted into the patient-provider interaction, research shows that physicians in office practices spend at least as much time looking into their computer screens as they do looking patients in the eyes.[60, 61] It's been well studied. These days, kids draw pictures of physicians looking at a screen instead of their patient. And, when asked to describe the job of a physician, kids will say that he or she is someone who "types in a computer" rather than someone who wears a white coat and stethoscope.

There is a thought-provoking *JAMA* article about a physician who was appalled by this very experience.[62] This physician had just returned from two years serving as a medical officer aboard an aircraft carrier in the Persian Gulf making life-or-death decisions for a crew of 2,500 military personnel. He performed amputations and once had to divert an entire aircraft carrier to ensure a patient arrived safely at a tertiary hospital. As a result of such experiences, he developed a deep sense of purpose and strong commitment to service.

Post-navy, during his residency training, he was recognized for being particularly gifted at connecting with his pediatric patients. So he was shocked when a seven-year-old girl drew this picture of him typing at the keyboard with his back to the family:

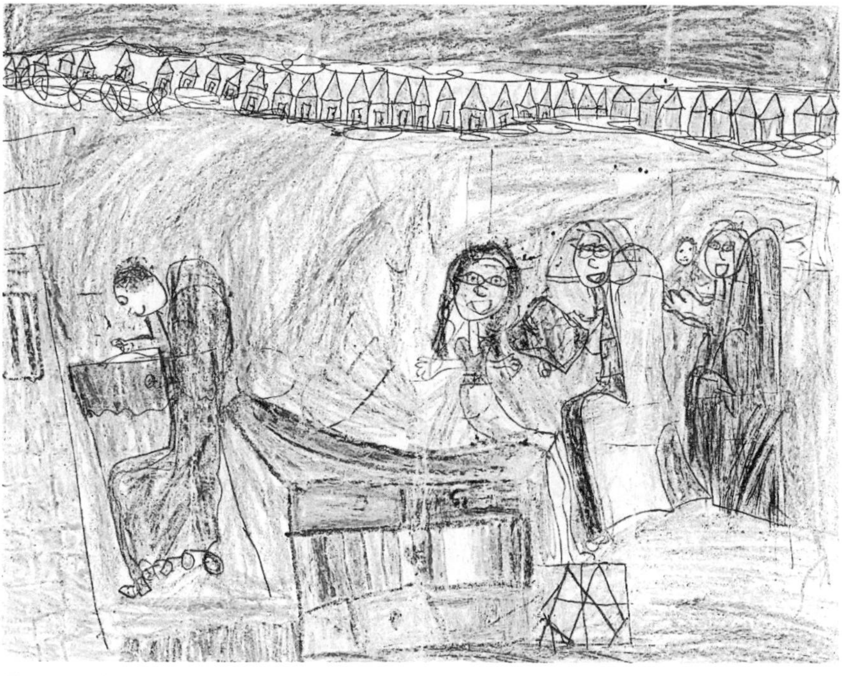

Figure 1.1: The resident physician whose patient drew this picture captioned it like this: "The economic stimulus bill has directed $20 billion to health care information technology, largely funding electronic medical record incentives. I wonder how much this technology will really cost?"
©2011 Thomas G. Murphy, MD

Do you see how this child has portrayed her doctor? His back is to the patient and family. Instead of growing up thinking of a pediatrician as a kindly person in a white coat who bends down to smile and look a small person in the eyes, the patient will think of him as a person who is *disconnected* from her experience...someone who is busy typing at a keyboard.

The physician was simply stunned that his patient saw him in this way. As the article notes, this child's picture aptly telegraphed the frustration felt by so many physicians who feel torn between the needs of today's EMRs and their patients.

Let's take a moment to contrast this child's picture from 2012 with another famous rendering from way back in 1891:

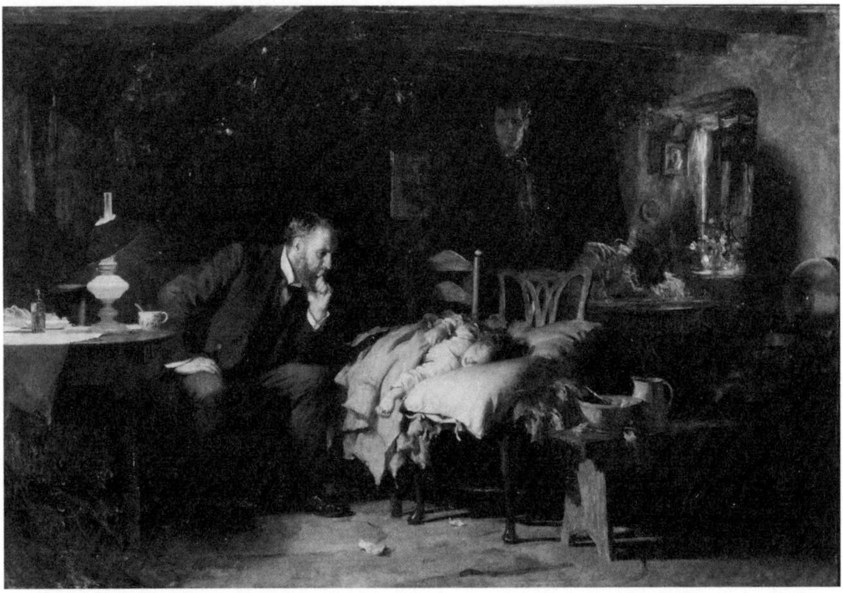

Figure 1.2: "The Doctor" by Sir Luke Fildes, 1891

Take a moment to carefully contemplate this famous Victorian painting, titled "The Doctor", painted by Sir Luke Fildes. Do you see how this physician is fully engaged with his young patient? This child has one hundred percent of her physician's attention. He is totally "locked in." Nothing could distract him.

Here's how this painting came to be: Sir Henry Tate—sugar tycoon and founder of the famous Tate Gallery in London—commissioned a painting from Fildes, leaving the subject of the painting up to the painter. Fildes chose to paint this poignant moment that occurred during his own personal tragedy, before his young child died at home.

But why? A comment from Fildes' biographer (who was one of his other children) lends insight. He wrote, "The character and bearing of their doctor throughout the time of their anxiety made a deep impression on my parents. Dr. Murray became a symbol of professional devotion."[63]

So it's a serious sign of the times when youngsters are sketching their doctors staring at a screen. The human connection in the patient-physician encounter is sacred; it facilitates healing. And yet, the EMR is not optional. Many physicians feel they must now give priority to data over attention to patients.

Resident physicians on inpatient services spend only *12 percent* of their time seeing their patients at the bedside in direct patient care.

Athena Health ran an interesting television ad campaign recently on this theme with a video where a child was busy typing on a laptop as he "played doctor" while his loving parents looked on. When they tried to express their approval, he gave them a stern look and held up a finger to chastise them for interrupting his work on the computer by speaking. (You can watch the video on YouTube by searching "When I Grow Up—Athena Health".)

The same problem exists in the hospital. A Johns Hopkins study found that resident physicians on inpatient services spend only *12 percent* of their time seeing their patients at the bedside in direct patient care, compared to 40 percent of their time doing computer work away from the patients.[64]

Again, it's not just a U.S. problem. A recent Swiss study found the same thing: resident physicians spent about half of the workday away from patients (5.2 hours) working on a computer and only 1.7 hours with patients.[65] It's hard to connect with patients if one is working on a computer, let alone working in a different room.

Providers may be doing work on behalf of patients while they are on the computer, but patients do not feel such attention. Nurses face the same struggle. It's worrisome.

It's true that many physicians might opt to go back to a paper medical record if they could. However, there's no question that the EMR is necessary to respond to the greater regulatory demands for documentation in health care today. EMRs have also improved patient safety and communication between physicians to review labs and procedures for patients and have delivered a host of additional benefits for health care systems.

But all this comes at a price. Sometimes physicians can feel like glorified typists. They're required to look at a screen instead of at the patient, and that changes the nature of their interaction with patients. Since the EMR won't be going away anytime soon, there must be a way to do better. It has to be fixed.

Why Do Providers Miss So Many Opportunities for Compassion?

Is it really just because of the EMR? Taken together, there is abundant data in the scientific literature that health care providers miss most opportunities to respond to patients with compassion. But *why?*

1. "I don't *see* it."

Lack of insight is complicated. Does a provider just not notice these opportunities? Or does he willingly ignore them? It's hard to know.

It could be a lack of emotional intelligence, or not being comfortable addressing emotional needs. Maybe it's being more self-focused instead of other-focused, as that University of Michigan study suggested.

2. "I don't have *time*."

The idea that providers don't believe they have time for compassion dovetails with the results of the Princeton study of the seminarians. It's a critical aspect to the compassion crisis. As a result, you'll find that a full chapter is specifically dedicated to this crucial topic.

3. "I don't *care*."

The idea that providers don't care about providing compassion to patients relates to health care provider burnout, or the emotional culture of the environment in which one practices. In the pages to follow, both of these important topics will be addressed.

4. "I don't know *how*."

This is the belief that compassion is not in one's nature (e.g., "I am not a touchy-feely person"). The question is whether or not compassionate behaviors can, in fact, be learned through training (i.e., nature versus nurture). This will also be addressed in a later chapter.

5. "I don't believe it *really matters*."

And last is the question of whether or not providers believe compassion makes a difference. Debunking the myth that compassion is merely a "nice to have," rather than essential for good outcomes, is one of the foremost aims in writing this book. It is a theme that will be running through all of the pages that follow.

Change Is Slow in Health Care

The reality is that it takes time to change norms in medicine. In the chapters to follow, you will see the data that compassion matters—for patients, for patient care, and for those who care for patients. But compassionomics is a new field of study. The scientific evidence behind practicing compassionate care isn't widely recognized or appreciated...*yet.* But this is the story behind so many advances in medicine. It just takes time.

Consider Ignaz Semmelweis, for instance. He was a grumpy Hungarian physician who is today widely credited with discovering the value of hand washing and aseptic technique in health care. But this wasn't always the case. He faced a lot of detractors in his day.

In fact, physicians didn't begin to understand the value of hand washing until 1847. Before that time, the maternal death rate of women who delivered babies in hospitals in Vienna was ten to twenty times higher than those who delivered at home with a midwife.

Dr. Semmelweis, who was Hungarian and Jewish, applied to work as a surgeon in the prestigious Vienna General Hospital, but was denied due to his nationality and religion. As a result, he was relegated to obstetrics where he routinely heard from patients begging to be discharged because they believed doctors to be harbingers of death.

He began to question why women who delivered babies in the hospital were so much more likely to die of postpartum infections (i.e., puerperal sepsis or "childbed fever") compared to women who were attended by midwives and delivered at home. He noted that physicians began their hospital rounds each morning by conducting autopsies on women who had just died and then moved on to delivering live babies next.

Semmelweis deduced that doctors were transferring some kind of "morbid poison" between the corpses and the laboring women. (Today, that poison is recognized as pathogenic bacteria.) He then ordered physicians working with him to wash their hands in a chlorinated lime solution until the "stench" of the corpses was gone.

Sure enough, the mortality rate of his patients fell dramatically. However, many of his colleagues stubbornly resisted the idea that they could have caused their patients' deaths. They pushed back in the fiercest way. Semmelweis was an ornery person to begin with, and he became increasingly angry in the face of so much resistance to hand washing as an effective practice. Eventually, he lost his position in Vienna, and he hightailed it back to Budapest.

It wasn't until 1861 when he finally got around to publishing an academic paper on the subject (a paper that also included savage attacks on his critics). And even then, his mental health rapidly deteriorated until he was finally committed to a psychiatric hospital where he soon died.

Semmelweis' timing was bad. The medical profession just wasn't ready to accept such a radical idea back in 1847. It wasn't until Louis Pasteur began to set forth the most important tenets of his germ theory of disease in the early 1860s that the idea began to have context and take hold. In fact, it was in 1867 that the Scottish surgeon Joseph Lister—who hadn't ever heard of Semmelweis—set forth his own theory of aseptic technique in surgery.[66]

Will compassionomics have a better start than Dr. Semmelweis did? The majority of patients already connect with most of the concepts, as do many health care providers.

However, medicine is slow to change, and the lesson of Semmelweis is not one to forget. Hopefully these authors do not suffer the same fate as Semmelweis did, but shining a light on the compassion crisis in health care is important. Even if some people disagree.

CHAPTER 2: Does Compassion Matter?

"Without data, you're just another person with an opinion."

—W. Edwards Deming

Seeing all the data on the compassion crisis in health care begs an important next question: so what?

Does compassion *really* matter?

Most of us probably agree that health care providers *ought* to be compassionate—that treating patients with compassion is the right thing to do. It's a responsibility and a duty, a moral imperative.

For the record, though, not everyone agrees that compassion is an "ought" to do, or that it is even a moral imperative in treating patients. For example, in response to the call to action for more compassion in the National Health Service in the United Kingdom (mentioned in Chapter 1), one high profile ethics professor went on the record as saying that compassion is not a necessary component of health care from any perspective.[27, 67]

However, the overwhelming majority of health care providers and health care leaders in the U.S.—and around the world—have typically taken the position that a good bedside manner and treating patients with compassion is something that health care providers and health care institutions ought to do.

But is compassion just an "ought," or are there also evidence-based effects that would make compassion a vital and necessary part of the effectiveness of health care?

Studies show that people believe compassion is vitally important for quality health care. Remember the Harvard study from Chapter 1 that was published in *Health Affairs,* where half of patients said both individual health care providers and the U.S. health system as a whole were not compassionate?[1] In that same study, researchers also asked the 1,300 study subjects—including both patients and physicians—if they believed that compassion matters in health care.

Three-quarters of both patients and physicians said "yes." They also said it matters so much that it could actually mean the difference between *life and death.*

However, those are just opinions. In medical science, and in health care, opinions are not enough. We need hard data to determine whether or not compassion matters in measurable, quantifiable ways…if it actually affects the health and well-being of patients.

So the question becomes: can the effects of compassion actually be *measured?*

The Hypothesis: Compassion Matters

In the same way that a quantitative, evidence-based approach was needed to determine that there is a compassion crisis in health care, a scientifically rigorous approach to examining the impact of compassion in health care must also be employed—measuring both the effects of its presence and the results of its absence.

The goal was to determine whether or not it matters based on the evidence. Not just based on survey results that capture patients' perceptions about their care, but also data from rigorous scientific studies showing the effects.

To determine if compassion really matters or not, the question must be approached like an experienced researcher would approach it. At the beginning of answering any research question, the most important first step is always to establish the hypothesis.

A hypothesis is a supposition or proposed explanation of the nature of things that is made on the basis of limited evidence as a starting point for further investigation. Then, the aim of the further investigation is to test the hypothesis in order to determine if it is true. It is important that the researcher is prepared to accept the path where the data leads, whether it supports or rejects the hypothesis. Researchers are not advocates for their hypothesis in the way lawyers are advocates for their clients.

Researchers must remain free of bias as they test a hypothesis because the goal of research is never to prove a point. Rather, it is to test a hypothesis to find an *answer*. So it's vital to be unbiased at the inception of scientific investigation.

This kind of unbiased approach is necessary for the scientific method and to ensure that researchers won't be led astray to false conclusions by any preconceived notions or biases, either conscious or subconscious. There is as much value in rejecting a hypothesis as confirming; either way, the body of scientific evidence grows.

In these pages is the story of testing one overarching hypothesis: Compassion *matters*. Specifically, the hypothesis is that providing health care in a compassionate manner is more effective than providing health care without compassion by virtue of the fact that human connection can confer distinct and measurable benefits.

Just to be super clear about bias: When we set out to determine whether compassion matters we were more than willing to conclude that it does not. As was explained in the preface that was exactly what we expected to find.

Really, there are three interrelated hypotheses here: that compassion matters (1) for patients (through better patient outcomes); (2) for patient care (through higher quality, lower costs, and better financial sustainability); and (3) for those who care for patients (by promoting the resilience of health care providers and staff as well as lowering burnout).

So these pages share the scientific evidence for compassion and its effects on health, health care, and health care providers. The clinical research data come from the real-world practice of medicine—quantitative and qualitative research that spans the spectrum from the primary care clinic all the way to the ICU and even extending to the hospital and organizational level.

The Science versus the Art of Medicine

Early on in medical school, physicians-in-training are taught about the science and the art of medicine. Nurses are trained in a similar fashion. The science of medicine is how to *treat* patients; the art of medicine is how to *take care* of them.

The science of medicine is the collection of facts that comprise the knowledge base for how to make diagnoses and formulate treatment plans. But the art of medicine is different. The art of medicine is about building rapport and a caring connection with patients; some refer to this as "bedside manner." It is undeniable that compassion for patients is an integral component of the art of medicine.

However, in thinking that compassion is limited only to the art of medicine, one might be tempted to consider it distinct from providing medical care. That's like thinking about compassion in the same way you think about dessert after the main entrée...a delicious "extra" to indulge in, but only after a great meal if you're not already full.

Following that kind of thinking, a physician's most important job is to save someone's life clinically, but, if there's time, being compassionate to a patient is also nice. It's just optional, a "nice to have." (As emergency department nurses sometimes like to say, "I'm here to save your ass. Not kiss it!")

Where does such thinking come from? It comes from conventional medical training, where the science and the art of medicine are both considered vitally important, but very different. They are purported as separate and distinct from each other—mutually exclusive. Apples and oranges.

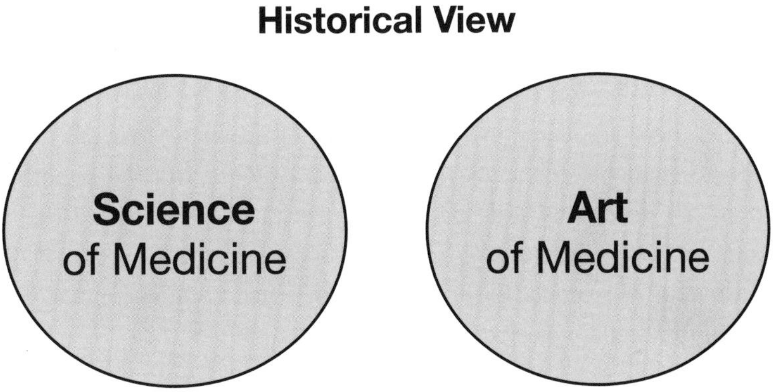

Figure 2.1: The historical view: the science and the art of medicine are distinct.

But what if the evidence shows there is actually *overlap* between the science and art of medicine? That is the hypothesis that is being tested here. Perhaps there is science in the art of medicine—a convergence.

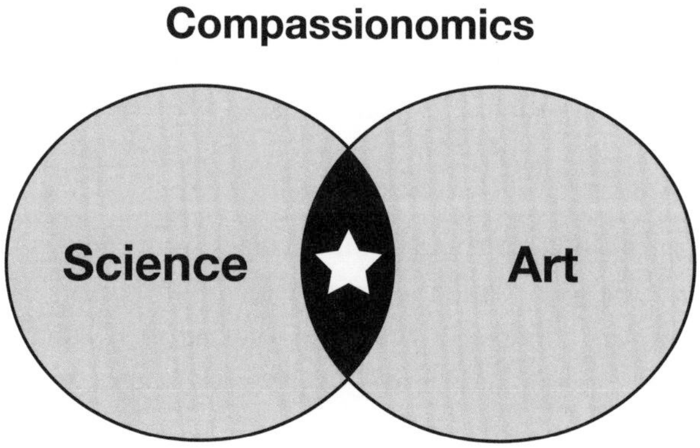

Figure 2.2: The compassionomics hypothesis: there is science in the art of medicine.

Obviously, there are elements of the science of medicine that are distinctly science and elements of the art that are distinctly art. But the hypothesis is that there are situations and conditions in health care in which the art of medicine has not only meaningful, but also measurable, effects that belong in the domain of science. If that is the case, then compassion for patients belongs in the domain of evidence-based medicine.

If compassion for patients is found to be a highly effective therapy that changes outcomes—one that is so much more cost-effective than many other therapies utilized instead—it would become part of every caregiver's toolbox. You would use it at every opportunity you have, rather than considering it as optional.

Such a therapy could radically improve patient lives, lengthen fulfilling careers for health care providers, and possibly help reverse the U.S. health care system cost crisis. But only if that is what the evidence shows. Just as researchers must be unbiased when testing a hypothesis, so should readers of this book be open to the possibility that compassion does *not* matter in measurable ways. Proof should be demanded.

But similarly, many readers have been trained in the conventional thinking that the science and the art of medicine are distinct and mutually exclusive.

That can also be a bias that, either consciously or subconsciously—no matter how much evidence is presented—could make a reader unable to consider the possibility that the hypotheses presented here are true.

Bias is notoriously difficult to overcome. It's okay to be skeptical, but don't let it cloud your consideration. *Dare* to open your mind. Open your mind to the possibility that compassion is actually more powerful than you ever dreamed. Demand proof, of course. But do it with an unbiased mindset that is open to possibility. After all, that is what the scientific method is all about.

The Journey through the Data

Before showing you the evidence, let's look first at the methodology used to test this hypothesis to learn how the scientific evidence was compiled from the biomedical literature and understand how the data were synthesized. Then, after evaluating all of the scientific evidence, you can decide for yourself whether or not compassion really matters. You be the judge.

The data presented in these pages are not the product of "cherry picking" certain studies from the scientific literature that show compassion matters. Rather, the data were compiled using a *bona fide* research methodology called "systematic review."

The genesis of this book is not a look at what *some* or a *few* of the studies on compassion in health care showed. Rather, it's systematically what the *compilation* of the studies on compassion revealed after they all were chased down and reviewed.

A systematic review is a type of scientific literature review that uses a systematic methodology to collect, critically appraise, and synthesize all of the data available in the world's literature on a specific question. It is the process to cast the widest net to capture all the information on a single topic. Systematic review is considered to be one of the most important tools for establishing the state-of-the-art in medical science.

The purpose of a systematic review is to provide a complete, exhaustive summary of current literature relevant to a research question. The purpose in this case: does compassion really matter?

This general approach is outlined in the *Cochrane Handbook for Systematic Reviews of Interventions*, which is considered the "bible" of systematic review containing all the rules for examining a health care question.[68] Essentially, every relevant article and available piece of data was reviewed to examine the hypothesis that compassion matters.

However, examining a special topic like compassion in medicine requires a special approach. Conventional systematic review methodology is not sufficient. The conventional method for systematic review is to use a protocol-driven search strategy of an electronic database of evidence (e.g., the search engine PubMed from the National Library of Medicine).

But compassion is a topic that falls into a special category of systematic review called "complex evidence."[69] Complex evidence is that which addresses broad questions—like health policy, for example—and synthesizes both qualitative and quantitative evidence from multiple and disparate types of sources.

Research shows that conventional protocol-driven database searches will miss *more than half* of the relevant data when examining topics of complex evidence.[69] As a result, conventional search methodology is inadequate.

> This systematic review is the first time all of the data on compassion's impact on health and health care has appeared together in one place.

Here's an example: If the search term "pneumonia" was typed into PubMed, all of the articles that contain information about infections in the lungs would be mapped to that term. A researcher could feel confident, as could the rest of the scientific community, that no relevant research would be missed.

However, the data for compassion science has not been mapped to a single search term or curated in the same fashion. You can't just enter the search term "compassion" and get all of the relevant studies. As a result, this systematic review is the first time all of the data on compassion's impact on health and health care has appeared together in one place.

Think of the early days of the internet and search engines. Until technology improved and a company like Google came along to map terms more extensively, searches were much less accurate. So if you wanted to search for everyone in the country named Charlie Brown, you would be relying on a search engine to know that people may go by Charlie, even if their name is Charles or Chuck or Charlene or Charlotte.

Or maybe they are just listed as "C." Or perhaps Charlie is their middle name. Fortunately, search engines are now sophisticated enough to figure this out for us. But what if they couldn't? In that case, you'd be forced to know all of the forms of every word, in every instance, to make sure you didn't miss someone.

Since compassion science has not been mapped (yet) in publication databases, one cannot simply type the search term "compassion" into PubMed and get all the relevant studies. It's not that simple, unfortunately.

Compassion science is a field so new that there is no single adequate search term. As a result, relevant research studies may be mapped to very different search terms in databases—terms like "doctor-patient relationship" or "rapport," perhaps "humanism" or even "bedside manner."

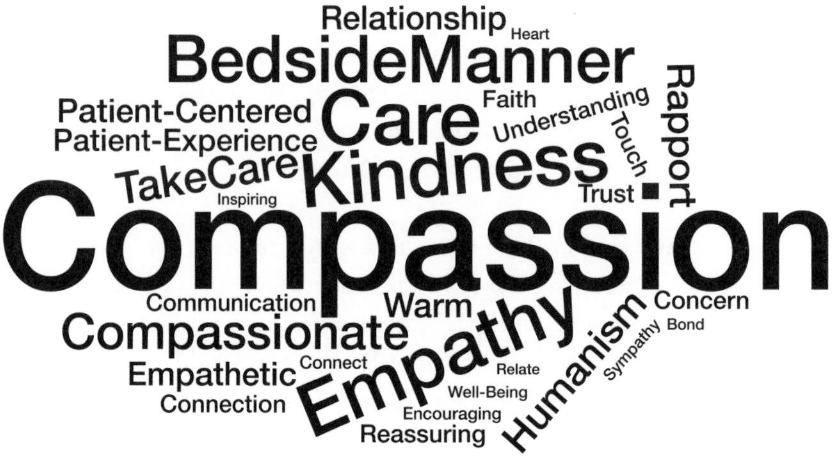

Figure 2.3: Compassionomics is a field so new that there is no single search term.

Studies that are mapped to these search terms in electronic databases and search engines may contain data that are very relevant to an examination of the effects of compassion in health care. The conventional systematic review methodology would likely miss much of the pertinent data. Therefore, for the systematic review of the evidence on compassion, a much more laborious methodology was needed.

The Sherlock Holmes Approach to Getting Answers

In accordance with the recommended methodology for systematic reviews of complex evidence,[69] this systematic review of compassion took a much more hands on (and painstaking!) approach. It's called a "references of references" methodology.

So, instead of simply typing terms into a search engine, this review started with a small collection of the studies considered to be quintessential papers on the effects of compassion in medicine and then worked *backward*. By going to the references section of each of these classic studies, every paper listed in the references section was then, itself, reviewed for pertinent data.

Then the reference section of each of those papers was reviewed. And each of *those* papers were pulled. And *their* references were reviewed. And so on, and so on...until there was no longer any relevant data to be found. You can think of this methodology as a "family tree" of sorts, ever growing and branching out...until every last reference was exhausted.

> More than 1,000 scientific abstracts were examined and reviewed as well as more than 250 research papers.

In total, more than 1,000 scientific abstracts were examined and reviewed—by hand—as well as more than 250 research papers. What was particularly valuable about this methodology was that it captured key scientific studies that had been flying under the radar for years, even decades. To capture *all* of the relevant studies is vital because it allows a thorough review of the data in aggregate over a long time span for greater validity.

Surprisingly, some of these "under the radar" studies were even conducted by some of the most respected institutions—like Harvard Medical School—and published in some of the best journals—like *The New England Journal of Medicine*. How is it that such high-profile publications can go missing? These studies likely garnered a lot of attention at the time of publication, but over the years they were not connected to other studies in a way that produced a pattern. They didn't influence medical practice in the same way that change was occurring in other fields of medicine, where studies and scientific findings were continuously building upon each other over time.

At the time of publication, people likely found these papers on the power of compassion incredibly interesting and perhaps also very impactful. They made ripples in the water, and some studies probably made a substantial splash.

But they did not connect with other studies to make a *wave* that could transform health care. But with the methodology in this systematic review—that finally connects all of the key studies together—the ripples and splashes form an unmistakable tidal wave of data that will show you the true power of compassion and lead you to only one conclusion. (Spoiler alert: compassion matters.)

Given that some of these vital studies had been published up to fifty years earlier, this systematic review required cracking open the spines of journals physically located in the bowels of a library—dusty journals which, in some cases, probably hadn't been peered into for decades. That is why this systematic review on compassion science literally took *two years* to complete.

So rather than typing terms into a search engine and getting an instantaneous output with all the studies, this two-year systematic review was much more like using a library card catalog and the Dewey Decimal System to find books on a remote shelf in a library sometime before the internet. (Note: If you're a millennial or younger, you might need to take a moment to Google "card catalogs and the Dewey Decimal System" to understand what was involved in research pre-internet. It was an incredibly time-consuming endeavor.)

Essentially, this systematic review was a methodical "Sherlock Holmes" type of investigation searching for clues and evidence on the power of compassion. The "references of references" methodology was slow going, no doubt, but that is what a systematic review of complex evidence requires.[69]

Earlier, a distinction was drawn between the meaning of empathy (the feeling and understanding components) and compassion (the action component). It's important to note here that, for the purposes of synthesizing and presenting the available research in an understandable way, the word "compassion" may be used as we discuss some studies, even though the term "empathy" may be used in the title or body of the paper. The body of research shows that authors often use these two terms interchangeably.

The important thing is that studies were included in this systematic review if they met the threshold of this working definition of compassion—an emotional *response* to another's pain or suffering involving an authentic desire to help—whether or not the study authors called it compassion.[7] If what the study was examining met this definition, then in this systematic review (and throughout the rest of this book) it will be referred to as compassion.

Think of it this way: Since empathy is the feeling or understanding of another's pain or suffering—and compassion is the action that flows from empathy—then anytime a study examines health care provider *behavior* toward a patient, the study *must* involve compassion.

Empathy is like a one-way street running toward the health care provider: detecting, processing, understanding, and even feeling the incoming emotional cues from the patient. Compassion, on the other hand, is a street that runs in the other direction, a responsive action toward the one who is suffering. Empathy can happen through a one-way mirror. Compassion cannot.

So if a study involves behaviors toward a patient, it has to be (by definition) a study of compassion, even if the authors of the study chose to use the term "empathy" instead. Accordingly, throughout these pages, anytime a study involves behaviors toward a patient, we will (for our purposes) refer to it as compassion.

An interesting side note: The data also show that there's been a spike recently in the number of researchers studying compassion.[70] This is in stark contrast to, say, the number of researchers currently studying the bubonic plague.

No spike there. Why? There is no bubonic plague crisis any longer. It doesn't matter anymore. However, interest in studying compassion for others seems to be at a fever pitch. There is a worldwide compassion crisis at the moment. Right now. And it matters.

How Compassion Works

Whenever researchers hypothesize that there is a link between two things—a factor under investigation and the outcome measure of interest—they always postulate a mechanism of action: By what mechanism did the factor affect the outcome? What mechanism causes the effect?

For example, with medications for treating mental health conditions, the mechanism of action may be a drug binding to specific receptors in the brain or modulating the levels of neurotransmitters in the brain. For medications to treat high blood pressure, the mechanism may be a drug binding to receptors in blood vessels throughout the body.

But in the case of compassion, how is it that compassion can have meaningful effects? What are the mechanisms of action? There has to be a mechanism of action in order for there to be a meaningful effect.

During this systematic review of the scientific evidence, more than twenty distinct mechanisms of action for compassion on patients came to light by which compassion can have meaningful, beneficial effects on patient outcomes.[14] These can be grouped into four main areas: physiological effects, psychological effects, enhanced patient self-care, and increased quality of care.

What do those encompass exactly? Here are a few examples as a preview of the data to come: When providers have compassion for a patient, they are more likely to be meticulous about their care, have higher quality standards, and are therefore less likely to make a major medical error.

But there are also physiological effects. For example, compassion can buffer stress-mediated disease. Compassion can also modulate a patient's perception of pain.

There are also endocrine effects, like improved blood sugar control in patients with diabetes and enhancement of immune system function. The psychological benefits of compassion can also be immense (which is probably not surprising). But you may be surprised to learn that compassion for patients can also motivate patients to better self-care, i.e., how patients take care of their own health. And that is critically important.

For example, when providers care deeply about patients—and patients feel that—they are more likely to take their medicine. These mechanisms are the "how" when it comes to understanding the enormous power of compassion.

A very important caveat to keep in mind as you consider this evidence: the main driver of clinical outcomes is clinical excellence. Period.

Of course, compassion is not a panacea; it's not a substitute for quality clinical care. If a surgeon botches the technical aspects of a surgery, or a physician makes an error by prescribing the wrong drug, there is no way that compassion can make up for that.

But when compassion is used in conjunction with excellent clinical care, it can be incredibly powerful. Don't think of clinical excellence and compassion as an "either/or" situation. It should be an "and," as in "clinical excellence *and* compassion—when used *together*—deliver the best outcomes."

Also, it is important to consider the entire spectrum of outcomes. You will see some impressive data that demonstrate the power of compassion, including decreases in mortality. However, it is important from the outset to set expectations, with respect to the concept of "curing" disease.

For example, in these pages, you will not see any evidence that compassion shrinks tumors in patients with cancer. However, you will see a body of very compelling evidence that compassion can have a major effect on how a cancer patient *experiences* their disease (e.g., the severity of their symptoms).

Is that an important goal? Just go ask a cancer patient. Unfortunately, in some cancer patients with incurable disease, the patient's experience is the only goal that can be impacted. Accordingly, achieving a "cure" is not the only important outcome measure in medicine.

Now that you understand the methodology of this systematic review of the scientific literature, let's look next at the actual data on the effects of compassion for patients. The main thing to remember is this: It's important to stop thinking about compassion in a sentimental or emotional way. Rather, start thinking about compassion in a *scientific* way. It's all about examining odds ratios, confidence intervals, and p-values in making the case for compassion.

If you don't know what these statistical terms are, don't worry about it. Just realize that the scientific bar for evidence in the systematic review in the pages to follow is very high. It's the same bar for the evidence used to prove the benefit of any medication you took this morning, or the surgical procedure that your family member underwent recently. If you are a health care provider, it's the same bar used to establish the standards of medical care in your specialty.

If, after seeing all the data in the pages to come, you still believe compassion is just a "nice to have," then you're likely not using evidence-based thinking. That's like continuing to believe in leeches, bloodletting, and the ancient Greeks' system of the "four humors," where interactions of certain bodily fluids—blood, yellow bile, black bile, and phlegm—were believed to explain differences in everything from gender and age to emotions.

That kind of thinking just isn't supported by science.

But let's be clear: beliefs that seem silly now used to be considered state-of-the-art. So the intention isn't to belittle the medical practices of the past. The body of knowledge in medicine is continuously growing and changing. The state-of-the-art continuously evolves, as it should.

But once new evidence becomes irrefutable, there's a responsibility to act on it. Otherwise, health care providers might still be giving patients tobacco enemas.

Wait...tobacco enemas? In the late 1700s, the medical world was divided on the best way to revive a patient who had stopped breathing. You've likely heard the expression, "He's just blowing smoke up your arse." Meaning, he's flattering you...giving an insincere compliment.

But back in the day, literally blowing smoke up a patient's rectum through a long tube was considered a legitimate medical procedure performed by doctors.[71, 72, 73] Actually, it was considered a standard treatment for drowning victims. In fact, some of the greatest minds in the healing arts were fervent believers in the value of this practice. (Although, to be fair, many physicians believed it was better to blow air directly into the mouths of patients—even back then.)

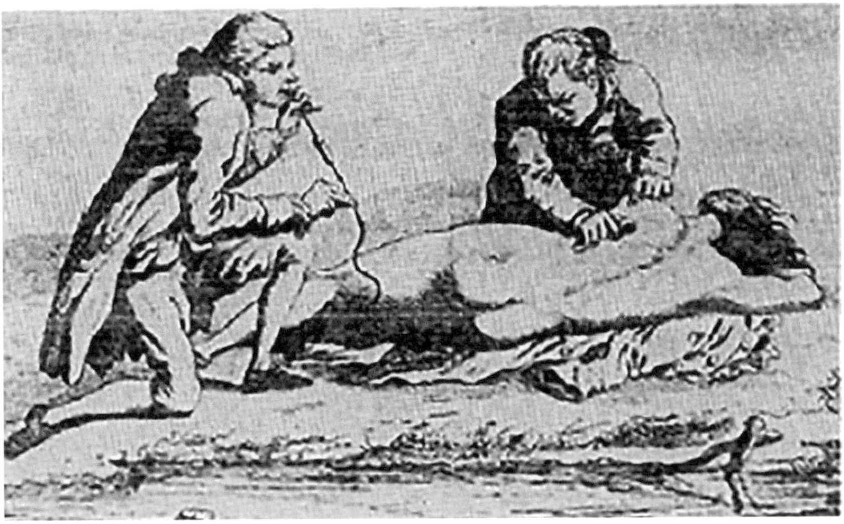

Figure 2.4: Smoke Enema: Depiction of how patients were resuscitated in the 1700's.

Clearly, it's universally accepted today that the best practice for resuscitation is to use assisted ventilation to pump air into people's lungs when they stop breathing. No one would try to use a tobacco enema to get a patient breathing again now. Of course, science doesn't support that approach.

In the same way, some people still believe compassion is a nice to have, even though there is abundant data that shows it's *essential* for quality health care. So what about you? Will you forgo the use of compassion despite the evidence? Or will you join those that embrace the need for it?

It's up to you to decide after you review the evidence in the pages to come. It is important to recognize that the data to follow are not what we think, nor what we believe. Rather, it is what we *found*.

CHAPTER 3: The Physiological Health Benefits of Compassion

"In God we trust; all others must bring data."

—W. Edwards Deming

Before considering the evidence for health care provider compassion and its effects on individual patients, let's first take a high-level look—a thirty-thousand-foot view—at the data on human connection and health outcomes to examine trends in the general population. Much like an epidemiologist (a scientist who studies the incidence of disease in populations) might approach the topic.

If there appears to be a link between meaningful interpersonal relationships and health in the general population, it makes sense that there could also be similar effects from human connection and relationships with patients in the health care environment. So we will begin our journey through the data by starting at the macro level, and then we will zoom in on the effects at the patient level.

The Link between Human Connection and Health

Compelling data on the health benefits of interpersonal relationships can be traced back decades. In 1988 researchers from the University of Michigan published a landmark paper entitled "Social Relationships and Health" in the prestigious journal *Science*.[74]

They analyzed the available evidence from population-based studies and concluded that, after taking into account people's baseline health status, there was an increased risk of death among persons who have a low quantity (or low quality) of personal relationships. They also concluded that social isolation is a major risk factor for dying from a wide variety of causes:

> *"Social relationships, or the relative lack thereof, constitute a major risk factor for health–rivaling the effect of well-established health risk factors such as cigarette smoking, blood pressure, blood lipids (cholesterol), obesity and physical activity"*
>
> —House et al. 1988

For the first time, it was beginning to become clear: *loneliness kills.*

Loneliness kills.

Put another way by a scientist who studies emotions, "Such an existence is too expensive to bear. When launching a life raft, the prudent survivalist will not toss food overboard while retaining the deck furniture. If somebody must jettison a part of life, time with a mate should be last on the list: [one] needs that connection to *live*."[75]

Loneliness and social isolation are not necessarily the same thing. Some people can be socially isolated and not feel lonely. For instance, some may consciously choose a hermit-like existence. Conversely, one can be surrounded by lots of people and feel desperately lonely, especially if the relationships one has are not meaningful.

Loneliness, therefore, is the subjective experience of isolation (i.e., perceived isolation). It's the discrepancy between one's desired and actual level of human connection.[76] So it's not just the quantity of relationships, it's also the quality that matters.

Since that sentinel publication in *Science* back in the late 80s, numerous other rigorous, large-scale analytical studies have confirmed the link between human connection and risk of death from all causes.[77, 78, 79, 80] For example, researchers from Brigham Young University analyzed 148 published research studies (involving more than 300,000 participants across a wide variety of health conditions) and found that having meaningful relationships was associated with 50 percent higher odds of survival.[77]

They also found that in terms of mortality risk, a lack of meaningful relationships was comparable to the risks of smoking and alcohol abuse and worse than obesity and high blood pressure. In another study analyzing 70 published papers specifically focused on the risks of loneliness, the same research team found that being lonely was associated with 26 percent higher odds of early death.[78]

In a longitudinal study supported by the National Institutes of Health (NIH) of 1,604 elderly persons, with six years of follow-up, researchers from the University of California San Francisco found that being lonely was associated with a 50 percent higher risk of decline in functional status (e.g., activities of daily living) and death.[80] In yet another study of an elderly population, researchers from Harvard Medical School learned that being lonely was associated with a subsequent decline in cognitive function.[81]

We can have confidence in these results because all of these studies used rigorous methodology and adjusted the analyses for factors that could be potential confounders, i.e., factors that might give rise to alternative explanations to the conclusion. This minimizes the chance that confounders impacted the results of these studies in a meaningful way. So it wasn't just a case of the subjects being alone and, for example, less safe, thereby increasing the chances that they would die. Their decline—and death—didn't occur because they were *alone*, it was because they were *lonely*.

There are also compelling data in the heart disease literature to support these findings about the relationship between emotional support and death. A Yale study published in *Annals of Internal Medicine* studied this in 194 patients who survived a heart attack.[82] Prior to discharge from the hospital, the researchers interviewed the patients and collected data on their emotional support at home.

Recovery from a heart attack can certainly be tough, both physically and emotionally. The researchers' hypothesis was that having emotional support from close relationships would enhance recovery from the heart attack and help keep them alive long-term.

> Heart attack patients with a lack of emotional support had three times higher odds of death.

What they found is that 39 percent of all the patients they studied died within six months of the heart attack, and patients with a lack of emotional support had *three times higher* odds of death compared to patients who had emotional support. And that was after adjusting the analysis for demographics, marital status, living arrangements, medical history, physical health status, and the presence of depression.

Emotional support appears to be essential...even for survival. It takes close relationships—ones that are meaningful—to help heal a heart that is literally broken.

Loneliness is a Threat to Public Health

The evidence is overwhelming. From a public health viewpoint, loneliness needs to be included on the list of health risk factors for the population, along with physical inactivity, obesity, poverty, environmental exposures, violence, and lack of access to health care. It's a legitimate public health problem.

Accordingly, the World Health Organization now considers "social support networks" to be a vital determinant of health.[83] A recent article in the *New York Times* called the health effects of loneliness "a growing *epidemic*."[84]

In perhaps the most striking sign of the degree of alarm in the public health world, the U.K. government just appointed a Minister for Loneliness.[85] No, we're not joking. The threat is real and growing.

But it's not all bad news. In fact, it's quite the opposite. Just as there is strong evidence that loneliness can be harmful to one's health, there is also evidence that meaningful human connection can have beneficial effects.

In what is likely the longest running scientific study ever conducted (eighty years and still ongoing), the Harvard Study of Adult Development began tracking the health of 268 Harvard sophomores, as well as a group of Boston teenagers, beginning in 1938 and checking in with them regularly over time. (Note: all the original study subjects were men because Harvard was still all male back then).

The researchers followed the trajectory of their lives, with the aim of identifying the key factors responsible for good health and happiness. Only a few of the people initially enrolled in the study are still alive, but the results over the years paint a clear picture of the importance of human connection in health, vitality, and longevity.

Dr. Robert Waldinger, the current study director and the fourth to hold that title, who is a psychiatrist at Massachusetts General Hospital and professor at Harvard Medical School, summarizes it like this:

> *"Good relationships keep us happier and healthier…and loneliness kills. When we gathered together everything we knew about them about at age 50, it wasn't their middle-age cholesterol levels that predicted how they were going to grow old,*

it was how satisfied they were in their relationships. The people who were the most satisfied in their relationships at age 50 were the healthiest at age 80."[86]

Meaningful human connection was in fact *protective.* But how? Although many might agree that humans are by nature a social species, what is the mechanism by which human connection can impact our health?

The short answer is that we don't know yet, at least not entirely. The mechanisms appear to be extremely complex, but many researchers have identified at least one common thread: *stress.*

Being lonely causes a similar response in the body as being under extreme stress all the time. For example, it raises the level of a stress hormone called cortisol circulating in the blood, which can play a role in chronic inflammation and subsequent development of cardiovascular disease.

Also, without meaningful human connection to balance one's stress, loneliness results in activation of the part of the nervous system called the sympathetic nervous system. It is the "fight or flight" response that gets turned on when you are experiencing a threat of harm.[87]

This makes sense because research from the University of Chicago has also shown that loneliness predicts a rise in blood pressure over time, and a recent meta-analysis of 23 research studies found that loneliness is associated with a 29 percent higher risk of coronary artery disease and a 32 percent increase in the risk of stroke.[88, 89]

Here is another mechanism of loneliness: its effect on the immune system. In a study sponsored by the NIH, researchers from Carnegie Mellon University studied the immune response to influenza (flu) vaccine among freshmen undergraduate students and its relationship to students' level of loneliness.[90] They did this both at the beginning of the study and over the course of the semester in which they received the flu vaccine.

Then they measured the level of antibodies against the flu virus in the students' blood, which is a readout of building immunity to the flu in response to the vaccine. What they found was striking: Students who were lonely had the lowest levels of antibodies against the flu virus. In other words, they had the weakest immune response to the vaccination; their bodies were less likely to fight off the flu virus.

The lonely students also reported greater psychological stress and had higher levels of circulating cortisol. But the results of the research are clear: After accounting for all other potential confounding factors, being lonely was associated with worse immune function and could hurt one's resistance to infection.

These data on immune function are corroborated by the findings in another Carnegie Mellon University study published in *JAMA*.[91] In this study, researchers assessed the social relationships of 276 volunteers by measuring the number of activities with a spouse, parent, friend, workmate, or other close connections.

Then the participants were given nasal drops containing rhinovirus (i.e., the common cold virus) and were monitored to see if they developed a cold. The researchers also measured physiological response to the cold virus, such as how much mucous they produced and how well the subjects were clearing the virus from their nasal passages.

> A lack of human connection can increase susceptibility to the common cold.

What they found is that, compared to people with robust social connections, people with social isolation (i.e., the least human connection) had increased susceptibility to the common cold, more mucous production, and a lower clearance of the virus from their nasal passages. Those lacking in human connection were not as resistant to illness.

Eye-opening research from the University of California Los Angeles has found that loneliness can also affect our genetics. Specifically, these researchers looked at gene expression in circulating white blood cells, which are involved in the immune response.

By upregulating (i.e., "turning on") and downregulating (i.e., "turning off") various genes in the immune system, loneliness can produce a state of chronic systemic inflammation (activation of inflammation throughout the body).[92] Chronic systemic inflammation has been linked with a myriad of adverse health effects, not only the development of cardiovascular disease, but also arthritis, diabetes, dementia, and many others.

Human Connection Matters

So yes, loneliness can have devastating effects on health. But compassion can be the antidote. The scientific evidence suggests that the chronic inflammation we just talked about (and perhaps the health effects that can result from that over time) can actually be reduced by someone who cares.

Research from Northwestern University that studied 247 adolescents and their parents found that high parental compassion is not only associated with their children having lower emotional distress, but their children also had significantly lower circulating blood markers of systemic inflammation![93]

How often have you heard about how stress can worsen health conditions? Probably quite often. You may have already been aware of the connection between stress—specifically emotional distress—and its potential adverse effects on your health. This has been known for decades, perhaps most notably in cardiovascular disease.[94]

So the notion of a "mind-body" connection, where one's thoughts, beliefs, and experiences (e.g., their experience of loneliness) affects their biology and physical health, is probably not hard to believe. But one thing you may not know is that while the link with adverse health effects has been known about for decades, it was only recently that researchers could actually *see* this connection. They saw it on brain scans.

Here's how it happened: In a Harvard study funded by the NIH and published in *The Lancet*, researchers used functional MRI brain scans to measure the activity in a region of peoples' brains called the amygdala, and then they followed up with them over time to see what was happening with their physical health.[95]

The amygdala is a structure deep inside the brain, about the size of an almond, where we process emotions, and it's also an "alarm system" involved in the fight-or-flight response. It's activated under conditions of extreme stress, including emotional distress, and loneliness can be one of these triggers.

How does the functional MRI fit in here? It takes a look inside the brain to see what areas light up due to subtle increases in blood flow. It shows researchers which areas of a patient's brain are firing at any given moment.

The people recruited for the study were healthy at the time and not under any particular distress at the moment, so whatever brain activation they had in the amygdala was presumably the baseline stress (or distress) that they carry around with them every day. (As we noted in Chapter 1, you never really know what kind of pain people are carrying around, and of course we can't do functional MRI on every person we meet to try to figure that out.)

What this Harvard study found was striking. The baseline activation in the amygdala region of the brain predicted not only the amount of inflammation they had going on in the blood vessels throughout their body (the researchers measured it), but it also predicted the subsequent development of serious cardiovascular disease events, like heart attacks and strokes, over time.

So it may not take much to convince you that there is a mind-body connection, due to decades of reports about the health outcomes, but now we have brain scans that can help explain and actually visualize the neurobiology behind it all.

And here is the most dramatic example of the mind-body connection that exists: It's a condition called Takotsubo cardiomyopathy (also known as "stress cardiomyopathy" or "broken heart syndrome"). It's a very serious cardiac emergency that (thankfully) is uncommon, but seeing a case of it can be among the most unforgettable events in one's medical career.

You will read about an especially dramatic case of this condition later, but here's how it works: Takotsubo cardiomyopathy is commonly triggered by extreme emotional stress, like a relationship ending or a death in the family. The name Takotsubo comes from the Japanese word for octopus trap (which is apparently what the heart looks like on echocardiography during this condition).

Here's what happens to people: When doctors use an echocardiogram to look at the heart pumping in a Takotsubo cardiomyopathy patient, they see that the main chamber of the heart—the one that is responsible for pumping blood out to rest of the body—takes on an abnormal shape, thought to resemble a fishing pot by those who first described it in the medical literature.

In this condition, the heart suddenly becomes unable to pump blood effectively, and the patient suddenly goes into a state of heart failure and life-threatening shock. When this happens, the first thing that the doctors typically think of is the most common cause of sudden heart failure: a heart attack.

But when they look for clogged heart arteries they do not find any. The blood vessels are wide open. How and why it occurs is not totally understood yet, but one piece of it appears to be a spike in circulating hormones called epinephrine and norepinephrine that are released by the body in response to stress, such as severe emotional stress.

It can be rapidly fatal. Literally, the person can suddenly collapse or even drop dead. Have you ever heard that, after the death of a loved one, someone suddenly "died of a broken heart?" That's why Takotsubo cardiomyopathy is also nicknamed "broken heart syndrome." It actually happens, and it has been well described in the medical literature (e.g., the *New England Journal of Medicine*).[96]

So, you might now ask: "What does all this data on loneliness and the mind-body connection have to do with compassion?"

The answer is: *everything.*

The most obvious reason is that reaching out to lonely people with compassion fosters human connection that can make a lonely person feel less alone. In one of the most striking compassion research studies you will read about later, a randomized trial of a compassion intervention for cancer patients at Johns Hopkins University, one of the key elements of the intervention was this message from the physician to the patient.

> *"I know this is a tough experience to go through and I want you to know that I am here with you. We are here together, and we will go through this together. I will be with you each step along the way."*[97]

Seriously ill people go through very dark times and walk through dark places where they may feel all alone or abandoned. More than ever before in their life, they need to know that someone is willing to walk with them.

Now that you understand all the scientific data for the dramatic effects of loneliness on health outcomes and the effect it can have on their health (especially when someone is sick), will you be more willing to walk with a patient who feels all alone? Will you be willing to ask *if* they feel alone? We may never know if we neglect to ask. Hopefully, now you know how much it matters.

The data on the health effects of loneliness, human connection, and the mind-body connection provide the context. They set the stage for all of the data on compassion that will follow and lay the groundwork for the profound effect of human connection on human health.

It's important to see this "big picture" first, before reviewing the data that is specific to compassion for others. If human connection was not a determinant of health, then there would be no scientific rationale for believing that modulating human connection (through compassion) would be meaningful for health. But now that we know human connection is strongly associated with better health, it makes sense that augmenting human connection with a compassion intervention could result in meaningful change.

> For good health, human connection *matters.*

The data we've reviewed so far has laid an important foundation, a starting point to begin to open our minds to the possibility that how we relate to one another—how we connect or fail to connect—can, in fact, impact one's health in meaningful ways. For good health, human connection *matters.*

That's powerful. And it is obviously rooted in very rigorous scientific evidence. It's not mushy. It's not soft. It's science. It's part of that overlap between both the art and science of medicine, areas that previously were believed to be completely separate and distinct.

But now that we know human connection matters, what is the evidence that *compassion* matters? Next, let's zoom in specifically on the power of compassion for patients.

Compassion Heals

Dr. Alann Solina is an expert in putting people to sleep. To be fair, he's also an expert in waking them up. That's what anesthesiologists do.

As chief and chair of the Department of Anesthesiology at Cooper University Health Care and Cooper Medical School of Rowan University, Dr. Solina has provided anesthesia to more than 25,000 patients undergoing surgical procedures over the course of his career. The method by which anesthesiologists put people to sleep and make sure they have their pain minimized as much as possible is straightforward. They use drugs. At least that's what they teach aspiring anesthesiologists in their training.

There is no doubt that effective drugs are at the core of providing effective anesthesia for perioperative patients. But are drugs the only effective therapy? In Dr. Solina's experience, the answer is most definitely, "No."

Dr. Solina's leadership of the Department of Anesthesiology is characterized by being an "in the trenches" leader. That is, while carrying a huge administrative load in running the department, he also continues to maintain a very active clinical practice on the front lines of medicine. Why? "Among all that I do, taking care of patients at the bedside is what gives me the most fulfillment," he says.

When asked what specific aspect of clinical practice brings him the most fulfillment, his answer is simple: "Connecting with patients prior to surgery, building rapport, providing them with reassurance, and, most of all, treating them with compassion." Why? Because he sees the profound effect that it can have.

If you are a patient, having surgery can be hard. There can be tremendous anxiety in the days leading up to surgery, and that can skyrocket when you are in the pre-op area waiting to be wheeled into the operating room. In addition, patients having surgery may have an underlying condition associated with major suffering, so they're looking for relief. That moment of waiting for surgery can be one of the most vulnerable times in a person's life.

In that moment, Dr. Solina has observed, compassion is essential. And it works.

Works? What does that mean? Works *how*?

Dr. Solina has made an astute observation, one that is consistently borne out time and time again, in his decades of experience. "When I am able to build a bond with a patient ahead of surgery, where I show that I care about them and they put their trust in me, I find that they actually need a lower amount of sedatives ahead of surgery and oftentimes none at all. When we wheel them into the operating room, they are much more likely to be peaceful and calm."

He has come to this conclusion after decades of close personal observation. "It's not just about the drugs and the anesthetic agents; it's also about the anesthesiologist," he reports. When he makes a compassionate connection with a patient who is about to be wheeled into the operating room, he actually becomes *part of the therapy*.

Is Dr. Solina overreaching? Are his observations a bias towards overvaluing his relationships and interactions with patients?

What do the scientific data say? There are rigorous experimental data (actually, clinical trials published in two of the most highly regarded medical journals worldwide) supporting exactly what Dr. Solina has been observing over the course of his career in academic medicine.

The Role of the Healer as Therapy

In the 1960s, at Massachusetts General Hospital in Boston, researchers in anesthesiology from Harvard Medical School conducted two experiments in patients awaiting surgery. They published the results in *The New England Journal of Medicine* and *JAMA*.[98, 99]

In these studies, the researchers tested an unconventional hypothesis, one that was decades ahead of its time: Could the anesthesiologist be the agent of therapy? Could he or she actually *be* the treatment? They tested the hypothesis that a compassionate connection from the anesthesiologist would have a meaningful and measurable effect on patients.

These studies were randomized controlled trials: a research design in which half of the patients were assigned, at random, to a new experimental therapy, and the other half of the patients did not get the experimental therapy (i.e., the control group). A randomized controlled trial is considered the most rigorous type of study from a scientific perspective, because it is the best way to minimize the risk of bias or confounding of the study results.

What was striking about these two studies, however, was that the experimental therapy was not some new anesthesia drug or high-tech approach. Actually, it could be considered "old school."

In these studies, half of the patients were randomly assigned the experimental therapy that consisted of a special (extra) visit prior to surgery from—you guessed it—the anesthesiologist. The purpose of the extra visit was explicitly to build doctor-patient rapport.

The anesthesiologist's compassion for the patients was a cornerstone of the reassuring and bonding experience. In fact, the researchers called these patients the "special care" group. One of these studies compared the effects of the anesthesiologist's special care versus the effects of a powerful sedative (a drug called pentobarbital) administered just prior to surgery.

The results were striking. The researchers found that the patients who were administered pentobarbital were drowsy just prior to surgery, but they were not calm. On the other hand, patients in the special care group were calm, but not drowsy.[98]

How reliable were these results? The research used a predefined methodology to standardize the assessment of calm and drowsy, used a randomized trial design, and was published one of the leading biomedical journals in the world.

The results were highly statistically significant. Therefore, we can have high confidence in the findings.

So this experiment demonstrated through science that a rapport-building, compassionate connection with an anesthesiologist before surgery can make patients calmer as they are about to undergo surgery, necessitating less sedatives. In fact, the researchers found that to achieve what they prospectively defined as "adequate sedation," the effect of the special care pre-operative visit from the anesthesiologist was *more than double* the effect of administering pentobarbital. You will recall that this is exactly what Dr. Solina has observed about the power of compassion for patients over decades in real-world practice!

But that's not all. In the second of the two experiments at Mass General, they tested the effects of the special care intervention (i.e., the same pre-operative visit from the anesthesiologist) on patients' post-operative pain.[99]

Equally as striking as the results of the first experiment, in the second experiment they found that patients randomized to the special care visit from the anesthesiologist prior to surgery had *50 percent lower* requirement for opiate pain medication (e.g., morphine) following surgery. Interestingly, the patients who were randomly assigned to special care also had a statistically significant decrease in their length of stay in the hospital following surgery.

In 2015, another randomized, controlled trial found essentially the same effects on post-operative pain.[100] Researchers randomized 104 patients about to undergo surgery to one of two treatment arms, either the usual pre-operative care, or pre-operative care with enhanced compassion.

In this study, rather than an anesthesiologist, the people delivering the pre-operative care were surgical nurses. For the enhanced compassion intervention, the nurses underwent specific training to give compassionate responses to patients' emotions through explicit compassion-focused behaviors.

On the first post-operative day, the researchers found that patients randomly assigned to a compassion intervention had *50 percent lower* scores on pain ratings compared to patients randomly assigned to usual care. Very similar results to what they found at Mass General way back in the 1960s.

In these randomized trials of vulnerable patients about to undergo surgery, the health care providers *themselves* made a major difference in the patients' care. The compassionate pre-operative visit reduced the need for drugs, both sedatives and pain medication. These were the effects observed with the experimental application of a "new" therapy...a compassionate human connection!

Perhaps the results here should not be that surprising, because there is abundant data to support the physiology of the calming effect of compassion on patients. So the notion that compassion for patients could combat not only stress, but also stress-mediated disease, should not be that difficult to believe.

Compassion Calms Physiological Response to Stress

Compassion acts in a powerful way on the autonomic nervous system, which is responsible for all of the body functions that happen automatically, without you having to consciously think about it. For example, you do not have to consciously think about your heart beating, and you don't have to remember to breathe. They just happen.

The autonomic nervous system has two components: the sympathetic nervous system and the parasympathetic nervous system. Earlier in this chapter, we talked about activation of the sympathetic nervous system, i.e., the "fight or flight" response to threat, danger, and stress in general. Sustained activation of the fight or flight response due to prolonged stress and anxiety can cause all kinds of physical symptoms that aren't conducive to healing.

But the other side of the autonomic nervous system is the parasympathetic nervous system, i.e., the "rest and digest" response. It directly counterbalances the response of the sympathetic nervous system, like a yin and yang phenomenon.

While the sympathetic nervous system involves a spike in circulating cortisol and adrenaline for the fight or flight response while you are under threat, activation of the parasympathetic nervous system is a response producing a feeling of peacefulness and calm.

Activation of the parasympathetic nervous system can also be thought of as the "relaxation response." And it is part of the scientific explanation of the positive emotion—the warm, calming effect that we feel—when someone cares deeply about us and shows us compassion. It not only lowers our stress, it quells our fears.[101]

Along with parasympathetic nervous system activation, there is also a rise in a circulating hormone called oxytocin, a molecule that serves numerous functions in the body including an increase in feelings of nurturing, bonding, and affiliation (i.e., gravitating toward close relationships with others). That is why some people refer to oxytocin as the "trust hormone", the "bonding hormone," or even the "love hormone."

Scientific evidence supports that human connection is a powerful activator of not only positive emotion, but also the parasympathetic nervous system.[102] This is especially true for compassion. For example, research from Wake Forest University shows that compassion can change the physiology of the receiver of compassion by harnessing the power of the parasympathetic nervous system.[103, 104] In these experiments conducted in a health care clinic, the researchers found that treating another person with compassion not only improved the receiver's subjective sense of well-being and lowered their stress, but it also improved the receivers' physiological measures of autonomic nervous system activity.

The receivers' respiratory rate and heart rate decreased, while their heart rate variability increased. This is a good thing: it's a sign of cardiovascular well-being when an individual's heart rate varies based on changing conditions.

The measurement of heart rate variability is a measure of variation within beat-to-beat intervals that is measured with a heart rhythm monitor. When heart rate variability is high, this indicates that the body's natural "pacemaker"—the link between the nervous system and the cardiovascular system—is functioning properly.

Although it is not something that is routinely measured in doctor's offices (at least not yet), scientists are well aware that lack of heart rate variability can be a "canary in the coal mine" for nervous system and cardiovascular system dysfunction (i.e., indicator of physiologic instability). The important take-home point here is that compassion for others not only improves the receivers' subjective experience (i.e., feeling of warmth), but it can actually have measurable effects on how the receivers' nervous system and cardiovascular system function.

This effect can cut both ways. While the beneficial physiological effects of compassion are mediated largely through activation of the parasympathetic nervous system, negative interpersonal interactions can cause the opposite reaction through activation of the sympathetic nervous system.

Although it is intuitive that a negative interpersonal interaction can be upsetting and can exacerbate one's stress, there is ample scientific evidence that it can also trigger a reduction in one's heart rate variability.[105]

Compassion Lowers Blood Pressure

If the effect of compassion on one's respiratory rate, heart rate, and heart rate variability isn't compelling enough evidence for you that compassion can have meaningful physiological effects, what about blood pressure? While understanding the value of heart rate variability may be new to you, you probably already know that a rise in blood pressure over time is bad thing.

> Compassionate touch from a supportive other can lower the receiver's blood pressure.

Research from Brigham Young University shows that compassionate touch from a supportive other can lower the receiver's blood pressure over time.[106] The mechanism is thought to be buffering (i.e., reducing the effects of) stress-mediated rises in blood pressure.

These data are corroborated by numerous other research studies that have shown a compassionate connection from a supportive other can buffer one's cardiovascular stress responses, when compared to the presence of a non-supportive other or experiencing the stress alone.[107, 108] This may be why that University of Chicago study mentioned earlier in this chapter found that loneliness was associated with developing high blood pressure.

So the take-home message here is this: compassion is not just "in your head." Rigorous research shows that compassion for others (or lack thereof) can affect people's nervous system and cardiovascular system in measurable ways. (If you need a reminder of the most dramatic example, just look back at the section on Takotsubo cardiomyopathy, and how a person under severe emotional stress can die of a broken heart!)

Perhaps this is part of the explanation why the compassionate "special care" visit from the anesthesiologist in the Mass General study described earlier was more effective than drugs for inducing calm in patients headed for the operating room.[98]

We have already seen that a compassionate connection from a health care provider can have a profound effect on patients in an extreme health situation, like undergoing major surgery.[99] A University of Colorado study supported by a research grant from the NIH had a similar finding after analyzing data from 34 controlled experimental studies of patients recovering from a medical crisis (specifically, heart attack or surgery).[109]

In the vast majority (85 percent) of the outcome measures examined across these 34 studies, the researchers found a positive association between psychological and emotional support from health care providers and favorable clinical outcomes. Compared to "ordinary care," they found that psychological and emotional support was associated with an improvement in the patients' recovery. Again, compassion mattered in measurable ways.

Compassion Promotes Healing from Trauma

It appears that compassion also matters in patients who undergo major trauma.[110] In a study of 136 trauma patients admitted to a Level 1 trauma center, researchers assessed Patient Reported Outcome Measures (PROMs)—which are the patients' subjective assessment of their own recovery—at six weeks and one year following discharge from the hospital.

Using a validated compassionate care scale, they also measured the patients' assessment of the compassion of the physicians caring for them at the trauma center. They analyzed the data with a mathematical model that adjusted for demographic, socioeconomic, and injury-related factors and found that high physician compassion was independently associated with a good outcome at the one year mark.

> In a study of trauma patients, the odds of a patient-reported good outcome were four times higher when the physician was rated as having high compassion.

In fact, the odds of a patient-reported good outcome were *four times higher*. So if you were a trauma patient in this study, the odds of you reporting a good outcome one year later were four times higher if the physician that treated you was particularly compassionate in handling your care.

Compassion Improves Quality of Life in Palliative Care

Another extreme health situation is which compassion appears to make a measurable difference is end-of-life care. Palliative care is a specialty within medicine that focuses on relief of symptoms and quality of life among patients who have a terminal diagnosis. The goal of palliative care is not to cure the disease, but rather to improve the quality of life in the time that a patient has left.

A cornerstone of palliative care is compassion for patients and their families.[111] A study from Mass General (in collaboration with Columbia University and Yale University) published in *The New England Journal of Medicine* tested the effects of compassionate palliative care in terminally ill patients with lung cancer.[112] They randomized the patients to receive standard cancer care versus standard care plus early palliative care and tested the effects on quality of life.

The results confirmed the hypothesis; patients receiving palliative care had better quality of life. That was expected. What was unexpected was that there was also an effect on *survival*. Patients randomly assigned to receive compassionate palliative care actually survived, on average, 30 percent longer!

Think about this: a study designed to show that compassion increases quality of life in people with limited time left to live actually found that it increased how long they lived. We wonder if the authors of the study even contemplated that was a possibility. In some sense, these patients were surviving on compassion.

But what about less dire circumstances? Does compassion only matter in an emergency or major (life or death) crisis, or does it also matter in everyday health?

We have seen how compassion can have a measurable effect on a patient's physiological parameters (i.e., measures of nervous system and cardiovascular system homeostasis). But what about in the context of a routine visit to the doctor's office?

The answer is *yes*. Let's walk through some of the most common reasons for visits to the doctor and see examples of how compassion can make a difference there as well.

Compassion Reduces Perception of Pain

What about the impact of compassion on a patient's perception of pain? You will recall from the Harvard anesthesiology research that a compassionate connection from the anesthesiologist before surgery reduced the requirement of opiate pain medication after surgery.[99] Is there evidence of this type of effect in other health care domains?

First a disclaimer: there is no evidence that compassion for patients eliminates pain. It doesn't. That's not the question. The question is this: can compassion *reduce* pain? Can it buffer a patient's experience of pain in a way that makes it more bearable?

Another thing before we look at the data: The science of feeling and treating pain is extraordinarily complex. So much so that there is now an entire specialty in medicine devoted to the subject (i.e., pain management specialists).

In fact, there are sub-specialists of specialists that now specialize in pain. All of these specialties—anesthesiologists, family medicine physicians, internal medicine physicians, neurologists, psychiatrists, emergency medicine physicians, physical medicine/rehabilitation physicians (and the list is growing)—now have pathways to advanced training in pain management.

There are numerous physiological, pathophysiological, and psychological factors that influence one's experience of pain and pain relief. The data to follow is not meant to be overly simplistic or minimize a very complex set of factors that culminate in a patient's experience of pain.

But, that said, there is a clear signal in the data. Human connection can in fact modulate the pain that people experience in measurable ways.

> Human connection can modulate the pain that people experience in measurable ways.

But how? Although the physiological mechanisms are complex and incompletely understood at the present time, it is clear that endogenous opioids play a large role. Endogenous opioids are molecules produced naturally by the body in response to a number of potential triggers, one of which is receiving compassion from others.

One example of endogenous opioids produced by the body are endorphins, the molecules responsible for what happens to runners when they experience a "runner's high." That's when a runner becomes numb to the pain of extremely strenuous running and actually experiences a euphoric feeling.

The biological effects of endogenous opioids are similar to the effects of exogenous opioids (e.g., giving powerful drugs like morphine); they bind to similar opioid receptors in the brain to give an analgesic (pain reducing) effect or reduce sensitivity to pain. For years, scientists have known from experimental studies that a compassionate connection with a supportive other can affect one's experience of pain. An experimental study refers to experimentally-induced pain (i.e., deliberately inducing pain in a human subject).

Of course, this has to be done in healthy volunteers because it would be unethical to expose a sick patient to more pain than they already have for the sake of an experiment! But there is abundant experimental data from laboratory studies conducted in healthy volunteers.

Touch Matters

In one study from the University of Haifa in Israel, researchers applied a painful heat stimulus to volunteers' forearms and then tested their subjective pain scores when either a stranger or a trusted other (e.g., a spouse or life partner) held the subject's hand.[113] Pain wasn't affected at all with hand holding from the stranger.

But you know what? When it was a loved one doing the hand holding, there was statistically significant reduction in the rating of pain—by more than

50 percent. Trust is powerful. But so is the compassion of the trusted other providing support. The researchers found a statistically significant inverse correlation between the assessment of the hand holders' compassion and the pain rating (i.e., higher compassion = lower pain). This study shows that the touch of trusted others can in fact reduce one's perception of pain, and there is a synergistic effect of compassion and the magnitude of the effect.

In another interesting and elegant study from the same group, the researchers found that during experimentally-induced pain, the compassionate touch of a trusted other results in physiological "coupling."[114] The cardiovascular system and respiratory system of the trusted other literally gets in sync with the cardiovascular system and the respiratory system of the one receiving the painful stimulus.

The researchers found that there is coupling of both the heart rates and the respiratory rates of the two people, a synchronous harmony of the heartbeats and breathing that mirrors each other. Their autonomic nervous systems actually align.

Even their brain waves mirror each other![115] Further, it is in this physiological coupling that the effect of compassionate touch on pain reduction occurs. In fact, the research showed that a compassionate response from a trusted other was only effective if touch occurred.

Touch matters. Maybe you have felt the effects of that synchrony and connectedness before, when someone who cares deeply about you lends a hand. Compelling data on this phenomenon are also available from the laboratory of Dr. James Coan at the University of Virginia, but this research relates to the threat (i.e., the expectation) of experimentally-induced pain, in the form of an electric shock.[116, 117]

In this laboratory, volunteers gazed at a screen in front of them. Whenever they saw a red "X", there was a one in five chance that they would receive an electric shock in the next few seconds. Whenever they saw an "O" on the screen, that meant they were safe. Coan and colleagues wanted to see how people's brains reacted to the threat of pain and, in particular, whether the brain behaved differently whether a person was facing the threat alone, holding the hand of a stranger (one of the lab technicians), or that of someone they knew and trusted.

The zaps of the electric shocks hurt…a lot. After the first jolt, the volunteers felt a sort of panicked dread every time they saw a red X. They were hugely relieved when the experiment ended.

What Coan and colleagues found using brain imaging is that when a person was alone or holding a stranger's hand as he or she anticipated the shock, the regions of the brain that process danger lit up like a Christmas tree. But when holding the hand of a trusted person, the brain grew quiet.

The researchers believe that having a trusted other with you alters the perception of that threat. The volunteers can "take it" (i.e., do not perceive threat or danger) because they do not feel alone.[118]

This research may not be surprising to you because, intuitively, having people walk with us through difficult times can lessen the pain. We know this clinically as well. A University of Toronto randomized controlled trial published in *The New England Journal of Medicine* found that, for patients with metastatic breast cancer, participating in supportive-expressive group therapy (i.e., a support group) significantly reduced patients' reports of pain over time, especially if the baseline pain level was high at the time of study entry.[119]

Compassion Builds Trust

Do all of the data on the effects of having a trusted other have important implications for health care? What if health care providers are meeting a patient for the first time? Can they really play such a meaningful role for a patient?

Actually, yes. When seeking health care, most patients confer trust in physicians, nurses, and other caregivers when they make the choice to place their health and well-being in their hands. Without trust, why would a patient ever take a health care provider's advice or adhere to his or her recommendations? Patients want to give trust to their providers.

But here is the catch: Trust is not automatic. A health care provider must build that trust, and one of the ways to rapidly build trust is through compassion. There is ample evidence on this in the biomedical literature.

For example, in a study of 550 outpatients, researchers at Michigan State University found that patient perception of physician compassion was associated with higher trust in the physician.[120] In a NIH-supported study of hospitalized patients, researchers at University of California San Francisco found that compassionate responses to patients by the physician had a measurable and statistically significant effect on patient rating of trust in the physician.[48]

Multiple studies have shown an association between better patient experience and connecting with or trusting the physician. So a health care provider that is compassionate can readily become a trusted other for a patient. And therefore, a health care provider may be a person whose compassion and emotional support can affect patients' experience of pain. The trust may not be automatic, but the bar is fairly low to earn it.

In one of the first studies that demonstrated a health care provider's compassion can actually change what is happening in a patient's brain, researchers at Michigan State University performed a functional MRI to measure brain activity in people that underwent an experimental painful stimulus.[121] The subjects were recruited from the waiting room of a primary care clinic.

All of the study participants underwent a medical interview from a physician and were randomized to one of two study groups. In the first group, the medical interview was patient-centered, with an emotional support focus and included a 21-point compassionate care procedure from the physician.

In the second group, it was a medical interview without any expression of compassion from the physician. Then the subjects were given a painful stimulus (electrical stimulation) while simultaneously being shown an image of the physician at the same time that a brain scan (functional MRI) was done.

What they found was that the compassion group experienced less pain, as evidenced by *47 percent* less activation in the region of the brain for experiencing pain. So the connection they made with the compassionate physician—who they just met—actually buffered the pain.

What does this mean? Compassion from the physician imprinted upon the study subjects. The trusted other didn't need to provide real-time compassion, such as hand holding. The compassion literally echoed from the initial visit into the later (painful) part of the experiment.

You may ask: Besides all the experimental studies, and the study of the compassionate care of the anesthesiologist for surgical patients, are there other studies showing that compassion can buffer a patients' pain in a real-world clinical setting? The answer is *yes.*

Compassion Reduces Back Pain

Low back pain is one of the most common reasons for seeking medical care in the U.S. Eighty percent of people will experience significant low back pain at some point in their lifetime, with 10 to 20 percent of those at risk for developing chronic low back pain and disability. Thus the scope of the problem is huge, and the toll that it takes on people is immense. Those individuals often are so debilitated by pain that they need to stop working, turning to workers' compensation funds or disability benefits to get by.[122]

Here are some noteworthy study results to consider: In a rehabilitation medicine randomized controlled trial in patients with chronic low back pain, researchers randomly assigned patients to receive either conventional physical therapy or physical therapy plus an "enhanced therapeutic alliance," in which the therapist intentionally used a compassionate tone of voice and nonverbal behaviors—like eye contact and touch—plus statements of compassion such as, "I can understand how difficult low back pain must be for you."[123]

The outcome measures for the study were a well-validated scale of pain intensity, reported by the patients prior to and after therapy, as well as "pressure pain sensitivity," which is the standard quantitative method for measuring low back muscle tenderness in pain research. Basically, it is a calibrated instrument that precisely measures how hard you can press on sore back muscles before the patient reports having pain.

What the researchers found is that patients randomly assigned to the compassionate therapeutic alliance had *more than double* the pain relief from physical therapy, compared to physical therapy without the compassion enhancement. Further, following therapy, researchers could also press significantly harder on the patients' sore backs without eliciting pain if they were in the enhanced compassion group.

In another rehabilitation medicine study of two hundred patients, researchers tested the association between the quality of the patient-doctor interaction (from the patients' perspective) and the amount of pain patients were still in six months later.[124] Specifically, they measured the physicians' affective (or emotional) quality of the interaction, a key part of which was physician compassion.

They measured the patients' pain and disability at the beginning of the study and again at six months. What they found was that when patients perceived high quality interaction with the physician, the improvements in pain intensity, pain frequency, and the level of functional impairment specifically due to pain were all more than *double* the improvements experienced by patients who perceived low quality interaction with the physician.

So if health care providers can make a sizeable dent in all that pain, suffering, and lost productivity with compassionate care, shouldn't they do it?

Compassion Reduces Headache and IBS Pain

If the evidence of the effect of compassion on back pain isn't convincing enough, then consider the data on headaches.

In another interesting pain study, researchers tested the association between physician compassion, as assessed by patients, and the pain experienced by patients who suffer from migraine headaches.[125] They recruited patients going to neurology clinics for migraine treatment and measured the patients' degree of disability from migraines at the time of seeing the physician and then again ninety days later, using a standardized, well-validated scale.

They also measured the patients' assessment of the physicians' compassion using another well-validated survey that is the most commonly used survey instrument in compassion science research to date. It's called the CARE measure (the acronym stands for Consultation And Relational Empathy).

What they found was a very high level of correlation between the physicians' performance on the CARE measure and the decrease in migraine headache-related disability experienced by the patients. So the more compassion, the lower the pain. Specifically, there was a high level of correlation between the CARE measure and the number of days with a headache, as well as intensity of the headache pain.

One of the most interesting studies pertaining to impact on pain is in a disease called irritable bowel syndrome, or IBS. This is a chronic, potentially debilitating intestinal disorder that causes abdominal pain (along with gas, diarrhea, and constipation). It's a fairly common problem; for example, it's the reason for nearly a third of patient referrals to gastroenterologists.

People with IBS can experience great suffering. There are few treatments and those that exist are only partially effective. As a result, and in an attempt to get some sort of relief, patients often turn to "complementary medicine" treatments (sometimes also called "alternative medicine") such as acupuncture.

But what if compassion is actually more powerful than either conventional or alternative therapies? In a randomized controlled trial from Harvard Medical School, researchers randomly assigned 262 patients with IBS to one of three treatment groups: (1) nothing (control group)—observation only; (2) acupuncture; or (3) an "augmented patient-provider relationship," (i.e., augmented by human connection through warmth, attention, and compassion).[126] For example, compassionate statements included "I can understand how difficult IBS must be for you."

In this third arm of the study, the providers were not allowed to give any other potentially effective treatment, like extra education, counseling, or use of a technique called "cognitive behavioral therapy." The only things in the intervention were human connection and compassion.

Then they measured the effects of each of these interventions on the patients' symptom relief, symptom severity, and quality of life. Compared to observation alone, acupuncture helped a bit. But the really striking results were in the group that experienced the augmented relationship with the health care provider.

The warmth and compassion from providers made an enormous difference! Three weeks later, the proportion of patients in the augmented human connection group that had adequate relief of symptoms, including abdominal pain, was *double* the proportion of patients with adequate relief in the observation-only control group. For these patients with IBS, compassionate care was a game changer.

Another Thought to Consider

Considering all of the data just reviewed in this chapter regarding compassion and pain—from experimentally induced pain, to post-operative pain, to back pain, to headache and IBS—showing such dramatic impact and published in distinguished scientific journals, how is it that these findings are not better known? With the number of deaths annually in the U.S. from opioid overdoses now surpassing the deaths from car crashes, deaths from guns, and deaths from the peak of the HIV crisis, shouldn't medicine be taking a closer look at caregiver compassion as a possible component of the treatment modalities to lower opioid use, as in the studies described above?[127]

So why haven't all of these studies on compassion and pain been pulled together before? This is an example of the purpose of this book. Despite all these data being previously available in the scientific literature, all the dots had not been connected together to paint the overall picture.

Compassion Improves Functional Impairment

Intractable pain can certainly limit a person's ability to function properly. So it's not surprising that the studies above—those that showed caregiver compassion can impact the pain that patients experience—also showed that compassion improved patients' overall functional status. That's what they found in the back pain study, the rehabilitation medicine study, the migraine headache study, and the irritable bowel syndrome study.[123, 124, 125,126]

But there is also research on the impact of compassion on functional impairment for reasons other than pain. A synthesis of all the available data on the topic of the therapist-patient relationship in physical rehabilitation research found that a therapeutic alliance that includes an affective (i.e., emotional) bond is associated with better functional outcomes for patients.[128]

> Compassion for others is not just what you *say.*

Among these, one study stands out from the crowd in both scientific rigor and wow factor—and it shows that compassion for others is not just what you *say*. This research was supported by a grant from the National Science Foundation and was a collaborative effort between researchers at Harvard and Stanford Universities.[129]

In it, they studied the impact of *non*-verbal communication (i.e., "body language") of physical therapists on functional outcomes for elderly patients admitted to the hospital. An admission to the hospital can be a major setback for anybody, but especially for elderly patients. After a bout of illness or injury, elderly patients often need some physical therapy in the hospital so that they can function well enough to be discharged. This study tested the impact of therapist compassion (or lack thereof) in that scenario.

The study was rock solid in terms of scientific methodology. The researchers videotaped the elderly patients' physical therapy sessions. Trained judges watched the video clips of the therapists' behaviors and analyzed every move they made using validated scales for categorizing body language.

They assessed the functional status of the patients too, not just their physical functioning—such as their ability to do activities of daily living without assistance (e.g., walking, getting to the bathroom)—but also their cognitive functioning at the time of admission to the hospital, the time of hospital discharge, and three months after hospital discharge.

Here's what they found after analyzing the data: Non-verbal "immediacy" (e.g., leaning in toward the patient, less interpersonal distance, making direct eye contact, and facial expressiveness, such as smiling and nodding) had a significant association with better patient functional outcomes on both physical and cognitive functioning. Likewise, non-verbal "distancing" behaviors (e.g., keeping at a distance, looking away, no eye contact, and a lack of facial expressiveness) by the therapists were associated with worse physical and cognitive functioning in the elderly patients.

When we show people compassion and make an interpersonal connection, our non-verbal communication has to be one of immediacy rather than distancing. That's how compassion works. You cannot show compassion for others if you seem distant.

Clearly, compassion is not just about what you say, but also what you are communicating to people without using words. And this research shows that the effects can be profound.

Compassion Improves Endocrine Function

What's the most common cause of amputation? It may surprise you to learn that traumatic injuries are only responsible for 5.8 percent of lower limb amputations in the U.S.[130] The most common cause of amputations is actually diabetes.[131]

Diabetes is one of the foremost public health challenges facing health care today. An estimated thirty million people have diabetes in the U.S. alone (approximately nine percent of the population).[132] The estimated health care costs of diabetes in the U.S. are $327 billion annually.[133]

But diabetes is equally devastating at the personal level. The human toll of diabetes includes the development of heart attacks, stroke, and kidney failure, in addition to complications from diabetes itself, which require frequent admissions to the hospital.

Due to the effects of uncontrolled blood sugar on the nervous system, patients with diabetes are prone to developing very painful conditions in their legs. Uncontrolled blood sugar can also damage blood vessels over time and impair blood flow to the lower legs, sometimes requiring amputations. Diabetes is a common cause of major disability, and it is often an underlying cause of early death. In fact, in 2015 diabetes was the seventh leading cause of death in the U.S.[134]

If it isn't clear enough from these facts, it's important to do what you can to prevent yourself or your loved ones from developing diabetes. For those that have diabetes, it's vitally important to treat it appropriately to make sure you avoid the complications that can arise.

Unfortunately, diabetes can be very challenging to treat. Although there is no cure for diabetes, control of the disease (and, specifically, control of the patients' blood sugar) is possible. But doctors need all the help they can get. If there was a simple and inexpensive way to aid blood sugar control in patients with diabetes—even if the effects were only modest—it would certainly be worth a try. So can compassion make a difference? Yet again, the answer is *yes*.

Although many of the studies in the pages to follow will include measurements of health care provider compassion from the patient perspective, it also can be informative to measure health care providers' own beliefs about compassion, because their values and beliefs most definitely influence their behavior toward patients. Accordingly, researcher Dr. Mohammadreza Hojat and his colleagues from Sidney Kimmel Medical College at Thomas Jefferson University in Philadelphia developed an interesting research tool (survey) to measure the importance of compassion from the health care provider perspective.[135]

Although the researchers called it the "Jefferson Scale of Empathy" (rather than compassion), what they were measuring definitely fits our working definition of compassion, as described in Chapter 2. So we'll consider it to be a compassion scale from here on.

Here's how the tool works: It's a 20-question survey given to health care providers that assesses their beliefs about the importance of understanding patients' feelings and whether or not compassionate attentiveness to patients' emotional states can influence treatment success and other outcomes (including making the patient feel better). It also measures capacity to communicate the understanding of patients' emotional state with an intention to help.

Basically, this research methodology measures whether or not health care providers believe that a caring relationship with patients makes a meaningful difference. The scale is very methodologically sound, and it has been well-validated.

Now let's look at two of their studies that measured the compassion scale in physicians who were treating patients with diabetes, to see if there was a link with better outcomes. In their first study, they examined data for 891 patients with diabetes under the care of 29 different family physicians at Thomas Jefferson University.[136] All of the physicians completed the compassion scale survey. Then, based on the results, the researchers placed the physicians into one of three groups: high, moderate, or low compassion.

They then reviewed the data for blood sugar control among these patients with diabetes, specifically the patients' hemoglobin A1c levels in the blood. It's a blood test that shows what a patient's average blood sugar level has been over the past few months.

> Among patients with diabetes, the odds of optimal blood sugar control were 80 percent higher with high compassion physicians.

What they found was that patients of high compassion physicians were significantly more likely to have optimal blood sugar control, compared to patients of low compassion physicians. In fact, the odds of optimal blood sugar control were an astounding *80 percent higher*! Statistically, the researchers ran tests on the data to make sure that the association between compassion and better blood sugar control was not influenced by patient factors like age, gender, or health insurance status. So we can have confidence in the results.

Interestingly, that wasn't all. In these 891 patients with diabetes, the researchers found that high physician compassion also had *80 percent higher* odds of optimal blood cholesterol control.

Their second study in patients with diabetes was a bit different but, remarkably, even more compelling.[137] In this study, these U.S. researchers took their physician compassion scale all the way to Parma, Italy. Why? To do a study of enormous scale.

Italy has a national health service in which all people in the region around Parma who receive health services from the government have to select a primary care physician in the Local Health Authority. The researchers were able to tap into the Local Health Authority to enroll 242 physicians who completed the physician compassion scale. This allowed them to analyze data for all of their patients with diabetes: a whopping 20,961 patients in all.

What they found was striking indeed. After breaking physicians down into high, moderate, and low compassion groups like they did in their earlier study, the researchers then analyzed the association between physician compassion and the most serious complications of poor blood sugar control—emergency conditions like diabetic ketoacidosis, or diabetic coma, that require admission to the hospital.

> Patients of high compassion physicians had 41 percent lower odds of serious diabetes complications.

They found that compared to patients of low compassion physicians, patients of high compassion physicians had *41 percent lower* odds of serious diabetes complications! So this large-scale study showed results that were even more remarkable than the Jefferson study. These were not just blood sugar levels that were better, these were the actual complications from high blood sugar. The reason why physicians track the blood sugar levels are to prevent complications. Complications are the endpoints that matter most.

So what could the possible mechanisms be to explain effects on blood sugar? The short answer is that no one is precisely certain. But one possibility is that compassion affects patients' physiology in such a way that it also affects how the nervous system influences endocrine function. (Refer back to our earlier discussion on how compassion can affect the nervous system and cardiovascular system.)

That is, it can have a direct effect on the body in such a way that it minimizes extreme spikes in blood sugar, possibly through an effect on the levels of circulating stress hormones. Another potential mechanism is what we will discuss in Chapter 5 (better patient self-care).

It's possible that compassion for patients builds better rapport between doctors and patients, and this motivates patients to adhere to their medication regimen (e.g., insulin) more closely.[138, 139] For example, sometimes patients will say that one of their motivations to adhering to what their physician prescribed is that they do not want to "let down" their doctor by not sticking to his or her treatment plan.

Or sometimes compassion can help patients believe that better health is actually possible (rather than feeling hopeless), and this results in better adherence to prescribed therapy.[138] All of these mechanisms could be responsible for the effects of compassion that we see in patients with diabetes, at least in part.

But regardless of the mechanism, whether it is a direct effect on the body or it is causing patients to take better care of themselves, the association between compassion for patients and better control of diabetes is clear. Given the magnitude of the diabetes problem and the inherent challenges in treating diabetes, using more compassion in the care of diabetes patients should be a no-brainer.

Compassion Helps Wounds Heal Faster

For decades, scientists have known that psychosocial stress can slow the rate at which wounds heal. It was first demonstrated in a study published in *The Lancet* back in 1995.[140] How does that work? In wounds, immune function and local tissue inflammation play a big role in regeneration and repair of injured tissues. Psychological stressors can work against proper immune function at the site of injury (called cellular immunity) and slow the healing process. In this sentinel research paper, the researchers from Ohio State University demonstrated this in a very scientifically rigorous way.

Ten years later, in a follow-up study from the same group supported by a research grant from the NIH, the researchers tested whether emotional support from a trusted other could impact the rate of wound healing.[141]

Here's how they did it: They recruited 42 married couples who were free of any medical issues and admitted them to a research unit for 24 consecutive hours on two separate occasions. They used a standardized well-validated method to study early wound healing.

First, they created the wounds by attaching suction cups to the forearms of the married couples and hooking the suction cups up to vacuum pressure for an hour. This created blisters on the forearm. Then the researchers popped the blisters. They checked the healing of the blisters once a day using a standardized validated technique.

Basically, the blister wound was considered significantly healed when it stopped leaking fluid. Also, this method allowed the researchers to measure molecules in the blister fluid called cytokines that are part of the natural healing process.

In the first 24-hour admission to the research unit, the married couples participated in a structured social support activity. They were encouraged to be emotionally connected with each other and talk about how they could grow their relationship. Then they were asked to tell the researchers the "story" of their relationship. (Sounds sort of like a marriage retreat?)

In the second 24-hour admission, the tables were turned. This time they were asked to hash through the most conflict-producing topics in their marriage. They did not have any structured emotional support time; it was focused only on conflict. And it worked. The researchers were keeping track of "hostile" behavior by the married couples, and it was off the charts!

What they found was that the time to wound healing was significantly shorter, specifically 17 percent shorter (five days to heal instead of six days), with the social support visit compared to the conflict visit. And that's not all: The measured levels of cytokines in their blister fluid favored healing with the social support visit, but not with conflict. That helps to explain why the speed of healing was different. (It's very interesting what people will subject themselves to in the name of science, isn't it?)

But what's the evidence of human connection affecting wound healing in clinical medicine? Remember that randomized controlled trial of pre-operative compassion discussed earlier in this chapter? The one where the researchers randomly assigned pre-operative patients to usual care versus an enhanced compassion intervention from surgical nurses prior to having surgery?

That's the one where the patients' pain scale ratings were cut by 50 percent in the patients randomly assigned to enhanced compassion.[100] Well, they also measured wound healing, one month following surgery. They used a pre-defined, standardized, and well-validated scoring scale to assess proper wound healing.

At one end of the scale was proper scar tissue formation, and on the other end of the spectrum was devitalized tissue indicating wound breakdown. The researchers found that patients randomly assigned to enhanced compassion had statistically better wound healing scores than patients randomly assigned to usual care. The pain that patients were experiencing at the site of the wound was also found to be statistically lower in the enhanced compassion group.

Compassion Even Improves Symptoms of the Common Cold

Earlier in the chapter, we reviewed the data on how human connection can impact the immune system and resistance to infectious disease. Specifically, we read how in the general population, human connection can be a factor in the immune response to the flu vaccine, gene expression producing chronic inflammation, and even resistance to the cold virus.[90, 91, 92] Here's another compelling study on the power of...*hugs*?

In another NIH-funded study from Carnegie Mellon University that was published in the flagship journal of the Association for Psychological Science, researchers tested the power of hugs to combat the common cold.[142]

It was a study of 406 healthy volunteers that assessed participants' social support and, specifically, the number of hugs that they received over the preceding 14 days. Then they took a syringe containing the cold virus and shot it up their noses.

Then they quarantined the volunteers and monitored them for the development of cold symptoms. What they found was that people with high stress and conflict in their life were more likely to develop an infection (as evidenced by viral replication, antibodies to the cold virus, and symptoms).

That may not be surprising, based on the studies we reviewed earlier. But what *was* surprising was that the volunteer's level of social support and, specifically, the number of hugs they received in the preceding 14 days, protected against the development of infection. In fact, 32 percent of the protective effect of social support against infection was directly attributable to hugs!

But what is the clinical evidence that health care provider compassion for patients has a meaningful effect on their immune function?

To answer this question, researchers from the University of Wisconsin-Madison, with support of the NIH, conducted a study in patients with, again, the common cold.[143] A few pages back, we talked about the CARE measure, which is the well-validated survey that measures the compassion of the health care provider from the patient's perspective.

These researchers enrolled 350 patients presenting to a primary care office with the common cold. They asked the patients to complete the CARE measure for their physician and followed patients over time, measuring the duration and severity of their symptoms as well as a marker of the immune response (called interleukin-8) in their nasal passages.

> High physician compassion was associated with enhanced immune response, a one day decrease in duration of cold symptoms, and 15 percent decrease in cold symptom severity.

Then they compared the outcomes for patients of the physicians with the highest compassion scores versus the patients of lower compassion physicians, as rated by patients. After accounting for possible confounding factors, they found that high physician compassion was associated with a doubling of interleukin-8 levels (indicating enhanced immune response), a one day decrease in duration of cold symptoms, and a 15 percent decrease in cold symptom severity. It appears that caring makes a difference…even with the common cold!

Compassion Can Literally Keep You Breathing

By now, you are beginning to see that science demonstrates the power of compassion for patients. Patients with medical crises like surgery, trauma, or a heart attack may have better outcomes. Patients with pain may experience relief. Patients with impaired function may recover more quickly. Patients with chronic conditions (e.g. diabetes) may have better control of their disease. Patients may heal faster. Patients may be less prone to infection.

But one story really illustrates the power of compassion on a patient's physiology: the ability to *breathe*. And, like all the data that appeared earlier, this story also comes from the medical literature. In fact, it was published as a case report.[144]

On May 16, 1972, a 34-year-old man who was a few days out from abdominal surgery suddenly developed critical illness due to septic shock (i.e., a severe life-threatening infection) and was admitted to the ICU. He was clinging to life, literally. His organ systems were failing. He needed life support with mechanical ventilation.

Surprisingly, he pulled through the acute phase in the ICU, but the fight of his life was just beginning. Although the sepsis did not kill him in those first few days, it dealt such a blow to his lungs and his strength that he simply could not breathe on his own, even after the sepsis resolved.

He was stuck on the ventilator, totally dependent. Imagine laying in an ICU bed, flat on your back, not moving, not even being strong enough to take breaths for yourself. He had to have a tracheostomy (a potentially permanent breathing tube) surgically placed in his neck.

He was unable to speak. His eyes watered. His lips quivered. His health was shattered. So was his spirit. In his mind he was consumed with thoughts of death and dying. He thought he would never breathe on his own again, permanently dependent on the machine.

But, thankfully, he did make it off the ventilator. He even made it out of the hospital…120 days later. Eventually, he made a complete recovery.

So what was the difference-maker that allowed him to pull through – to be strong enough to breathe on his own again? The answer was simple: the nurses.

But not just any nurse, and not every nurse. It was a few special nurses that he considered his "angels." After recovery, the man told his story:

> *"After weeks of being on a ventilator in the ICU, I could tell right away when a new nurse came on duty at the change of shift and entered my room. I could tell within one minute whether or not the nurse cared.*
>
> *If it was a nurse who did not care, my heart would sink. My spirit was crushed. I lost my will, and I did not believe I would ever get off the ventilator. But if it was a nurse who cared, one of my 'angels,' I would instantly feel stronger. I believed I could*

beat this and breathe on my own again. Without my angels, I never would have made it. Their compassion is what saved me."[145]

Caring made a difference.

Who was the man stuck on the ventilator who told his story in this published case report?

It was Dr. Edward D. Viner, who was chair of the Department of Medicine at Cooper University Health Care for more than 20 years and now is the founding director of the Center for Humanism at Cooper Medical School of Rowan University.

Dr. Viner has become a mentor to both of us. In fact, he helped plant the seed in our minds that we ought to study the effects of compassion in a scientifically rigorous way and make sure it is taught to medical students and physicians—to *"science this up."* He is one of the reasons this book came to be.

Dr. Viner found, through firsthand experience, that compassion for patients affects their physiology. Compassion can literally help patients have the strength to breathe, as it did for him.

But, equally important, the nurses' compassion also affected him profoundly in his *mind*. It gave him the belief that he could, in fact, recover. And this leads us to a discussion of our next topic: the psychological health effects of compassion.

CHAPTER 4:
The Psychological Health Benefits of Compassion

"Our sorrows and wounds are healed only when we touch them with compassion."

—Buddha

Psychiatrist Dr. Helen Riess is the director of the Empathy and Relational Science Program at Massachusetts General Hospital and a professor at Harvard Medical School. In brief, her research is focused on the science of human connection.

In her TED talk, entitled "The Power of Empathy", she explains that one of her most fascinating scientific discoveries was propelled by an observation that she made, of all places, on an airplane.[146] She was just settling in for a long flight from Boston, bound for the west coast. The cabin was completely quiet as the plane ascended to cruising altitude, when suddenly a piercing sound broke the silence…the shriek of a baby crying hysterically!

We have all been on that flight before. People respond differently: some passengers try to move to another seat, some get visibly annoyed and agitated, and some brave passengers take an entirely different approach.

Understanding how stressful it must be for the parent who is struggling to console the crying baby, these passengers offer words of support to the mom or dad. Many even do so loud enough—intentionally—so that anyone sitting nearby is encouraged to be compassionate as well.

But a passenger response that Dr. Riess witnessed on this particular flight was not only amazing but totally unexpected. As the inconsolable baby ramped up his ear-splitting cries to echo throughout the cabin, a little boy who was barely three years old wiggled out of his seat, toddled over to the screaming baby, and offered him *his own* pacifier!

"Wow," thought Dr. Riess, "that little boy really heard and *felt* that baby's distress." And then that little boy decided to do something about it. That's the essence of compassion.[146] But what happens, scientifically, when two human beings connect in that kind of moment?

Compassion Relieves Psychological Pain

In Chapter 3, you learned about the effect that compassionate care can have on the autonomic nervous system. Research shows that the giver of compassion can activate the parasympathetic nervous system (for a calming effect) in the receiver of compassion, and even that their brain waves can begin to "mirror" each other.[102, 103, 104, 115] But the work by Riess and her colleagues takes this concept one step further, through the use of psychotherapy.[147]

Psychotherapy is sometimes called "talk therapy." In psychotherapy, a professional therapist treats individuals with psychological disorders through specific communication techniques designed to provide insight and change attitudes and behaviors, rather than by using medications. In psychotherapy, human connection matters. Big time.

There is much to be learned about the power of empathy by studying Dr. Riess' work. For instance, a young woman ("Jane") came to see Dr. Riess as a patient because she needed help with weight loss.

She was seventy pounds over her ideal body weight. For years, other weight loss methods had not worked, so she was seeing Dr. Riess on the recommendation of a nutritional counselor, in hopes that psychotherapy could help. However, the results—even after two years of therapy—were very disappointing. She just wasn't making any progress.

About that time, one of Riess' students wanted to begin a research study, one that Riess now admits she wasn't too crazy about at the time. But like a good research mentor, Riess decided to support her student's research idea anyway.[147] That decision ended up being career-changing for Dr. Riess. Literally.

The student wanted to measure how the autonomic nervous system of the patient and the therapist mirrored each other during psychotherapy. So they elected to use measurements of skin conductance (also called electrodermal activity) where electrodes are placed on the skin.

These generate a tracing that shows how much activation of the sympathetic nervous system and psychological or emotional distress there is at any point in time, for both the patient and the therapist. The existence of these skin changes had already been well-studied in other medical fields. This student wanted to take it to the next level to understand the response and reaction during psychotherapy specifically.[147]

Jane agreed to participate in the study. After Jane's next therapy session, the student examined the data and immediately called Dr. Riess. "You've gotta see this," he said. They reviewed the data together.

Both of them were blown away.

If you'd been sitting in Dr. Riess' chair, you would've found this to be a very calm, "vanilla," nothing-out-of-the-ordinary psychotherapy session. But if you considered the skin conductance data, you would have found it to be anything *but* normal.

While Riess' skin conductance showed that her emotions were even-keeled throughout, Jane's were "off the charts" at multiple times throughout the session, indicating extremely high levels of anxiety and distress.

But here's the thing: You wouldn't know it. Even Dr. Riess did not detect it (and she's a psychiatrist trained to understand the human mind who was solely focused on Jane in that session).

Jane was a professional with a high-powered career. She appeared to be very self-confident, calm, and composed. On the outside, anyway. But on the inside, Jane was suffering from crippling anxiety. And it never fully came to the surface, even after two years of therapy. The skin conductance data uncovered that she had been suffering...in *silence.*

When Riess showed Jane the tracing and explained what the data meant, Riess was shocked by Jane's response. "I am not surprised by this at all. I live with this every day," she said. "But no one has ever *seen* my pain. Until now." This experience moved Riess to the core. Clearly, she had been missing something with Jane.

All the research therapy sessions were videotaped, so Riess went back and watched the video again and again, examining every detail, this time as an emotion "detective." Riess discovered that the highest peaks on Jane's tracings, indicating the most distress, coincided with some of Jane's very subtle motor movements like flicking her hair or looking down at the floor, or a change in tone of voice.

Riess began to clue in to these subtleties and their significance. Dr. Riess began to meet Jane in those moments, using a tried and true intervention—empathy.

Every psychiatrist and psychologist understands that empathy is an integral component of effective psychotherapy.[148] From that point on in therapy sessions, when Riess detected Jane's subtle outward signs of psychological pain, she responded to them consistently—with *compassion*—and the two would go deeper.

For the first time, Jane unburdened herself emotionally. She let go of many painful, never-before discussed experiences from her past. And that was when everything began to change for Jane.

She began to exercise regularly. Her eating habits changed. And the woman who had never been able to successfully lose weight actually lost nearly fifty pounds in the following year![146, 147]

Compassion changed Jane's life. But it changed Dr. Riess' life too. Riess learned that with careful attention to signs that people are in psychological or emotional pain—and the ability to meet people in that pain with compassionate care—it could change *everything* for a patient. As a result, she is now committed to advance her empathy training to reach health care providers broadly through her organization, Empathetics.[149]

We will take a closer look at Riess' research on empathy training in Chapter 9, but for now, the take-home message is this: Empathy and compassion can impact people's psychological health. It certainly did for Jane. And it will for countless others, too.

That brings us to a crucial message about the psychological health benefits of compassion. In contrast to the last chapter on physiological effects, where most of the data were rooted in a clinical context—and therefore mostly applicable to the relationship between a health care provider and a patient—the data we are considering now applies to *everybody.*

Everyone knows somebody who is struggling, and some people are struggling much more than others. The scope of mental health needs (for example, anxiety and depression) in society is massive and growing.[150]

Although the data in the pages to follow on the psychological health benefits of compassion are taken from clinical research in the context of clinical care by a psychiatrist or psychologist, these data are just as applicable to those who are struggling with mental health all around us: our family, friends, neighbors, classmates, and coworkers. Research shows that one in five people that we meet have some sort of mental health struggle.[150]

> You can have a tremendous impact on someone's psychological health.

So when you read the data below, please don't think that they only apply to psychiatrists and psychologists. They do not. Even though that may be where the data come from, you don't have to be a psychiatrist or psychologist to treat someone with compassion when they are in psychological distress. Remember: you too can have a tremendous impact on someone's psychological health.

It may be intuitive to you that walking with people during dark times in their life and showing them compassion can alleviate their psychological pain and suffering, at least to some extent. But is there also scientific evidence for this in the literature? The answer is *yes*.

Diving in to the Data

A recent systematic review published in the *Harvard Review of Psychiatry* found that compassion-based interventions in psychiatry were highly effective in the treatment of patients with psychotic disorders, eating disorders, post-traumatic stress disorder, major depression, and even patients who recently attempted suicide.[151, 152, 153, 154, 155, 156, 157, 158, 159, 160, 161] One of the major mechanisms of these beneficial effects is that compassion-based interventions can reduce patients' self-criticism and shame related to their mental health condition.

A recent, very rigorously conducted meta-analysis of the psychology literature—a study of studies, essentially—pooled the data for 21 published randomized controlled trials (1,285 participants) of compassion-based interventions.[162] Here's what these researchers found: there was a statistically significant effect of compassion-based interventions on relief from depression, anxiety, and psychological distress, as well as an increase in well-being.

By statistical criteria, the effect sizes were substantial and also clinically meaningful. It's important to note that these were studies where people were trained not only to be compassionate to others but also to themselves (note: more to come on the topic of self-compassion in Chapter 10). Then they tested the effects of compassion interventions on their psychological health.[151, 162]

This is distinctly different from a study of physician or therapist compassion towards patients and testing the impact on patients' psychological health. Rather, it's about the profound effect each of us can have when we treat ourselves, and those we meet in our daily lives, with compassion.

Moreover, this research provides important context because it strongly supports the concept that compassion can heal psychological wounds and help promote psychological well-being.

So if compassion can achieve all of that, let's now dive into the data that demonstrates these effects, both for patients with mental health conditions as well as for patients who have psychological distress related to physical disease (e.g., depression in patients with cancer).

You'll also learn about the effects of compassion on depression and anxiety specifically, as well as the effects on patient-reported quality of life and well-being. But as a starting point and common thread for weaving together all the data, it is important to first establish one thing. Of all the things that can impact one's psychological health, there is something that rises to the top as one of the most, if not the most powerful thing: *human connection.*

That's not to say pharmacotherapy (i.e., drugs) isn't helpful. There have been monumental advances in pharmacotherapy for mental health conditions.

These scientific advances have been unquestionably life-changing for millions and millions of people.

For some people, drug therapies have been life-saving. Drug therapies can be a godsend for those struggling with mental health disorders. But there is also scientific research showing that human connection can make a meaningful difference in one's psychological health. In battling diagnoses like major depressive disorder and generalized anxiety disorder, or in helping someone get through a period of serious psychological distress, we need all the help we can get. But what is the evidence?

Reopening a Scientific "Cold Case"

You have probably heard of a "cold case" before. There was even a popular television show called *Cold Case* that ran for seven seasons back in the 2000s. A cold case is a crime that has not yet been fully solved but is no longer the subject of an active criminal investigation.

But if new information emerges from new witness testimony, reexamined archives, new material evidence, innovative techniques to examine retained material evidence, or fresh activities of a suspect, a cold case can be "reopened." It's a very real thing that occurs in law enforcement, and, consequently, it makes for great television.

But it's also a real thing in science.

Sometimes study results are published in the scientific literature, but there are unsolved aspects of the problem that the researchers are studying. The data don't totally make sense or pieces of the scientific puzzle just don't fit together perfectly. Certain phenomena may not be fully explained by the data.

These things can leave scientists scratching their heads, sometimes for years. Then a new scientific approach becomes available, or maybe the scientists just realize that they need to analyze the data in a different way, accounting for factors that they did not account for the first time around.

When this becomes necessary, they go back into the cold case files—sometimes blowing the dust off of data archives that have been dormant for years and years. They reopen the investigation to take another look.

That's what happened with the Treatment of Depression Collaborative Research Program (TDCRP) study that was first commissioned by the National Institute of Mental Health (part of the NIH) way back in 1985.[163] One of the aims of the research was to compare the effectiveness of different approaches to psychotherapy in treating patients with depression.

But another aim of the research was to compare the effectiveness of psychotherapy to the effectiveness of a drug therapy already known to be effective: specifically imipramine hydrochloride, a drug that is still on the market today. Ultimately, the TDCRP researchers concluded that, compared to psychotherapy, the biggest effects on depression came from the drug.[164]

But that conclusion did not sit well with a group of researchers from the University of Wisconsin-Madison (UW-Madison). Why? Because the original TDCRP researchers ignored the potential effect that individual psychiatrists can have on eventual patient outcomes. The research assumed (mistakenly, as postulated by the UW-Madison researchers) that all psychiatrists are equally effective at treating depression with psychotherapy.

So, nearly twenty years later, the researchers got access to the original TDCRP data and reopened the cold case.[165] They analyzed the same data, but in a different way. There were multiple different psychiatrists providing care to the patients in the TDCRP study. The UW-Madison researchers factored into the data who the psychiatrist was (i.e., the *person* of the psychiatrist himself or herself) while assessing the treatment outcomes of the patients.

In doing this, they saw—for the first time—an unmistakable pattern in the data. The original TDCRP researchers missed it.

Although the variation in depression scores for patients in the study was affected by the drug (imipramine hydrochloride), the variation in depression scores was explained even more by which psychiatrist the patients saw. The individual psychiatrist's effects were actually greater than the drug's effects!

By reopening this cold case, the researchers learned that both individual psychiatrists and drugs contribute to outcomes in treating depression. And they concluded that effective psychiatrists can actually increase the effects of drug therapy.

The *person* of the psychiatrist matters—in a major way.

Here's a quote from the conclusion section of the cold case study:

> *"The most effective psychiatrists augment the neurochemical effects of the drug. Based on these findings, it can be concluded that the person of the psychiatrist makes a difference in the response to antidepressant medication. Therefore, the health care community would be wise to consider the psychiatrist not only as a provider of treatment, but also as a means of treatment."*[165]

But what was it about the psychiatrist that made him or her more or less effective than other psychiatrists? Could it be…wait for it…their *compassion?*

Compassion for Others Can Alleviate Depression

The UW-Madison study was not the only scientific cold case investigation of the TDCRP data archives. There was another—this time by researchers from Yale University.[166] It offers insights into what it was about individual psychiatrists that made them more or less effective in treating patients with depression.

As part of all the research activity in the original TDCRP study, one thing that they measured was called a "relationship inventory" from the patients' perspective. This is the piece of data that the Yale researchers went back and focused on.

It was a survey that measured the patients' assessment of therapists' (1) compassionate understanding, (2) "congruence" (i.e., whether or not the therapist made an *authentic connection* with the patient), and (3) "unconditional positive regard" (i.e., genuine *caring* about the patient). Using the patient ratings on the relationship inventory, the Yale researchers found that a compassionate connection from the therapist was a major factor in depressed patients' response to therapy! Makes sense, right?

Here's another interesting finding: A University of Pennsylvania study of 185 patients undergoing cognitive-behavioral therapy for depression tested the relationship between therapist compassion and recovery from depression.[167] The researchers used a well-validated compassion scale (i.e., research survey) that allowed patients to rate how warm, caring, and compassionate their therapist was.

They also used a well-validated scale for measuring the severity of depression symptoms. The researchers were very rigorous in the analytical approach—controlling for the initial severity of depression and even accounting for the fact that severe depression could make a patient less likely to judge their therapist as compassionate—to ensure that neither of these things was a factor in the results.

> **Therapist compassion had a moderate to large effect on reducing depression symptoms.**

What they found was a robust, statistically significant association between high therapist compassion and recovery from depression. Based on the magnitude of the associations observed, the researchers concluded that therapist compassion had a *moderate to large effect* on reducing depression symptoms.

So this was the effect of the therapist themselves (and specifically the effect of the therapist's compassion), not the cognitive-behavioral therapy techniques that were employed. This result is not about the treatment protocol, it was *how* the protocol was applied (i.e., with or without a compassionate, caring approach).

But how? How does compassion impact depression?

Scientists from Duke University have found that compassion can reduce feelings of hopelessness, combating *demoralization*.[168] People who suffer from depression often perceive an inability to extricate themselves from the distressing condition, and compassionate care can help build positive expectancies for recovery.

Accordingly, it has been said that compassion can help alleviate a patient's "depression about depression." In Chapter 5, you'll learn more about how compassion can motivate patients to take better care of themselves, and depression is a prime example.

Compassionate care can raise patient self-efficacy, which is defined as a patient's belief that their treatment will be successful and that they will, in fact, recover and achieve good health. We know from research in cancer patients that compassionate care builds patient self-efficacy, activation, and enablement (i.e., a patient's active involvement and participation in his or her own treatment).[169] Each of these things is associated with improvement in emotional distress related to having cancer.[170]

In cases where medications are used for treating depression, self-efficacy can even raise patients' adherence to therapy. In a University of Colorado study supported by a grant from the National Institutes of Health (NIH), researchers studied patients newly diagnosed with depression who were prescribed antidepressant medication for the first time by a primary care provider.[171]

The aim of the research was to assess primary care providers' communication and the effect of what they said on whether or not the depressed patients actually took their medicine. The researchers audio-recorded the primary care office visits, and a trained researcher coded the language of the provider (i.e., compassionate or not) using validated research techniques. The researchers also assessed adherence to antidepressant therapy by measuring the proportion of days the patients actually took the medicine over the next six months.

What they found was that, after accounting for potential confounding variables in the statistical analysis, compassionate language from the primary care clinician was independently associated with adherence to antidepressant therapy. Compassionate language was an independent predictor of whether or not the patient even went to the pharmacy to get the prescription filled in the first place![171]

Compassion can also alleviate depression that comes as a result of debilitating physical health conditions. In a study that we looked at back in Chapter 3, compassion of the physician was associated with greater reduction in patients' pain during physical rehabilitation.[124] But they also measured depression symptoms in that study and found that compassion of the physician was also associated with significantly lower depression at the time of discharge from the rehabilitation program and persisting six months later.

Remember that physical therapy study from Chapter 3 that resulted from a Harvard and Stanford collaboration?[129] It studied elderly patients requiring admission to the hospital. That was the study where "distancing" non-verbal communication by the physical therapist (e.g., physical distance, no eye contact or facial expressiveness) was associated with worse functional and cognitive outcomes for the elderly patients. Compassionate non-verbal communication (e.g., leaning in, closeness, eye contact, smiling) was associated with better functional and cognitive outcomes. Guess what? The researchers also measured depression. They found that therapists' distancing behavior was also associated with the patients' level of depression at hospital discharge. So, again, it's not just what you *say* that matters.

And you do not have to be a physician or therapist to make a difference. *Everyone* on the care team has the opportunity to make an important positive impact on a patient with compassionate care.

In a study from the U.S. National Institute of Mental Health, researchers tested the association between the compassion of nursing home staff (specifically, nursing aides) and self-reported depression symptoms of elderly, cognitively intact nursing home residents.[172]

Being a resident in a nursing home can be very hard, not only physically but also emotionally and psychologically. Depression among nursing home residents is extremely common. Here's what that study found: the compassion of the nursing aides *mattered.*

> Compassion of the nursing aides was associated with lower depression in nursing home residents.

High compassion of the nursing aides was associated with lower depression in nursing home residents. That's fascinating, indeed. But what was most interesting is that the results depended on the perspective of how compassion was measured.

The perspective of the nursing aides (i.e., how compassionate they thought they were) and the perspective of the nursing aide supervisors (i.e., how compassionate the supervisors thought their staff were) had no association with the nursing home residents' depression. Only the nursing home residents' perspective on the compassion of the nursing aides mattered.

In other words, the perspectives of the nursing aides and their supervisors did not line up with the perspectives of the nursing home residents, and only the perception of compassion from the person who received the compassion—the nursing home resident—was actually associated with relief of depression symptoms.

This has big implications on the use of compassion if the results are generalizable to other contexts. Providers may think they are providing compassionate care, but if patients do not agree (i.e., do not actually feel it), the impact on depression is not realized.

These findings underscore three important things. First, for people suffering with depression, compassion matters. Second, givers of compassion are sometimes not very good at appraising the quality of their own compassion for others. The receiver's perspective is actually what matters.

And third, let's remember that these were nursing aides who had the impact. When one thinks of a health care provider having a meaningful impact on patients, one typically thinks of a physician or a nurse. But here, the nursing aide wielded incredible power and had the capacity to make a meaningful difference for a patient.

The nursing aide was *powerful.* The power of compassion doesn't come from the resumé of the person providing it, it comes from the *person* of the person providing it. The power is in the connection, not the credentials.

And this makes sense for the power of compassion: it doesn't matter who holds the gun, it only matters if you get shot. Accordingly, anyone on the care team can make an impact by treating a patient with compassion.

In another study of nursing aides in nursing homes from the University of Utah, researchers found that compassionate care by nursing aides was effective in counteracting one of the most extreme manifestations of depression among elderly nursing home residents: learned *helplessness.*[173]

For people suffering from depression, compassion is definitely powerful. Anyone has the power to make a meaningful difference. Please don't misunderstand the message here. People who have serious mental health conditions, including depression, should be under the care of an appropriately trained and credentialed professional. That's a given. Compassion is not a substitute for quality care.

The message here is different. The message is that *in addition to* the care of those professionals in a formal role, the rest of us also have a tremendous opportunity to impact one's psychological health. And the data backs that up.

Think of the most severe—the most lethal—manifestation of depression: suicide. Now think back to the story from Chapter 1 about the suicidal man walking to the bridge. In his suicide note, he said that if just one person, any person, would show him compassion with nothing more than a smile, he would not go through with it. He would not jump. Again, this was what it said in his suicide note:

> *"I'm going to walk to the bridge. If one person smiles at me on the way, I will not jump."*[52]

It didn't have to be a licensed psychiatrist or other mental health professional that saved him with an act of compassion, it could have been *anyone*. When it comes to the suffering of depression, anyone (and everyone) has the power to change a life.

Compassion Can Alleviate Anxiety

> *"...and as I left his office, he said, 'You know, you have a very bad disease, but we are going to take care of you.' The doctor-patient relationship was incredibly therapeutic and reassuring. I had no qualms, no doubts with putting my life in his hands. I had full confidence in his expertise, his concern and emotional support."*
>
> —Breast cancer survivor[97]

In Chapter 3, you learned how a giver of compassion can harness the autonomic nervous system of the receiver of compassion, activating a receiver's parasympathetic nervous system, and therefore inducing a calming effect.[102, 103, 105] But those were experimental studies in healthy volunteers.

What is the evidence that compassion reduces anxiety in patients?

Researchers from Johns Hopkins University studied this phenomenon through a randomized controlled trial in 210 women, the majority of whom were breast cancer survivors.[97] The study participants were given a consultation from an oncologist. Then the researchers used a validated scale of patient anxiety as their main outcome measure. (If you've ever had a cancer diagnosis—or known someone who has—you'll understand why that's a pretty important outcome measure.)

The researchers wanted to be extremely rigorous about the research, so they made sure that all the research participants were receiving the exact same intervention (i.e., a standardized consultation from an oncologist). They scripted an informational consultation session with an oncologist and videotaped the oncologist presenting the information.

The information the oncologist shared was about metastatic breast cancer and included a discussion of what it means to go on chemotherapy treatment: reviewing its risks and benefits, the probabilities of short- and long-term survival, and the probability of side effects. It was just the facts—all business. No emotional support component. No compassion. That is the video that the control group (i.e., "standard care" group) watched.

But then they scripted and videotaped a consultation session—with the same oncologist who shared the exact same information—that was also infused with compassionate language, interspersed before and after all the technical information. That's the video that the intervention group (i.e., the "enhanced compassion" group) watched. The researchers measured the study subjects' anxiety levels before and after the consultations and then compared the effects of standard care versus enhanced compassion.

The first finding from this study was that the women who participated had a huge amount of anxiety inside them, no matter how calm they may have appeared on the outside. In fact, 57 percent of study subjects enrolled in this research scored above the 75th percentile for anxiety (compared to the general population), and 18 percent of them scored in the 99th percentile. Understandable, of course, given what a patient with breast cancer goes through.

As expected, participants in the enhanced compassion group were more likely to believe that the oncologist cared deeply. But here is the more noteworthy finding: at the end of the videotaped consultation, the participants randomized to the enhanced compassion group were measurably and statistically significantly less anxious than those in the standard care group!

There are other fascinating findings from this study that we'll share later, but for now it's important to understand that compassionate statements from a health care provider can reduce patient anxiety in not only meaningful, but measurable ways. Numerous other studies consistently support this, including studies in physical medicine and rehabilitation, studies on breaking bad news to patients, and studies in primary care.[124, 174, 175, 176]

One study calculated the cumulative value of every single compassionate statement from the physician in terms of impact on patient anxiety.[48] It was a NIH-sponsored study from the University of California San Francisco.

The patients in this study had been admitted to the hospital and were under the care of a hospitalist (i.e., a physician who specializes in hospital medicine). Using a validated scale to measure patient anxiety and a validated methodology for measuring the number of compassionate statements to patients by the physician, what they found was eye-opening.

First of all, the anxiety level for patients admitted to the hospital was very high, which is not at all unexpected. Regardless of how much anxiety they were exhibiting on the outside, they were definitely feeling it on the inside.

But second, and most importantly, the researchers found that for each compassionate statement from the hospitalist to patients, the patients' level of anxiety decreased by 4.2 percent. So, for example, if a hospitalist made three compassionate statements to a hospitalized patient, the patient's anxiety level (on average) decreased by 12.6 percent. Therefore, every statement of compassion can have a measurable, incremental effect.

> The power of compassion is not a binary thing; the power of compassion is cumulative.

The research shows that the power of compassion is not a binary thing; the power of compassion is *cumulative!* More compassion equals more power.

Compassion Can Alleviate Distress and Improve Quality of Life

If you are a patient with cancer, not only can compassion reduce anxiety in measurable ways, as we saw in the Johns Hopkins randomized trial that was focused on breast cancer patients, but it can also alleviate patients' psychological *distress*. Unfortunately, in some cancer patients who have a poor prognosis for survival, this may be the only outcome they can hope to improve.

In research studies, there are validated survey instruments to measure the amount of psychological distress that a patient is experiencing. In a study of 454 cancer patients receiving treatment in an outpatient oncology practice, researchers found that higher physician scores for compassion during the consultation (as rated by patients) were associated with lower patient emotional distress following the consultation.[170]

A 2012 systematic review of 39 studies in cancer patients found that high clinician compassion was associated with lower psychological distress, and one of the mechanisms for lower psychological distress was better psychological adjustment to a cancer diagnosis.[177, 178, 179]

Psychological adjustment (or adaptation) to cancer has been defined as an ongoing process in which the patient tries to manage emotional distress, solve specific cancer-related problems, and gain mastery or control over cancer-related life events. Adjustment to cancer is not a single event, but rather a series of ongoing coping responses to the multiple tasks associated with living with cancer.[180]

A compassionate physician-patient relationship is known to be an important factor in a patient's adjustment to a cancer diagnosis, and subsequently this is associated with less psychological distress.[170, 177, 178, 179, 181] This improved psychological adjustment can also result in improved emotional quality of life.[181]

Another study in cancer patients found that out of all aspects of the doctor-patient relationship, the patients' quality of life was most clearly predicted by the "affective" (i.e., emotional) quality of the relationship with the physician.[182] A German study of 710 cancer patients also found the same thing; physician compassion (as rated by the patients) was associated with less depression and improved psychological quality of life for patients with cancer.[169]

The effect of caregiver compassion on quality of life in cancer patients perhaps should not be surprising, in light of the decades of available data on the effects of patient support groups (i.e., supportive-expressive therapy that takes place in a group). Researchers from Stanford University who have published extensively on this topic have found that support groups result in improved mood and better coping, which are two of the major factors that make up psychological well-being and improved quality of life.[183] If compassionate relationships with peers in patient support groups make a difference for cancer patients, it is logical that compassionate relationships with health care providers over time could make a difference too.

But these patterns in the data are not just limited to patients with cancer. Compassionate communication by clinicians has been associated with lower emotional distress in patients in primary care as well.[184, 185]

For example, in a randomized trial from Johns Hopkins University that was conducted in 69 primary care physicians and 648 of their patients, researchers randomized physicians to an education program of "emotion handling" communication skills versus no education (control). They found that patients of physicians randomized to enhanced emotion handling had significantly lower emotional distress that was sustained out to six months.[185]

In a U.K. study of patients with low socioeconomic status in a primary care clinic, the researchers found that primary care physician compassion (as rated by patients) was associated with improved patient well-being up to one month following the visit.[186] There are very few medications and treatments that remain effective for so long after just one dose!

What about Post-Traumatic Stress Disorder (PTSD)?

Here's a thought: could compassion also be an effective way of preventing post-traumatic stress disorder (PTSD)? While this idea has not yet been proven, it is currently being investigated in promising new research.

PTSD is a relatively common psychiatric disorder characterized by distressing re-experiencing symptoms, effortful avoidance of trauma reminders, and physiological hyperarousal diagnosed in individuals who have been exposed to a traumatic event. It takes an enormous toll on sufferers. It is not only associated with reduced quality of life but also the development of additional serious health conditions over time.[187]

Furthermore, it is associated with greater health care costs and an inability to return to work. Accordingly, the World Health Organization has raised awareness of the clinical, social, and economic toll of PTSD and has called for innovative approaches to prevent it. In short, PTSD is a serious public health problem.

Historically, PTSD was described in soldiers exposed to the trauma of combat. They would come back from war with deep psychological wounds that would manifest with a myriad of symptoms including behavioral changes (e.g., agitation, irritability, hostility, hypervigilance, self-destructive behavior, or social isolation), psychological changes (e.g., flashbacks, fear, or severe anxiety), mood changes (e.g., loss of interest or pleasure in activities, depression, or loneliness), sleep disturbances, unwanted thoughts, or emotional detachment.

More recently, researchers have made another very interesting discovery. Many other forms of psychological trauma (besides combat) can result in PTSD. For example, it is now well established that people who experience life-threatening medical emergencies and critical illness can also develop PTSD symptoms.[188, 189, 190] It's quite common.

This explains, at least in part, why people who go through serious illnesses can have deep, lasting psychological trauma from their experience. You may know someone who went through a serious medical crisis and, even though they eventually recovered from a physical standpoint, they were never quite the same from a psychological standpoint.

This is now an area of intense research focus for two researchers from Cooper University Health Care and Cooper Medical School of Rowan University. Dr. Brian W. Roberts, an emergency physician and NIH-funded clinical researcher, studies resuscitation, the science of essentially bringing patients back to life after their heart stops. Dr. Michael B. Roberts is a clinical psychologist with extensive experience in treating and researching PTSD. In case you're wondering—yes, they are related. Actually, they're brothers. And the Brothers Roberts have a fascinating hypothesis.

Like all good hypotheses, theirs started with a careful observation. First, they performed a systematic review of the medical literature on treatments for patients who develop PTSD after going through life-threatening emergencies and surviving critical illness.[187] What they found is that there are some effective psychological treatments for PTSD. But their more striking finding was this: the *earliest* interventions (i.e., interventions applied earliest in the hospital course) appeared to be the most effective.

But why would that be?

The Brothers Roberts believe they know the answer. The earlier a psychological intervention is applied—as close as possible to the psychological trauma, or, ideally, *during* the psychological trauma—the higher likelihood that the intervention can actually *prevent* the development of PTSD, rather than just treating it after the diagnosis is made.

In their systematic review, they found that all of the published research used psychological interventions to treat PTSD when the patient was in the recovery phase of their critical illness—well *after* they suffered the psychological trauma of the medical emergency. So the psychological trauma had already set in, and the treatments were aimed to reduce the PTSD symptoms. Maybe it was already too late. Perhaps the psychological damage was already done.

Imagine for a moment how terrifying it must be to be brought in to an emergency department with a life-threatening emergency. You might be wide awake and able to hear everything that is going on around you in frantic attempts to save your life. You may be acutely aware the entire time that your life is actually hanging in the balance.

The Brothers Roberts believe it is in that moment that much of the psychological trauma is occurring. Therefore, rather than waiting until the recovery phase of critical illness to do something about it, why not intervene *during* the psychological trauma, right there in the emergency department? Instead of treating PTSD after the fact, perhaps caregivers could intervene while the traumatic event is actually occurring in a way that makes the lifesaving emergency phase of therapy not as terrifying and traumatic for the patient.

Accordingly, the Brothers Roberts want to *prevent* PTSD, rather than just treat it, transforming a patient's experience of emergency care so that psychological trauma does not actually occur. Think of it as preventive medicine, but in a hospital's emergency department rather than a doctor's office.

But what type of early intervention in the emergency department could make a life-threatening medical emergency less traumatic for a patient's psyche? What about...*compassion?* For the compassion hypothesis, the Brothers Roberts made two more observations. First, they went back to the medical literature and found that there already is compelling data that compassion can be effective for the treatment of PTSD.

This is research from the psychology scientific literature in a different context. It focuses on training PTSD patients in self-compassion and compassion for others as a treatment for their own PTSD.[155, 156] Nonetheless, it supports the concept that in PTSD compassion can make a difference.

But the second observation was clinical, and it came from the practice of pediatric emergency care. When an ambulance brings a child to a busy emergency department due to critical injury or illness, the emergency care team often calls for a special type of consultation from a child life specialist.

A child life specialist is a highly trained medical professional who is an expert in working with children who are in terrifying circumstances. They are experts in the psyche of a child and how to make things less traumatic, so that they do not develop long-term psychological damage from what they are going through. One of the main methods by which child life specialists accomplish this is through tender care and compassion.

In the midst of all the craziness that goes on in a busy emergency department, child life specialists speak to the children in soft tones. They use gentle touch.

They reassure the children that the caregivers are going to take good care of them. They connect emotionally. They use compassion to soothe the child, alleviating their fear, and making the entire experience less scary.

It is intuitive that we would not want children to have nightmares of their traumatic event after they recover physically. That's why emergency care providers call in child life specialists. We don't need randomized controlled trials—it's just common sense.

So if it is intuitive to do this for children, why isn't it also intuitive to do this for *adults*? We already know that adults who face life-threatening emergencies and critical illness suffer nightmares. In adults, it's called PTSD.

The Brothers Roberts' hypothesis is that, for patients with life-threatening medical emergencies, compassion *during* the traumatic experience in the emergency department can reduce patients' perception of a life threat—reducing their *fear*—and ultimately preventing the development of PTSD.

They're testing that hypothesis right now in the emergency department at Cooper University Hospital. Specifically, they are testing whether or not a compassionate care intervention (i.e., a specially trained medical professional using a standard operating procedure for compassionate care) can reduce fear, perceived life threat, and the subsequent development of PTSD in adults going through a life-threatening medical emergency.

We won't know the results for a while. But if the hypothesis is confirmed, given that compassionate care is relatively simple and scalable (not to mention low cost), this novel line of research has the potential to change the approach to emergency care *worldwide*.

How Patients Do May Depend on How They *Believe* They Will Do

It's about *hope*. For patients, hope is a vital element of the process of recovery. Hope gives patients the strength to carry on in the face of adversity.

And hope is not just vital in terminal or life-threatening diseases, but in all serious conditions. For example, a patient with obesity must have hope that he or she can actually lose weight. A patient with uncontrolled diabetes must have hope that his or her diabetes can actually be controlled.

Patients give up when they lose hope, and that has major implications for health and disease. But let's be clear about one thing: we are not talking about *false* hope here. False hope is when a patient has hope for a good recovery when science says it's not at all possible. This scenario is actually very common in medicine.

Imagine a patient with cancer who finds out that her tumor has already spread throughout multiple organ systems and science says with 95 percent certainty that it will be fatal within a short time, but the patient still believes that a cure is possible. In that case, what should a physician do? It's actually somewhat controversial in medicine.

On one hand, if that false hope is keeping the patient's spirits up (and perhaps that's all they have left in terms of quality of life), then it could be in the patient's best interest not to dash the patient's hope. On the other hand, one could argue that talking to the patient to readjust their expectations for recovery might be the most ethical thing to do, because it could help them spend their time differently in whatever time they have left.

It's a challenging situation, and there are many valid opinions about what physicians should do. But one thing is clear: it would certainly be unethical for a physician to intentionally give a patient hope for recovery when science says it is impossible. Almost everyone can agree on that.

But that's not what we are talking about here. We are not talking about false hope; we are talking about *real* hope.

Just as every physician has had the experience where patients have false hope in the face of incurable disease, almost every physician has also had the *opposite* experience. Patients who have a very real chance of recovery from whatever they are facing, but have already given up hope. Often this hopelessness can be a manifestation of depression. That's understandable. Patients with serious physical health conditions often slip into depression, and it can sometimes make them believe (incorrectly) that recovery is not possible.

Like the false hope scenario, this "no hope" scenario (zero expectation for recovery in the face of treatable disease) is also quite common, actually.

Common? Yes. But does it *matter*?

Yes, it does. But before we take a look at data on recovery expectations (i.e., hope) and clinical outcomes, there is an important caveat to keep in mind. Since depression may affect recovery expectations, it is important for research studies to account for the presence of depression in their analyses. That way, they can be sure that their results are the effects of recovery expectations specifically, independent of any effect of depression. In other words, for there to be compelling data that recovery expectations matter (i.e., hope matters), it would have to be *over and above* any effect of depression on outcomes.

Just as importantly, the research would also have to adjust the analysis for things like age, disease severity, and presence of other medical conditions, so that those things are not a factor in the results, in order to specifically hone in on the effect of patients' hope for recovery.

That's the very careful approach that researchers from Duke University took in a fascinating study of coronary heart disease patients conducted over nearly two decades and published in 2011 in *Archives of Internal Medicine*.[191] The researchers enrolled 2,818 patients who were admitted to the hospital for a coronary event (e.g., heart attack) and underwent cardiac catheterization, a procedure where a cardiologist threads a wire into a patient's heart arteries to assess for blockages.

Prior to discharge from the hospital, the researchers assessed patients' expectations for recovery (i.e., hope for a good outcome) using a well-validated scale. What they found, with up to 17 years of follow-up assessment, is that expectation for recovery was strongly associated with *survival!*

At the ten-year mark, survival in the patients with the highest recovery expectations—the most hope for a good outcome—was *nearly double* the survival among patients with the lowest recovery expectations (the least hope for a good outcome).

> How patients believe they will do can be a major factor in how they actually do.

Keep in mind, these results were determined after using statistical tests to remove the influence of age, disease severity, concurrent medical conditions, and depression. In short, how patients *believe* they will do can be a major factor in how they actually do, including whether or not they survive!

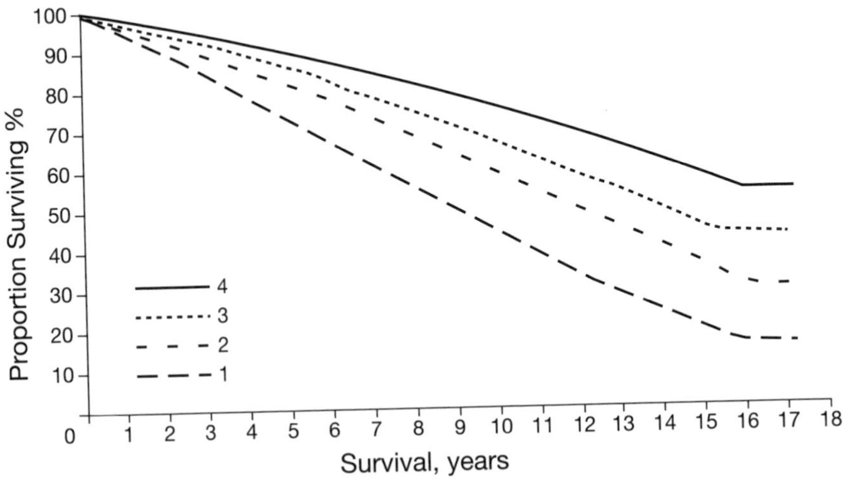

Figure 4.1: Recovery Expectations and Survival in Coronary Heart Disease: Patients who have the highest recovery expectations (i.e., most hopeful) are most likely to survive the longest. (curve 4=most hopeful; curve 1=least hopeful)
Source Archives of Internal Medicine
(Barefoot, Brummett et al. 2011)

In one systematic review of the medical literature, researchers from the University of Toronto identified that 94 percent (15 out of 16) of the published studies on patients' recovery expectations found an association between better recovery expectations and better clinical outcomes.[192]

Therefore, based on the available scientific data, one can conclude that hope *matters*. Belief in recovery *matters*. So what does all this have to do with compassionomics? The answer is: everything.

Compassion from health care providers can have a major impact on patients' hope for recovery. A randomized controlled trial conducted with primary care physicians found that when physicians' positive communication is specifically intended to raise recovery expectations, it is effective.[176] However, they found it is effective only if it is *compassionate* communication. Compared to a cold, impersonal communication style from the physician, the boosting of recovery expectations was far more effective when the physician was warm and compassionate.

It makes sense, right? As you learned in Chapter 3, when people show us compassion, it has physiological effects on our nervous system and quells our fears. And we know from experience, when people care deeply about us and show us compassion, we feel encouraged. It buoys us up with hope. It can shift our entire mindset.

When patients are struggling with hope, and are far more pessimistic about the trajectory of their health than the scientific facts of their illness would support, compassion can help patients "see it"...see their recovery as something *possible*.

Compassion can also motivate health care providers to go the extra mile to help patients understand their illness better. Sometimes patients' poor recovery expectations (having no hope for a good outcome) are the product of a lack of understanding, at least in part.

> **Sometimes taking the time to communicate better is the greatest act of compassion that a health care provider can give.**

Taking the time to sit down and explain the medicine in a way a patient can actually understand can make a major difference. Sometimes taking the time to communicate better is the greatest act of compassion that a health care provider can give.

Also, it is important to again emphasize that patients' poor recovery expectations may be a manifestation of depression. You've already seen data from many rigorously conducted scientific studies showing how compassion for patients can alleviate depression. So, by extension, compassion can also boost patients' hope for recovery.

We have seen the data for having no hope and how it can have a major negative effect on one's health, even survival. When patients have a reasonable chance for recovery, but have already given up hope, it is a health care provider's responsibility to do something about it, to go the extra mile to get patients the help that they need.

> **Science shows that hope matters. And science shows that compassionate care can be a powerful *restorer of hope*.**

Compassion Makes the Unbearable Bearable

Kenneth B. Schwartz was a special person. In fact, without ever knowing it or ever intending to, he started a *movement*.

After receiving a diagnosis of advanced lung cancer in November 1994, this 40-year-old, non-smoking, health care attorney with a wife and two-year-old son could have faced his diagnosis with bitterness or anger. Instead, he did something truly extraordinary—something that continues to echo throughout hospitals and health systems across the country and has impacted innumerable lives 25 years later.

It all started with an observation that he made. Then he wrote about it in a *Boston Globe Magazine* article, entitled "A Patient's Story."[193]

He observed that, as harrowing as his ordeal was, it was also punctuated by moments of exquisite compassion from his health care providers. He was struck by how that compassionate care could transform his experience and actually alleviate his suffering.

As he wrote in that *Boston Globe Magazine* article, compassion makes "the unbearable *bearable*." He described his caregivers as people who willingly and intentionally crossed the usual professional barrier between health care provider and patient (he called it the professional "rubicon") so they could know Schwartz as a person. They took a personal interest in him.

He also spoke of one physician scientist, Dr. Kurt Isselbacher, who was a renowned expert in clinical trials and director of the cancer center at Massachusetts General Hospital. Isselbacher was helping Schwartz navigate which experimental therapy might be the best to try in order to extend his life. He was a famous researcher, but he also cared about Schwartz and touched him with great compassion and gave him hope.

Not false hope, mind you, but real hope. The kind of hope that came from Isselbacher's real experience on the cutting edge of treating cancer.

Schwartz wrote this about him: "I was especially affected because such hopefulness was not coming from a faith healer, but a distinguished *researcher*."

To Isselbacher, science and compassion were not mutually exclusive. They were complementary, even synergistic. It was not an "either/or," it was an "and."

Schwartz also wrote this about his experience:

> *"In my new role as a patient, I have learned that medicine is not merely about performing tests or surgeries or administering drugs. These functions, important as they are, are just the beginning. For as skilled and knowledgeable as my caregivers are, what matters most is that they have empathized with me in a way that gives me hope and makes me feel like a human being, not just an illness. Again and again, I have been touched by the smallest kind gestures...a squeeze of my hand, a gentle touch, a reassuring word. In some ways, these quiet acts of humanity have given more healing than the high-dose radiation and chemotherapy that hold the hope of a cure."*

For Schwartz, compassion was not just a "nice to have." It was not just a moral imperative for caregivers. Not from his vantage point. To him, compassion was vital *medicine*. It changed everything.

Sadly, Schwartz died in September 1995, less than a year after his diagnosis. But his message was powerful, and it resonated with people. That powerful message would echo for decades—far beyond what Schwartz could have ever known—in "Schwartz Rounds" conducted in lecture halls and conference rooms in hospitals all across the country.

Schwartz Rounds are a regularly scheduled time where health care providers convene to discuss the social and emotional issues they face in caring for patients and families and to share their experiences and feelings on topics drawn from actual patient cases. Schwartz Rounds have been shown to improve health care providers' ability to give patients the compassionate care that they need.

Schwartz Rounds are made possible by the Schwartz Center for Compassionate Healthcare, which Schwartz founded just before his death. Today, the Schwartz Center has over 550 participating hospitals and health systems, not only in the U.S., but also in Canada and the U.K. The Center supports 200,000 health care professionals each year, by providing education and resources and convening regular conferences to advance compassionate care.

In summary, you've learned about the psychological health benefits of compassion in these recent pages. You saw compelling data that compassion can alleviate psychological distress and, specifically, that it can alleviate symptoms of depression and anxiety. You learned how compassion can improve quality of life and well-being and can foster hope...the kind of hope that people need to carry on.

But all of this scientific research for impact on psychological health really just comes down to the words of Kenneth Schwartz, which continue to echo today as much as they did back in 1995: Compassion "makes the unbearable *bearable*."

CHAPTER 5:
Compassion Motivates Patient Self-Care

"People don't care how much you know until they know how much you care."

—Theodore Roosevelt

Home health nurses work a little differently than nurses do in other settings. They provide care right in patients' homes. Guess what they typically do first when getting to know a new patient?

It's not bringing in equipment to make the patient's home more like the hospital or clinic. Nor is it setting up some kind of command center of monitoring or communication. What they do first is quite simple: they gather up all of the medication bottles throughout the house, put them all on one table, and reconcile the medications in the house with those prescribed to the patient.

Why is this so important? Because they need to see how many pills are left. So often, patients are not actually taking the medications that they have been prescribed. That's called "nonadherence" to prescribed treatment. It's a huge challenge in both medicine and public health.

Adherence is defined as the extent to which patients are able to follow treatment recommendations from health care providers. Nonadherence is, of course, the opposite: patients *not* following treatment recommendations.

The most common example of nonadherence is when a patient is supposed to be taking prescribed medication but is not taking his or her pills. But nonadherence can be about much more than just not taking medication. It's also a factor with other treatments, like patients with kidney failure who do not show up for scheduled dialysis treatments. Or when a physician recommends that a patient modifies a certain behavior—like quitting smoking, losing weight, or exercising regularly—but that patient doesn't follow through.

All of the things above add up to the concept of patient *self-care*. That is, the ways in which patients take care of themselves when they are not with a health care provider. Self-care is patients' ability to be diligent in caring for themselves in all the hours that health care providers aren't directly involved.

Think about it: A physician typically sees a patient for just a few hours in a year. But what about the other 99.99 percent of the time? The question becomes: how well will patients adhere to treatment recommendations during all the other hours when they are not face-to-face with their health care providers? For chronic diseases like diabetes or high blood pressure, succeeding in achieving health goals is all about a provider's ability to engage a patient in self-care.

Compassion Promotes Adherence

A physician can be the smartest doctor in the world and know just the right intervention to prescribe, whether it's a pill, a surgery, or a lifestyle change. But what good is it if the patient doesn't do it? If a patient doesn't take the medicine or follow through on a recommended therapy, how will he or she ever heal?

Former Surgeon General C. Everett Koop once summed it up like this:

"Drugs don't work in patients that don't take them."

A recent *New York Times* article called patient nonadherence to therapy an "out of control *epidemic*."[194] That's because the numbers are staggering. Rigorous research shows that people who are prescribed medications typically take only about *half* of their prescribed doses.[195]

Other research sponsored by the AHRQ and published in the *Annals of Internal Medicine* found that patients with chronic disease fail to take their medications as prescribed half the time.[196] They also found that 20 to 30 percent of medication prescriptions are never filled in the first place. In other words, the patient had no intention of *ever* taking them.

> Nonadherence to prescribed therapy in patients with chronic disease accounts for $100-300 *billion* in avoidable health care costs annually in the U.S. alone.

It's a huge problem, especially from a public health perspective. Because the downstream effects of people not taking their medicine are, to some extent, avoidable. Patient nonadherence results in poor control of disease which leads to avoidable complications and hospital admissions. In fact, research shows that nonadherence to prescribed therapy in patients with chronic disease accounts for $100-300 *billion* in avoidable health care costs annually in the U.S. alone.[196, 197, 198] We will dive more into costs in Chapter 7.

But the consequences of nonadherence are even more sobering when it comes to affecting patients' lives. Chronic diseases will progress if left unchecked, leading to worse long-term health outcomes, morbidity and even mortality.

It is important to recognize that patient nonadherence to therapy is an extremely complex and multidimensional health care problem. Researchers have identified numerous complex factors that contribute to nonadherence including socioeconomic factors, a patient's ability to pay for medications, patient beliefs about taking medications (e.g., "I'm not a 'pill person'"), and patient motivation.

Other things that factor in include cognitive impairment, a patient's lack of understanding about his or her disease, how complicated the instructions are, and side effects of the drug, among others. Every patient and situation is unique.

As a result, there is no one single "magic bullet" to effectively address the challenge of nonadherence.[198] However, there are tools and strategies to promote patient adherence to therapy that can help. Given the enormous magnitude of the problem—up to $300 billion in avoidable health care costs annually in the U.S. (and the corresponding human toll)—even small improvements in nonadherence can have enormous impact.

Let's look at the causes of nonadherence that are the most easily modifiable, especially the ones that can be widely disseminated at a low cost of implementation. Does such a low cost, easily implemented intervention exist that can modify such a high impact problem? Yes, it does: it's the patient's belief that *somebody cares.*

Alternatively, the belief that *nobody* cares leads to nonadherence. Without question, the belief that someone cares is a powerful driver of patient self-care. Primary care physicians are reminded of this on a regular basis. Patients with chronic diseases who are successful in adhering to their treatment regimen and achieving health goals often credit a spouse or other loved one as the main reason. They say, "I do it for my wife" or, "I do it for my son."

Or, they may express it as not wanting to let down or disappoint the loved one who cares about their health. Sometimes they express it as fear of their loved one's wrath if they slip up and fail to strictly adhere to therapy. But the common denominator is that they know somebody cares that they take their medicine. Science shows that social support is a key determinant of adherence to therapy in patients with chronic illness.[199, 200] When patients know they are not in it alone, it motivates them to take better care of themselves.

Here's the flip side: If patients believe nobody cares that they achieve a health goal—like control of a chronic disease—then they may be less motivated to heal. They may be less adherent to prescribed therapy. This can occur even in the absence of overt depression or loneliness. Even if patients intend to adhere to therapy, they may be less strict about actually doing so if they believe it doesn't really matter to anyone else.

It probably makes sense that care from loved ones makes a difference in patient self-care, but what about caring from health care providers? Are there data that health care providers' compassion for patients can also be a difference-maker for patient self-care?

Absolutely. If health care providers care deeply about patients, and the patients *feel* that, they are more likely to *take their medicine*.

Know Me as a Person

There have been remarkable scientific advances in the treatment of many diseases over the past thirty years, and one of the most striking of these is in the treatment of Human Immunodeficiency Virus (HIV). Once considered a death sentence, HIV is now very treatable with advances in antiretroviral therapies. With tight control of their disease, patients who are HIV-positive can now live to a ripe old age. When they die, the cause of death may be one of the common natural causes associated with old age, rather than HIV itself.

But the vital ingredient to success in controlling HIV disease is clear: it's patient adherence to antiretroviral therapy. They *have to* take their medicine every day. Even a little bit of nonadherence can allow their disease to get out of control, with serious health ramifications. But if they strictly adhere to their medication, the virus can be completely suppressed.

So, what do you think? Could a compassionate connection between a patient and their health care provider have a meaningful effect on HIV disease—a disease where patient adherence to therapy is especially vital to health outcomes? That's precisely what researchers from Johns Hopkins University wanted to find out. Specifically, they wanted to learn what happens when patients believe that their health care provider knows them *as a person.*

In a study of more than 1,700 patients with HIV, the researchers asked patients to respond "yes" or "no" to the question: "Does your HIV provider really know you *as a person?*"[201] They tested the association between three things: being known as a person, adherence to medications, and viral load (which is the number of copies of HIV virus that is measurable in the blood).

They tested this association because the viral load is the best indicator of whether or not a patient's HIV disease is controlled. If the virus is completely suppressed, their viral load will be undetectable in the blood (i.e., no copies of the HIV virus can be found). They adjusted the analysis for a number of potentially confounding factors, so we can have confidence in the results. What they found was nothing short of astounding.

> When providers knew their HIV patients "as a person", the patients had 33 percent higher odds of adherence to therapy and 20 percent higher odds of no detectable virus in the blood.

Being known as a person was independently associated with *33 percent higher* odds of adherence to antiretroviral therapy. But that's not all; being known as a person was also independently associated with *20 percent higher* odds of having no detectable HIV virus in the blood!

Why? In Chapter 4, you were introduced to the concept of self-efficacy. That's a patient's belief that a treatment can be effective and that health goals can really be achieved. It's a patient's belief that a therapy not only will work, but also that they can adhere to the therapy and successfully complete the treatment.

In the Johns Hopkins study, the researchers also measured patient self-efficacy. Specifically, they asked patients if they believed adherence to therapy could help them live longer. They found that patients who believed that their HIV provider knew them as a person also were more likely to believe that HIV medication could help them live longer. In fact, compared to patients who did not feel known as a person, the proportion of patients who believed the medications could help them live longer was *39 percent higher* among those who said their health care provider knew them as a person.

Those results on enhanced patient self-efficacy are corroborated in another study of patients with HIV conducted at the University of Virginia.[202] In this one, researchers recorded medical interviews of 435 patients with HIV by 45 physicians in four different outpatient centers to examine the relationship between the amount of compassion the physicians expressed and their patients' belief that they could successfully adhere to antiretroviral medication (i.e., self-efficacy). They found that, compared to patients of the physicians with the lowest compassion, patients of the physicians with the highest compassion had more than *double the odds* of believing that they could successfully adhere to the prescribed regimen.

So, in short, a compassionate bond in which the health care provider really knows a patient as a person can help HIV-positive patients believe their medication will work so that they really do take their medicine and clear the virus from their bloodstream. This compassionate bond between the health care provider and the patient is like the "glue" that binds it all together: self-efficacy, better adherence, and better outcomes.

But there's one more important thing to note from the Johns Hopkins study: in addition to better adherence and clearing the virus from the blood more effectively, being known as a person was also associated with HIV patients reporting higher scores for quality of life!

Wendy's Story

This improvement in quality of life was just the experience of Wendy, a transgender woman who was diagnosed with HIV many years ago.

Wendy experienced a tremendous amount of pain in her life. In transitioning from male to female, her family disowned her. To escape the pain of rejection, she moved from her home in California to the East Coast, but again she was treated very cruelly by many people who did not accept her.

Wendy even felt a lack of acceptance from her HIV health care providers who would often, very carelessly, refer to her as "he" when speaking to other staff members in the clinic. It cut her to the core every time it happened. As a result, Wendy did not feel connected to any provider, and she had no consistency in her HIV care. She must have seen dozens of different providers in different HIV clinics over the years.

The disrespectful way in which she was often treated in the clinic affected her behavior. It would not be unusual for her to act out in a disruptive manner in the waiting room if she felt that she had to wait too long. As a result, she was labeled as a "difficult" patient. She also didn't really believe that HIV medications could help her. For many, many years her viral load was sky high–totally out of control.

That's when Wendy came to Cooper University Health Care, where she met Dr. John Baxter. Dr. Baxter is the head of the Division of Infectious Diseases at Cooper. In addition to being known as a world-class researcher—where he has played a big role in some of the most important clinical trials in the field of HIV treatment—and an exceptional physician, Dr. Baxter is also known for his compassion. He cares deeply about his patients, and he has a special way of making patients feel that extra care.

The first thing that Dr. Baxter did was to listen to Wendy's story. He could tell that she was going through tremendous pain in the midst of her gender transition. He met her in her pain with compassion. He demonstrated the utmost respect to protect her dignity.

Dr. Baxter knew that always referring to her as "she" and acknowledging her female gender was the most basic, fundamental sign of respect and the first step in knowing Wendy as a person rather than just a "patient with HIV." He insisted that every single person working in the clinic do the same.

He knew that without ensuring this very basic expression of compassion, meaningful change in controlling Wendy's disease would not be possible. He made a point of setting the tone in the clinic and made sure that everyone interacting with Wendy treated her with the compassion and respect that she deserved.

The compassion from Dr. Baxter was something Wendy had never experienced in her prior health care encounters. It boosted her self-esteem in a major way. She was so thankful for him that her behavior completely turned around.

Wendy went from being labeled as a difficult patient who might act out in the waiting room to a patient who could not stop singing the praises of her physician. She would (very loudly) tell everyone in the waiting room how wonderful Dr. Baxter was. It was a remarkable change.

But that's not all. Wendy knew that Dr. Baxter cared deeply about controlling her HIV. He wanted her to live a long and healthy life, and that outcome was possible with strict adherence to state-of-the-art medications. Then he convinced Wendy that it was possible, and she believed him.

Wendy did not want to let Dr. Baxter down. He had high expectations. She vowed to make a change. For the first time, she started taking her medicine faithfully, as prescribed, never missing a dose. She did everything that Dr. Baxter said, to take better care of herself. For the first time, Wendy's disease came under control.

She soon went from a patient who was well known for not taking her medicine and a sky-high viral load to having *zero* copies of HIV in her blood. Today, Wendy has had an undetectable viral load for *more than three years!*

Harry and the Dreaded Hat

Here is another story of how a physician who knew his patient as a person had a powerful influence on his patient's self-care:

Harry was a kind man, devoted to his family, and CEO of a successful small business. Harry was also a real character. He loved to laugh. Practical jokes were his thing.

Harry was also someone who was "full of life." When he received the unexpected bad news that he had a rare urinary tract cancer, which carries an especially poor prognosis for long-term survival, he decided he wanted to maximize every meaningful moment in the life he had left.

That's when Harry met Dr. Mark Angelo. Harry had a lot of pain associated with the cancer, and so he was referred to Dr. Angelo, who is a palliative care specialist. (As mentioned in Chapter 3, palliative care is a branch of medicine focused on quality of life and symptom management for patients who have diseases that are no longer curable.)

Dr. Angelo came to know Harry quite well in the palliative care clinic, and the two of them built a strong bond. Angelo worked to control Harry's pain so that he could continue to work and get every last minute of joy out of his life. Even as he underwent chemotherapy, Harry attended every one of his kids' ball games and recitals. That was the most important thing in the world from Harry's perspective. You could consider it to be his purpose in life at that point in time.

One day, Harry visited Dr. Angelo complaining of abdominal pain so severe that he couldn't even sit down in a chair. He needed more pain meds and decided to stop working. Harry knew his time was short, so he confided in Dr. Angelo, "Doc, I think my run is coming to an end."

But Dr. Angelo expressed his hopefulness that he didn't think that was necessarily the case just yet. He suggested that maybe Harry was just feeling despondent due to the pain level…that if he could admit him to the hospital for intravenous pain medication, perhaps they could get control of the pain rather quickly and get him discharged in time to celebrate what Harry believed would be his last Thanksgiving at home. That was Harry's wish above all: to celebrate Thanksgiving at home with his family…perhaps for the last time.

Harry adamantly refused to be admitted. "No way," he said. He did not want to take the risk of missing Thanksgiving at home. At first, he was not even willing to talk about it. "I'd rather just take the pain meds when I really need them," he explained.

And that was the crux of the matter. Dr. Angelo began to understand that Harry was a very proud man who saw himself as some kind of "tough guy". He thought it was better to tough out the pain and only rely on the medication when the pain was extremely severe, rather than every several hours as prescribed.

But Angelo knew that if Harry agreed to be admitted to the hospital he could help get the pain under control quickly with intravenous medications and then, because he had a strong rapport with Harry, he could help him understand the importance of consistent dosing of oral pain medication at regular frequency once he was discharged so that Harry was not miserable for the holiday.

Because Dr. Angelo had a special bond with Harry, he could connect with him and help Harry understand that he did not have to be a "tough guy." In the condition Harry was in with incurable cancer, it was not a sign of weakness to take the medication. Knowing how important Thanksgiving was to Harry, Dr. Angelo begged him to first give inpatient therapy a chance.

Harry knew Dr. Angelo cared about him, and he trusted him, so ultimately Harry agreed to be admitted. If it were any other doctor, Harry would have refused. But if Dr. Angelo said to do it, Harry figured it must be the best thing for him.

As people who have cared for cancer patients understand, pain management can be very challenging—not just getting the pain controlled, but also managing nausea. Dr. Angelo was using intravenous pain meds to control Harry's pain and simultaneously working to control his nausea, so that Harry could tolerate pain medications by mouth. (That was the key part of getting him discharged in time to spend Thanksgiving at home.) Angelo visited Harry every day in the hospital, and their connection grew deeper.

And that is when Angelo noticed Harry's hat...a *Dallas Cowboys* hat. Harry was wearing that Cowboys hat every time Angelo went to see him in the hospital.

But here's the thing: Dr. Angelo was born and raised in Philadelphia and is a die-hard Philadelphia Eagles fan. And he was treating Harry at MD Anderson Cancer Center at Cooper in Camden, New Jersey, which is smack in the middle of Eagles country. Of course, Harry knew that hat would rile up Dr. Angelo.

If you are not a follower of the National Football League, let's just say that Philadelphia Eagles fans and Dallas Cowboys fans don't get along. It's generally not a good idea to wear a Cowboys hat in Eagles country.

As a guy from Philly, Angelo felt a little...shall we say...*taunted.* He was most definitely *not* a Cowboys fan. The two would trade jokes about the dreaded hat and Harry's insistence on wearing it. Angelo teased him (in jest, of course), but then did his best to ignore Harry's hat. But that just egged Harry on; remember, he was a practical joker who loved to laugh.

But on the day before Thanksgiving, when Dr. Angelo showed up at Harry's hospital room, Harry was in tears. He said he was done with it…all of it. He didn't care if he had pain. He just *had* to be home for Thanksgiving. So Dr. Angelo stopped the intravenous pain medications and switched him to oral meds, which thankfully worked very well. The next day, Thanksgiving Day, the plan was for Harry to go home.

Harry was thankful for that. But there was just one problem. When Thanksgiving Day came, his wife couldn't pick him up from the hospital because their young son had a high fever. She could not take him out of the house, and there was no one else to watch him. Since it was Thanksgiving Day, the usual medical transportation options were not available. It appeared that Harry was stuck.

That was when Dr. Angelo volunteered to drive Harry home…in his own car. He wanted to honor his promise to get Harry home for this important day.

It was perhaps not surprising that, when the hospital staff helped Harry into the passenger seat of Angelo's car, he was wearing his Dallas Cowboys hat. At which point Dr. Angelo joked, "Look, Harry. I'm happy to give you a ride home, but I am not giving that *hat* a ride home. Could you please put that thing away?"

Do you think Harry would take the hat off? No chance. He wore that Cowboys hat with pride the whole way home. Angelo just smiled.

As Dr. Angelo pulled into Harry's driveway, he saw Harry's son waving to them in his Spider-Man pajamas from the window. Harry's wife gave Angelo a big hug, thanking him profusely for delivering Harry home. She even offered him a glass of champagne and a seat at their Thanksgiving dinner table, although he declined so he could get home to his own family.

It was a very special Thanksgiving for Harry and his family. Daddy was home! And thanks to Dr. Angelo and the team at the hospital, Harry's pain and nausea were finally under control. Harry knew how much Dr. Angelo cared about him, so he did exactly as Dr. Angelo instructed. Instead of waiting for severe pain to hit him, Harry stayed ahead of the pain by taking the medication at the precise regular intervals Dr. Angelo prescribed. It worked. And Harry was able to truly *enjoy* Thanksgiving with his family. That meant everything to Harry, and his wife and kids.

Sadly, Harry was right...it *was* his last Thanksgiving. He made it to March of the following year when he died in an inpatient hospice unit (because he didn't want his children to see him die at home).

Soon after the news of Harry's death, as was his custom, Dr. Angelo called his wife to offer his condolences. As is often the case, he got her voicemail instead, where he offered condolences and explained she should not feel obligated to call back unless she wanted to.

He didn't get a return call until a couple months later when Harry's wife asked if she could come seem him. She wanted to bring Angelo something that Harry wanted him to have.

You may have already guessed what it was...his Dallas Cowboys hat, of course! In fact, Harry formally left it to Angelo in his Will. Harry's wife said that he was so moved by Dr. Angelo's gesture of compassion, especially driving him home on Thanksgiving when it meant so much to Harry, that he just felt Angelo should have his favorite hat.

Since that day, Harry's Dallas Cowboys hat enjoys a special place of honor in Dr. Angelo's office. Angelo smiles fondly when telling the story of Harry and the dreaded hat, because of Harry's keen sense of humor and because he understood that this was Harry's way of teasing his doc—a die-hard Philadelphia Eagles fan—even after Harry was gone.

So why are you hearing the story of Harry and the dreaded hat? So that you understand what it looks like when a caregiver knows a patient *as a person.* Dr. Angelo certainly knew Harry as a person. He knew exactly what was most important to Harry. Over the years, that meant making it to all of his kids' ball games and recitals. At the end, it was making it home for Thanksgiving one more time.

Dr. Angelo knew Harry as a person to such an extent that Harry got to know Dr. Angelo in the same way. So much so that Harry decided to play a fantastic practical joke on Angelo in his Last Will and Testament!

But let's focus in on one specific and very important aspect of Harry's story: Why did he agree to be admitted to the hospital? And why did he start strictly following his doctor's orders with regular dosing of pain meds once he was home? Those things were key to getting Harry's pain under control and allowing him to enjoy one last Thanksgiving with his family.

He only did what Dr. Angelo recommended because Harry trusted him. Dr. Angelo knew Harry as a person, and Harry knew Dr. Angelo cared. And that Thanksgiving, that was what made all the difference. That's why knowing a patient as a person can be so powerful in self-care.

Back to the Data

Now that you understand why it's so critical to know a patient as a person, let's take a closer look at more evidence for why compassionate communication from health care providers improves patient self-care.

Effective communication is essential in this regard, specifically when it comes to adherence to therapy. A rigorous meta-analysis supported by research grants from the National Institutes of Health (NIH) and the Robert Wood

Johnson Foundation that examined 127 studies published in the biomedical literature found that patient-centered communication from health care providers was associated with *62 percent higher* odds of patient adherence to treatment.[203] Given that compassion is a cornerstone of patient-centered communication, this makes sense.

Another meta-analytic study from Northeastern University found that more positive talk (and less negative talk) from health care providers was associated with better patient adherence to prescribed therapy.[204] Likewise, a study from Michigan State University provides yet more evidence that the compassion of health care providers is a key link between better physician communication and patient adherence to treatment recommendations.[120]

Researchers in this study gave a survey to 550 outpatients. The compassion questions asked patients if their physician showed caring and concern for their well-being, interest in knowing what their health care experience meant to them, and respect for their feelings. Other questions asked if their physician responded to them "mechanically."

What they found is that more compassion was associated with significantly better adherence to prescribed medications, through the mediating factors of better information exchange, perceived expertise, interpersonal trust, and partnership.

The association between compassion and better information exchange will be explored more in Chapter 6 on health care quality, where you'll learn that a health care provider's compassion is associated with both better patient disclosure of information and better patient recall of instructions.[174, 175, 202, 205] Since that is the case, it's perhaps no surprise that there is a link between compassion, better communication, and better adherence to therapy.

Another concept that is crucial to the issue of adherence to therapy is patient *motivation*. There are a plethora of data that support the link between caregiver compassion and patient activation, patient engagement, and patient enablement.

Let's consider each of these. First, patient *activation* is a patient's willingness and ability to take independent actions to manage his or her own health and health care.[206] It involves having (or gaining) the knowledge, skill, and confidence to manage one's own health.

Patient *engagement* is a broader concept that encompasses patient activation. Patient engagement involves the interventions designed to increase activation, and patients' resulting behavior, such as preventive care or health maintenance.[207] Implicit in the concepts of patient activation and engagement is the understanding that patients manage their health on their own the vast majority of the time, making decisions daily that affect their health in meaningful ways.

Research shows that compassionate patient care is associated with better patient activation and engagement and, as a result, better patient self-care.[169, 208] This makes sense. Physician compassion can drive patients to be more engaged in their health care and to want to have more information on both treatment options and health promotion. This has been associated with better long-term outcomes and enhanced quality of life.[169]

Patient *enablement* is a bit different: it's about *empowerment*. Patient enablement is the extent to which a patient feels empowered after a medical consultation, in terms of being able to cope with, understand, and manage his or her illness.[209] At a very basic level, it is encouragement (i.e., "You can do it"). But even if a condition is incurable or a desired outcome is not attainable, enablement is the encouragement that a patient can effectively cope with what comes. It's vital for optimal patient self-care.

The opposite of patient enablement or empowerment would be learned *helplessness*. You will recall that in Chapter 4 you read about a nursing home study where compassion from the nursing aides was associated with a reduction in learned helplessness among elderly nursing home residents.[173]

So perhaps it makes sense that multiple studies have found compassion for patients to be associated with better patient enablement.[186, 210, 211] In fact, in one study of more than 3,000 patients in primary care, researchers measured health care provider compassion from the patients' perspective (using the CARE measure, as described earlier) and patient enablement, using a well-validated scale.[211]

> Without compassion, patients will not feel fully empowered to cope with, understand, and manage their illness.

What they identified was that with low compassion from health care providers, maximum patient enablement was *never* found. They concluded that patient enablement *requires* compassion. Put simply, the researchers found that without compassion, patients will not feel fully empowered to cope with, understand, and manage their illness.[211]

The Importance of Trust

Another mechanism by which compassion for patients can improve patient self-care and patient adherence to therapy is through building trust.[138] Building trust, along with better patient activation and enablement, produces a stronger "working alliance" between the patient and health care provider.

A working alliance is agreement on goals of therapy and methods to achieve those goals, and the extent to which there is an emotional bond – characterized by liking and trust – between patients and their health care providers.[212] (Doesn't this perfectly describe Harry and Dr. Angelo?)

So rather than a patient acting as a passive bystander in his or her health care, a working alliance between patient and provider produces a special therapeutic bond that creates *synergy* toward better health. Research from Fordham University in New York shows that health care provider compassion produces just this type of better working alliance with patients.[213] Also, a better working alliance is associated with better patient adherence to treatment recommendations, as well as better health-related quality of life.[213, 214]

Now that we have described some of the mechanisms by which compassion for patients can affect patient adherence to therapy, let's look specifically at the data on the direct effects of a caring relationship on adherence. In scientific journals, those data can be traced all the way back to 1969.

Yes, much like the evidence described earlier on how compassion reduces patients' need for medications from anesthesiologists when having surgery, some of these data have been around for almost five decades. But, also as we also noted earlier, while these studies were published in the world's best journals and certainly were impactful in their day, it has not been until now that they have been pulled together here with all of the other studies to truly paint the picture of the power of compassion.

Let's consider some of these now. In a study from the University of Southern California published in *The New England Journal of Medicine*, researchers studied patients' response to medical advice among eight hundred outpatient visits to Children's Hospital of Los Angeles.[215] They examined the association between the quality of doctor-patient communication and adherence to treatment recommendations.

In this case, because the patients were children, the study was looking at the association between the pediatricians' communication and the parents' adherence to the child's treatment recommendations. All of the visits in this study were new (i.e., seeking care for a new illness), and it was the first time the pediatricians were meeting the children and their parents.

The researchers recorded the audio of visits with the pediatricians, and then two weeks later they held follow-up interviews with the parents to determine if they were following the pediatrician's treatment advice. Where applicable, the researchers performed "bottle checks" to see how much medication was left in the bottle at the time of the interview, to objectively test whether or not they were truly taking the medicine.

What they found was that a lack of "warmth" in the communication from the physician (as assessed by the parent) was associated with significantly lower adherence to the pediatrician's treatment recommendations. Actually, the proportion of patients with optimal adherence was *15 percent lower* when the parent believed that warmth was absent, compared to when they believed it was present.

And when parents had the highest level of dissatisfaction with the warmth of the pediatrician (i.e., the worst doctor-patient interaction) adherence was the worst. Only *17 percent* of patients in this category were following treatment recommendations closely!

In another study of 22 physicians and 370 of their patients in primary care, researchers measured the strength of the doctor-patient relationship using a validated scale of the patients' assessment of concordance (i.e., being "on the same page" as the physician).[216] They found that strong doctor-patient concordance was independently associated with *34 percent higher* odds of patient adherence to prescribed medications.

Another primary care study of patients with high blood pressure measured physician compassion (as rated by patients) and found that lower compassion from physicians was associated with significantly lower adherence to blood pressure medication.[217]

Similarly, a NIH-supported study from the University of California San Francisco published in *JAMA Internal Medicine* studied 9,377 patients with diabetes and found significantly higher adherence to medications with better interpersonal connection, specifically when patients had more trust in the health care provider.[139] Perhaps this explains, at least to some extent, why (as you saw in Chapter 3) research has found that health care provider compassion is associated with better blood glucose control and fewer complications requiring hospitalization among patients with diabetes![136, 137]

You will also recall from Chapter 4 that there was a NIH-supported study from the University of Colorado in which they studied the effect of compassionate language from the clinician in the treatment of patients with depression.[171] That's the one where compassionate language was found to be not only an independent predictor of adherence to antidepressant medications but also whether or not the patient even went to the pharmacy to get the prescription filled in the first place. This better self-care may explain, at least to some extent, the overall results described throughout Chapter 4, where compassion for patients with depression was associated with alleviation of depression symptoms.[166, 167]

So does this phenomenon only exist with primary care or mental health providers and their patients? Not according to the data.

The association between health care provider compassion and better patient adherence is also evident in the treatment of cancer. In a 2007 study from University of California Los Angeles, supported by a grant from the American Society of Clinical Oncology, researchers studied 881 women who had breast cancer and were undergoing chemotherapy with a drug called tamoxifen.[218]

In certain patients, the use of tamoxifen could reduce the risk of cancer relapse and death; however, it often requires a very long course of therapy (e.g., up to five years) to be maximally effective. Of course, it can be extremely challenging to adhere to such a long course of treatment. But if patients do not adhere to the chemotherapy, a relapse of cancer may be more likely.

In this study, researchers tested the association between emotional support from their health care providers over time (as rated by the patients, using a validated survey) and the patients' adherence to tamoxifen therapy. In the analysis, they accounted for many potential confounding factors, including tumor characteristics, cancer staging, other cancer treatments received, and any side effects that they experienced from tamoxifen, so we can have confidence in the results.

What they found is that four years after the cancer diagnosis, patients who perceived receiving "the right amount" of emotional support from their health care providers had significantly higher adherence to tamoxifen, compared to patients who reported "less than needed" emotional support from health care providers. In fact, the proportion of patients still adhering to therapy was *12 percent higher* (81 percent, versus 69 percent) in the patients who reported receiving enough support from health care providers, compared to not enough support.

Here's another one: Take a moment to recall the neurology study from Chapter 3, in which physician compassion was associated with less pain and disability among patients with migraine headaches.[125] Taking a deeper dive into that study, we can identify another potential mechanism of action for the pain relief that the patients experienced.

The researchers found that the compassion of the neurologist was associated with better patient adherence to prescribed therapy, both adherence to behavior modification and adherence to prescribed pharmacological therapy. So connecting the dots: more compassion leads to better adherence to the treatment plan, which delivers more relief from symptoms. Makes sense, right?

But self-care is not just about taking medicines and behavior modification. It's also about disease prevention, like following through on recommendations for cancer screening, for example. In a study of 1,205 women conducted at Georgetown University and funded by the National Cancer Institute, researchers found that a stronger relationship with primary care providers (as rated by patients) was associated with better patient adherence to primary care providers' recommendations for cancer screening.[219]

> Compared to patients of low compassion providers, the rate of cancer screening adherence among patients of high compassion providers was 13 to 30 percent higher.

Specifically, patients' assessment of the providers' compassion was associated with patients following through on cancer screening. Compared to patients of low compassion providers, the rate of cancer screening adherence (i.e., cervical cancer, breast cancer, and colon cancer) among patients of high compassion providers was, relatively speaking, *13 to 30 percent higher.*

Benjamin Franklin is credited with the famous saying: "An ounce of prevention is worth a pound of cure." These data on cancer prevention, coupled with the data for adherence to therapy that can stave off disease progression and complications, are scientific evidence that compassion for patients is not just a powerful therapy for treating serious disease, but also can be a meaningful intervention to keep patients *free* of disease in the first place.

Connecting to Purpose

"Those who have a 'why' to live, can bear with almost any 'how.'"

—Viktor Frankl

Think back to the story of Harry and the dreaded hat. Dr. Angelo really knew Harry as a person, and what was the result? He understood Harry's *purpose...* why Harry continued to get out of bed in the morning and fight for better health, despite his terminal diagnosis.

Harry's purpose in life was his family: being there for the kids' recitals and ball games and, ultimately, for one more Thanksgiving. That is what drove him. Ultimately, it was that purpose (and his trust in Dr. Angelo) that made Harry agree to be admitted to the hospital. Getting his pain under control was *not* Harry's purpose; that was just a goal. The real purpose was spending one more Thanksgiving at home.

It may be intuitive to you that a sense of purpose in life can be a powerful thing. In the concentration camps of World War II, Austrian psychiatrist and Holocaust survivor Viktor Frankl found that having a deep sense of meaning in one's life was a distinguishing factor of resiliency that allowed people to survive the atrocity.[220]

But now, emerging research in the biomedical literature is showing how powerful having a purpose in life can be for achieving better *health*. Researchers define purpose in life as a self-organizing aim of one's life that stimulates goals, manages behavior, and provides a sense of meaning.[221, 222] There are well-validated survey instruments in clinical studies that assess patients' degree of purpose in life.

Purpose in life is a strong motivator for patient self-care. If patients have a clear idea of who or what they are trying to get better for (or stay healthy for), then they have a purpose in life. Rigorous research shows that when patients know what they want to live for, they experience better health outcomes.

> Purpose in life was associated with significantly higher odds of adhering to health screening recommendations.

One study from the University of Michigan tested the association between purpose in life and the use of preventive health care services in more than 7,000 patients age fifty and older.[228] Their conclusion: Purpose in life was associated with significantly higher odds of adhering to health screening recommendations, including cholesterol screening, colonoscopy, mammography and cervical cancer screening among females, and prostate examination among males. Furthermore, they found that purpose in life was associated with significantly fewer nights spent as an inpatient in a hospital.

In large population-based studies, other researchers have found that purpose in life is a strong predictor of mortality—it lowers mortality risk—across adulthood.[223] These results on longevity have also been corroborated by researchers from the Icahn School of Medicine at Mount Sinai in New York, who found that purpose in life was associated with fewer cardiovascular events.[221] And when it comes to older adults, rigorous research has found that having purpose in life is associated with fewer heart attacks and strokes.[224, 225]

A Harvard T.H. Chan School of Public Health study of 1,461 elderly patients found that having purpose in life was associated with better functional status and, specifically, a *14 percent lower* risk of developing a slow walking speed in old age.[226] Literally, without purpose in life, people lose the "pep in their step".

People with purpose in life even sleep better at night. Research shows that purpose in life is associated with lower incidence of developing sleep disturbances.[227]

Science shows that purpose *matters*. Purpose is powerful.

So why are we telling you about the data for purpose in life in a book that is dedicated to the science of compassion? It's simple.

If health care providers do not care enough to find out a patient's purpose in life, they may never know what it is. And if they don't know what a patient's purpose in life is, they may be less effective in helping their patients connect to and fulfill their purpose. If health care providers do not know what their patients' purpose in life is, they may not understand what health goals their patients actually value.

Also, if patients do *not* have a clear sense of purpose in their life, or they have not yet found what it is, this can be a major risk factor for adverse long-term health outcomes.[221, 223, 224, 225, 228] So if health care providers do not care about their patients' purpose in life, they may never find out that their patients' lives *lack* that purpose. And if they do not care enough to ask, they certainly won't care enough to help their patients find purpose.

Here's where compassion comes in: compassion for patients makes health care providers more likely to connect in a more meaningful way, truly understand what their patients' purpose in life is, and—by extension—relate that purpose in life to establishing health goals with their patients.

At Cooper University Health Care, two very special primary care physicians have experienced firsthand the power that purpose in life can have in achieving health outcomes among the most challenging patients. Drs. Alexandra Lane and Jennifer Abraczinskas are physicians who practice in the Ambulatory Intensive Care Unit (ICU) at Cooper. This is a primary care clinic specializing in the care of patients with the most complex chronic care needs.

In the medical literature, the patients seen in the Ambulatory ICU are sometimes called "high-need patients", "high need, high cost patients", or "super-utilizers".[229, 230, 231] Sometimes health care providers even refer to them as "frequent fliers", because of the frequency with which they are admitted to the hospital.

You may be aware that in the U.S. a small fraction (~5 percent) of all patients have especially complex chronic care needs to such a degree that they account for around 50 percent of all health care spending.[232] This small segment of the total population is one of the highest priority challenges from a public health perspective.

These are precisely the patients that Drs. Lane and Abraczinskas specialize in. Due to severe chronic health conditions, these patients are extremely sick on any given day, always teetering on the edge of needing to be admitted to the hospital. Importantly, these patients typically also have very complex socioeconomic factors that complicate their health care, the most common of which are poverty and a lack of reliable support systems to assist with their care.

Some of them also have concurrent mental health conditions which further complicate their overall care. Treating these patients' severe chronic illnesses is extremely challenging, but when you add poverty, a lack of family support, and other complex factors, it becomes infinitely harder.

Nevertheless, Drs. Lane and Abraczinskas have been extremely effective in keeping their patients well (or at least well enough to stay out of the hospital). Caring for patients with the greatest, most complex needs has become a calling for them both, and it has given them a great sense of purpose.

They are deeply passionate about what they do, as evidenced by their amazing results: better health, better quality of life, and lower health care resource utilization (i.e., fewer hospital admissions and lower costs) among patients in the Ambulatory ICU.

But how? What is their secret?

There are many intricate aspects of their practice that contribute to their patients' successful achievement of health goals, but one factor stands out from the rest...*purpose in life!*

Drs. Lane and Abraczinskas care deeply about their patients. Their patients are very special, for all the reasons mentioned above, and they treat them accordingly. Lane and Abraczinskas are both known for their compassion for patients, and this is vitally important given the very extreme health and socioeconomic problems their patients are facing every day.

As a result of this compassion, and because they understand the scientific data on the significance of purpose in life, they connect with their patients in a special way. In their experience, they have observed that the high needs patients that are most likely to improve are those who have a clear sense of purpose in their lives and who are able to align their health goals with their purpose in life.

As a result, they make certain to understand their patients' purpose in life, and then connect to that purpose. They make certain to align the explicit goals of care with what their patients' value the most. Their results are truly remarkable, not only at the population level but also at the personal level.

Take Rasheed, for example.

Rasheed's Story

Rasheed was only 44 years old, but his admissions to the hospital were literally too numerous to count…totally off the charts. He typically spent multiple days per month admitted to the hospital.

Rasheed had severe high blood pressure, which would have been very difficult to control even if he had no socioeconomic challenges. But he was also living in extreme poverty. He had no family to speak of. He also suffered from crippling anxiety.

Much of this anxiety was the result of being repeatedly exposed to violence in his life and being the victim of violence himself. Complicating these matters was a long history of substance abuse. His drug dependence was a byproduct of trying to self-medicate his anxiety disorder for many years (due to a lack of consistent follow-up with mental health services).

Further complicating all of the above was a concurrent eye condition requiring him to wear dark sunglasses all the time, even indoors. As a result, many people considered him to be odd or even strange, which only increased his social isolation and compounded his anxiety. Rasheed had been unable to adhere to the eye doctor's recommendations in the past, so he was not considered to be a candidate for corrective surgery.

All of the factors above also resulted in poor adherence to his blood pressure medication. He also didn't adhere to his physician's recommendations for lifestyle modification to control his blood pressure.

For years, Rasheed's blood pressure was so out of control that he was frequently admitted to the hospital because of the stress it put on his heart, causing fluid to build up in his lungs or causing him severe chest pain. As a result, he developed congestive heart failure. Sometimes, his out of control blood pressure was so severe that it would even cause him to have neurological symptoms ("mini-strokes").

If something did not change soon, Rasheed was going to die.

But then Rasheed was referred to Drs. Lane and Abraczinskas in the Ambulatory ICU at Cooper. They did not see him as a super-utilizer; they saw him as a person. Yes, he was among the most complex of the complex patients, and the most challenging of the challenging. But they cared deeply about him and got to know him as a person, a person that was in need of their compassion. So they set to work exploring the root causes of his years of uncontrolled disease and substance abuse, and they sought to understand Rasheed's purpose in life.

Over months of regular check-ups in the Ambulatory ICU, Drs. Lane and Abraczinskas came to a striking (and sad) discovery. Rasheed had no sense of purpose in his life. They suspected that his lack of purpose in life was a major factor in his years of very poor health.

But how do you help someone find purpose in life when they have none?

Drs. Lane and Abraczinskas were aware of some very powerful data. That is, the data on living an "other-focused" life, a life that is focused on service to others. There is a robust body of scientific evidence that serving others can actually be beneficial for one's own health and well-being.

Could this result in meaningful change for Rasheed?

In Rasheed's local community, there were many people that were suffering from high complexity health challenges, just like Rasheed himself was experiencing, and many of them had diseases that were just as severe and uncontrolled. After gaining Rasheed's trust over time, and seeing small but meaningful improvements in his health, Drs. Lane and Abraczinskas encouraged Rasheed to get involved in his community, helping others around him to get control of their own health. They encouraged him to *serve*.

Feeling like he was at the end of his rope, and having essentially nothing to lose, Rasheed trusted his doctors and took their advice. This new beginning proved to be nothing short of miraculous for him.

First, Rasheed knew that the only way that he could be a credible inspiration for others was to take ownership of his own health. For the first time, he completely stopped using drugs. He went "cold turkey."

For the first time, he was strictly adhering to his prescribed medication regimen. He never missed a dose. For the first time, he kept all of his appointments with mental health providers. Rasheed became a model patient. He was finally able to have the eye surgery that he needed, so that he no longer needed to wear dark glasses all the time. He was a new person!

Rasheed became a health coach in his community. He even made a new career out of it, working part-time as a health coach in a local clinic. He loved helping others get control of their health. He found it so rewarding.

This motivated Rasheed to take the best possible care of himself. This, in turn, allowed him to be a shining example for all those around him in his community who were struggling with high complexity health conditions. It was a "virtuous" cycle.

Serving others, and helping others get control of their complex health conditions, became Rasheed's newfound purpose in life.

Drs. Lane and Abraczinskas helped Rasheed connect to that purpose by working diligently to help keep his health in check and by seeing him in the Ambulatory ICU clinic at a moment's notice if he needed any kind of attention. They understood it was vital to keep his health in the best possible condition, so that he could be an effective role model and available to serve others.

Since rededicating his life to serving others as a health coach, Rasheed has not been admitted overnight to the hospital. Not one time. His health—and his whole life—have made a complete "180."

Rasheed knows what it is like to struggle with complex health challenges, and because of this he has great compassion for others who are struggling with the same. This compassion is what drives him.

Rasheed sees his work in service to others as a way of paying it forward. That is, paying forward the great compassion shown to him by his physicians, Drs. Lane and Abraczinskas, who were the people who cared enough about him to help him find (and connect to) his new purpose in life!

CHAPTER 6:
Compassion is Vital for Health Care Quality

"(Compassion is)...one of the impulses that nature has implanted in us to do what our duty alone may not accomplish."

—Immanuel Kant

So far, we've examined the scientific evidence for a direct impact of compassion on patients physiologically, psychologically, and for their self-care. But what about its impact on the technical quality of care?

The effects of compassion on the health care environment and the system of care have a downstream effect on patients in meaningful ways. So in this chapter we will consider the effect of compassion on health care *itself* and the processes of care.

How Compassion Affects Quality

The National Academy of Medicine (formerly called the Institute of Medicine) defines health care quality as: "The degree to which health services for individuals and populations increase the likelihood of desired health outcomes and are consistent with current professional knowledge."[233]

This includes the use (or misuse) of health care resources—something you'll read more about in the next chapter, during our discussion about the effects of compassion on health care costs. But for the moment, let's hone in on just the effects on the clinical processes of caring for patients (i.e., clinical quality).

You will recall that embedded in the overarching hypothesis that compassion benefits patients is an additional hypothesis: compassion improves the quality of patient care and processes of care. There are two different signals in the data that could support this.

The first is any data showing that low compassion—or absence of compassion—is associated with worse quality of care. The second is any data showing that more compassion is associated with better quality of care. Collectively, either type of data would support the hypothesis that compassion is beneficial for health care quality.

In reality, our systematic review did identify compelling data about the latter (high compassion and higher quality) but found *a lot more* data on the former (low compassion and lower quality).

Why? It's largely because of the way in which hospitals and health systems measure the technical quality of care. Quality metrics are often based on rates of complications of care, such as medical errors. Rather than focusing on the vast majority of events that go exactly as planned, they are often focused on the small numbers of cases that go wrong.

The nature of quality metrics is often about tracking the bad things that can happen to patients. That's because the goal for hospitals and health systems is to have the incidence of bad things be as low as possible. That's mostly good news: hospitals and health systems should expect things to go well for patients and be interested in measuring and, therefore, preventing problems.

So, in tracking these bad outcomes or medical errors, the data to support the hypothesis that compassion benefits clinical quality would be data supporting that low compassion is associated with higher incidence of things going wrong. In other words, it would support the idea that low compassion makes patients less safe.

Why would that happen? One possibility is *carelessness*. Health care providers that don't really care about their patients may be more careless in the technical aspects of medical practice. On the flip side is *meticulousness*. Health care providers that care deeply about patients also may be more meticulous about the technical aspects of the medical care they provide.

For example, if health care providers care more, they may pay more attention to detail to make sure that nothing goes wrong (or that everything goes perfectly). They also may be more willing to go the extra mile for patients to help ensure the best possible medical care—not just acceptable care, but *exceptional* care.[234, 235] (But, as stated earlier, that's a harder signal to pick up in the health care quality data because it is commonly focused on the occurrence of adverse events.)

Now that you understand why there is a preponderance of this kind of data, let's examine this link between a lack of compassion and poor quality of care. Later, we'll consider the other possibility: how more compassion could increase health care quality.

A Lack of Compassion is a Threat to Patient Safety

Here's a rather dramatic, yet true, story that illustrates this point:

A 75-year-old woman is heroically saved at a major trauma center, only to be discharged and fatally struck by a car on her way home from the hospital. Could a lack of compassion from the hospital staff have contributed to her death?

Yes. Here's how it happened:

It seemed like any other morning to the resident physician, walking in to the hospital at 7 a.m. to begin a 24-hour shift as part of the trauma team. But when she arrived in the emergency department, it was clearly not a normal morning. It was downright eerie.

As the resident physician walked into a trauma resuscitation bay, there was blood everywhere, and an elderly female patient lying on the gurney had just been pronounced dead. This aspect of the morning, unfortunately, was not so unusual.

But what was odd was how the entire trauma bay was almost silent. Instead of the usual buzz of activity at the change of shift, the whole staff was very somber, despondent. They were whispering to each other and appeared crestfallen. They had pronounced patients dead on numerous occasions. But something was different this time.

Even worse was the expression on the face of a nurse holding the phone to her ear as the resident walked past. The nurse appeared to be in anguish and looked like she was going to pass out.

What was going on?

A colleague explained: The 75-year-old woman (we'll call her Mrs. Johnson) had actually arrived the night before, after falling down a flight of stairs at her home just a couple blocks away. She was rushed to the emergency department by ambulance and, after initial evaluation by the emergency medicine team, the trauma team was called to evaluate her.

Soon after her arrival at the hospital, her entire family arrived...about twenty people in total! Clearly, Mrs. Johnson was the matriarch of the family and everyone was really concerned.

Fortunately, the family received good news early on: she was alert and talking, and all of her testing, including a computed tomography (CT) scan, came back as showing no evidence of serious injury. So that was reassuring.

But Mrs. Johnson still complained of one thing: hip pain. Although there was no evidence of an obvious fracture on the initial set of imaging, the trauma team was concerned there could be a small hip fracture that the standard imaging was not picking up. So they ordered more tests. All the really serious injuries were already ruled out, but they needed to do more imaging of the hip, just to be sure.

Now it was already really late—the wee hours of the morning—by that time. The radiology department was backed up with other patients with more urgent, potentially life-threatening, conditions. It could be a couple more hours of waiting until everything was done, so the trauma team told the family they could go home.

Given her significant hip pain, all the health care providers assumed that they would find a small fracture and that she would be admitted to the hospital. The family agreed to go home and come back in the morning after getting some rest. But when all the testing and interpretation was finally complete, it was negative. All of it. Somehow, Mrs. Johnson had fallen down a flight of stairs but actually did not suffer any serious injuries, except bumps and bruises. The staff explained to her that she did not need to be admitted to the hospital and could go home.

By that time the sun was just coming up and, knowing her family had been awake most of the night with her in the emergency department, Mrs. Johnson was hesitant to wake her family to ask for a ride home. And then, when she finally did phone home, no one answered because they were all sleeping.

She explained to the staff that, even though her hip was still hurting, she thought she could make it home on her own. She lived just two blocks away from the hospital. It was a short walk.

But here's one question the staff did not ask: "In which direction?" On one side of the hospital was a residential community. On the other side of the hospital was a very busy four-lane road, one of the major arteries of the city, with a speed limit of forty miles per hour. It was true that her house was only two blocks away from the hospital, but it required crossing that very busy road.

Here's another question the staff did not ask: "Is there anyone else I can call for you to come and get you—a friend, maybe?" And yet another: "May I see you walk before you go, just to make sure you are steady on your feet and okay to walk?"

How about one more question that nobody asked: "I'm sure you're awfully tired. How about we discharge you and you can take a seat in the waiting room until your family wakes up and can drive you home?"

But since nobody asked any of those questions, Mrs. Johnson left on her own. She was hobbling very slowly. As soon as she stepped off the sidewalk to cross the street in front of the hospital, she was blindsided by a speeding car. This patient—just discharged—who was concerned about further troubling her family, was then admitted (for the second time in eight hours) into the very same emergency department she just left.

You already know the outcome. She died. In fact, her injuries were so severe from being struck by the car that it was obvious to the trauma team almost immediately on arrival that her injuries were not survivable. There were no signs of life. She was gone.

What about the nurse with the phone to her ear looking like she was going to pass out? The trauma team had just pronounced the elderly woman dead when that nurse's phone rang. It was Mrs. Johnson's daughter. She had just heard the voicemail from her mom saying she was going to be discharged home.

The daughter asked, *"Can I come pick her up now?"* The nurse was unable to speak. What an incredible tragedy.

So what was the lack of compassion here? This emergency department staff and trauma team provided sound clinical care when she was with them. It was impeccable, actually. She had all the appropriate tests and treatment. The team "checked all the boxes" as far as the medicine was concerned.

But they neglected to think of their patient as a *whole person*...to take the extra step of caring about how she would get home when the family wasn't available to pick her up. After all, she still had hip pain, and clearly (as evidenced by the outcome) it impaired her walking.

A little bit more care and consideration could have made all the difference for this patient. It could have saved her life. But instead, there was a fatal outcome that undid all the quality clinical care they provided earlier.

Imagine what it felt like to have to tell her family what happened to her. Imagine what it felt like for her family to hear what happened.

Days after the tragic incident, the physician who discharged the patient confided in the physician who was just coming on duty. He was despondent and devastated, feeling the burden of being the last person Mrs. Johnson spoke to before she died. He felt responsible.

"When I saw that all the testing came back negative, I moved on in my mind to the next case in the waiting room," he said. "She needed more help than just telling her the test results and handing her the discharge papers. I treated her as a 'hip pain', not as a person. The 'hip pain' did not need a ride home... but Mrs. Johnson *did*."

Making a Personal Connection Is Critical

Earlier, you learned about *depersonalization*. That's an inability to make a personal connection. Research on depersonalization comes from the studies on burnout in the helping professions, including health care providers. As described in our discussion of the compassion crisis in Chapter 1, depersonalization is one of the three components of burnout. (The other two are emotional exhaustion and the feeling that you can't really make a difference.)

In studying burnout, researchers use well-validated scales that measure all three components of the burnout syndrome. The questions about the depersonalization component of burnout hone in on one's ability (or inability) to make personal connections with others. For health care providers, that means personal connections with patients. Accordingly, burnout research in health care providers can specifically report on the degree of depersonalization among providers assessed for burnout.

> Depersonalization occurs when health care providers don't really care about patients, think of patients as objects or have become callous or hardened to patients' needs.

In the most commonly used research instrument for assessing burnout in health care providers, the Maslach Burnout Inventory, the measurement of depersonalization assesses whether or not a health care provider *really cares* about patients, ever thinks of patients as *objects* (versus knowing them as a person), or has become *callous or hardened* to patients' needs. By the way, because such surveys are always confidential in the research studies described below, we can be confident that respondents feel free to be honest.

An example of depersonalization from earlier in the book is when health care providers objectify a person's needs, such as thinking of the patient only as "the chest pain in room six," rather than thinking of the patient as "Mr. Hernandez in room six" and acknowledging that the patient is a person who needs help and has people who care about him.

Depersonalization is also an inability to make a personal connection that leads to a lack of understanding of how a patient's illness affects them as a *whole person*. A hand injury requiring surgery may seem non-life threatening, and therefore no big deal in the grand scheme of things, to an emergency department provider.

But then, if they take the time to make a personal connection, they might find out that the patient is a pianist struggling to make ends meet and just lost her livelihood for the foreseeable future. Her son just got into college; how will they afford the tuition now? Maybe that's why she's just staring into space in the exam room, not saying much.

Depersonalization—and the lack of a personal connection that flows from that—may also result in a lack of personal investment from the health care provider. That's the kind of lack of caring that can lead to a lack of meticulousness and attention to detail, and lower quality standards, where adverse events are more likely to occur.

Why is this important for compassion? A personal connection is integral to compassion. With depersonalization, there can be no compassion. It's not possible to have compassion for another person if there is an inability to see others' humanity on a personal level.

> Depersonalization prevents compassion.

Therefore, the presence of depersonalization among health care providers is a marker for an inability to have compassion and an absence of compassion. Although depersonalization and compassion are not opposites, depersonalization *prevents* compassion.

Accordingly, by examining the association between depersonalization and patient safety metrics, we can gain valuable insights on how a lack of compassion can affect the *system* of care and—by extension—patients.

Do No Harm: A Lack of Compassion Can Pose a Safety Risk to Patients

Let there be no mistake: As noted earlier, the main determinant of a good clinical outcome is clinical excellence. That is, the technical quality of care. No amount of compassion can make up for poor quality of care.

All the compassion in the world won't make up for getting a diagnosis wrong, prescribing the incorrect medication, or botching a surgical procedure.

That said, a lack of compassion can predispose health care providers to giving suboptimal care. A patient's risk of harm can actually be higher in the absence of compassion. To be clear, a health care provider who doesn't demonstrate compassion didn't just miss an opportunity to *improve* an outcome for his patient, but he or she is also more likely to *harm* a patient—to remove the chance for an acceptable outcome through this omission. And that's important.

There is tremendous focus in the health care industry on ensuring that preventable harms (i.e., medical mistakes) do not happen to patients. Actually, the U.S. government's Department of Health and Human Services' Center for Medicare and Medicaid Services (CMS) adjusts payments to hospitals based on harms to patients and rewards those hospitals with the fewest errors. And yet, there is just such a risk when compassion is absent during care.

Let's take a look at the data: The key linkage is the data on depersonalization among health care providers and quality of care provided. Earlier, you read that with depersonalization—that inability to make a personal connection—compassion for patients is impossible.

Of course, compassion is absent where there is no human connection. Without this connection, health care providers may not be as meticulous about the technical quality of care as they could be. There is robust evidence in the scientific literature that depersonalization represents a risk of harm to patients.

For example, in 2009 researchers from the Mayo Clinic published a longitudinal study in *JAMA* in which they studied 380 internal medicine resident physicians and tested the association between their scores for depersonalization and emotional exhaustion and the incidence of major medical errors committed by the physicians.[236]

In addition to depersonalization being an important marker for an absence of compassion, so is emotional exhaustion, because it can be an indicator of *compassion fatigue* among health care providers. In fact, it's probably intuitive that depersonalization plus emotional exhaustion is virtually guaranteed to result in compassion fatigue, at least to some degree.

In the study, residents were surveyed every three months for the duration of their three-year training program. The survey captured the physicians' self-reported *major* medical errors—only those medical errors which the physicians themselves considered to have serious consequences (or potentially serious consequences). The survey was anonymous, so it is highly unlikely that the physicians were concealing major errors. Nearly 40 percent of these physicians reported committing a major medical error at some point.

What they found was striking. Physicians who scored high for depersonalization were significantly more likely to commit a major medical error in the next three months. For any measurable increment of depersonalization on the scale (i.e., just one point higher), the odds of a major medical error were *9 percent higher*. That translates to at least *45 percent higher odds* of a major medical error in the next three months for the physicians scoring in the highest tier of depersonalization, compared to those who scored in the lowest tier.

Similarly, physicians who scored high for emotional exhaustion were also significantly more likely to commit a major medical error in the following three months. The odds were *6 percent higher* for any measurable increase in emotional exhaustion, which translates to at least *54 percent higher odds* of a major medical error for the physicians scoring in the highest tier of emotional exhaustion, compared to those who scored in the lowest tier. Again, the outcome measure for this study was a *major* medical error. Would you want to take a chance with one of those physicians?

In another study from the same Mayo Clinic researchers that was also published in *JAMA*, they used the same longitudinal study design surveying 184 resident physicians every three months.[237] They found similar results: compared to physicians in the lowest tier for depersonalization scores, physicians that scored in the *highest* tier for depersonalization had at least *50 percent higher odds* of a major medical error in the next three months.

Similarly, physicians that scored the highest for emotional exhaustion had at least *63 percent higher odds* of a major medical error in the next three months. But they specifically honed in on one more thing: the physicians' compassion. They used another well-validated survey instrument that measured the physicians' beliefs and values about their own compassion for patients.

> **Physician compassion was associated with lower odds of committing a major medical error in the next three months.**

What they found was that physician compassion was significantly associated with lower odds of committing a major medical error in the next three months. How much lower? That is a little harder to answer, because there is not yet a consensus on how to define "high" and "low" levels of compassion according to the scale that they used.

In the study above, for even the smallest measurable increment of higher compassion (i.e., just one point higher on a 28-point scale), there were *9 percent lower* odds of committing a major medical error in the next three months. So, even a little bit more compassion can make a meaningful (and measurable) difference! Accordingly, it appears that compassion may actually be protective; compassionate physicians might practice in such a way that they commit fewer medical errors.

Another study of 115 resident physicians from the University of Washington published in *Annals of Internal Medicine* sheds light on the relationship between depersonalization and quality standards among health care providers.[238] Using an anonymous survey, the researchers tested the association between physicians' level of depersonalization towards patients and their incidence of providing suboptimal care for patients admitted to the hospital.

Examples of suboptimal patient care that the physicians admitted to included: discharging patients from the hospital just to reduce physician workload, not fully discussing treatment options with a patient or fully answering questions, medication errors that were not due to lack of knowledge or inexperience, ordering restraints or medication for an agitated patient without evaluating the patient, skipping a diagnostic test because of a desire to discharge a patient, paying little attention to the social or personal impact of illness on a patient, and feeling guilty from a humanitarian standpoint about the care (or lack thereof) provided to a patient. This is essentially a list of items that you would never want to occur if you or a family member were in the hospital.

What they found was that depersonalization among the physicians was independently associated with higher incidence of self-reported substandard care at least monthly (and even weekly), which obviously is a reflection of having low quality standards. It turns out that the relationship between depersonalization and substandard care was "dose-dependent"; the higher the depersonalization score, the more likely the physicians were to provide substandard care. Compared to the physicians with the lowest scores for depersonalization, the physicians with high depersonalization scores had *more than four times higher odds* of substandard patient care practices.

If you're a health care provider, you may have encountered colleagues that suffer from depersonalization who are unable to make personal connections or who have really stopped caring about patients. Perhaps you have also observed them cutting corners in terms of quality standards?

The data are pretty clear that depersonalization among medical doctors is associated with increased risk of harm to patients, but what about surgeons? In a study of 7,905 surgeons across the U.S. led by researchers from the Mayo Clinic, they surveyed members of the American College of Surgeons and tested the association between depersonalization/emotional exhaustion and the occurrence of major surgical errors.[239]

Again, they used validated scales to measure depersonalization and emotional exhaustion as well as the occurrence of errors by surgeons. Errors were assessed by self-report, confidentially asking the surgeons if they made any major errors in the past three months.

They found that, overall, 9 percent of surgeons reported making a major surgical error. Both depersonalization and emotional exhaustion among surgeons were significantly associated with a higher incidence of major surgical errors. These results, stratified by levels of depersonalization and emotional exhaustion, appear in Figure 6.1.

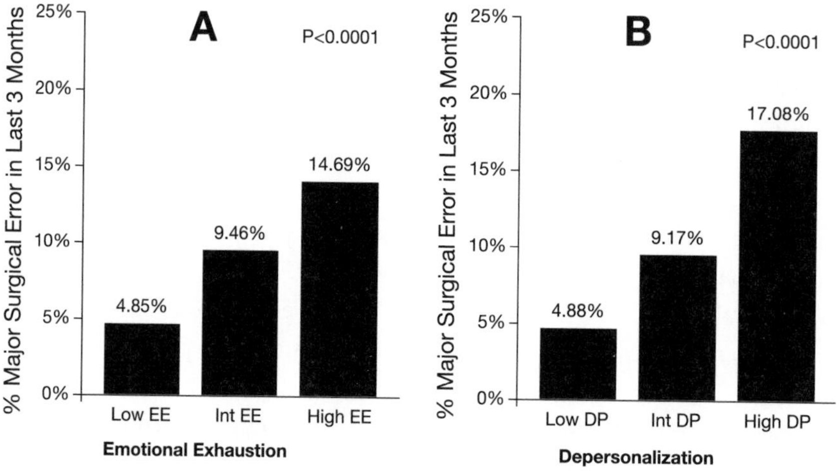

Figure 6.1: Proportions of surgeons (total n=7,905) reporting they made a major surgical error in the past three months, stratified by their level (i.e., from left to right: low, intermediate or high) of emotional exhaustion (EE) and depersonalization (DP).
Source Annals of Surgery
(Shanafelt, Balch et al. 2010)

It's a dramatic difference, isn't it? Compared to surgeons with low depersonalization or emotional exhaustion scores, surgeons with the most severe depersonalization and emotional exhaustion had a sharply higher error rate. The proportion of surgeons who committed a major error in the past three months was *three times higher!* The number one contributing factor in making the errors? According to the surgeons, it was a lapse in their clinical judgment.

In summary, surgeons scoring very high in depersonalization (which involves objectifying patients as well as being uncaring and callous towards them) and surgeons scoring high in emotional exhaustion (which leads to compassion fatigue) are prone to a lapse in clinical judgment that can result in a major error.

Concerning? Yes. Surprising? Probably not. (Here's a thought: maybe you should ask your surgeon how he or she is feeling before you go under the knife?)

Numerous other clinical studies have similarly supported that health care providers' inability to build meaningful relationships with patients can lead to low quality of care and is a risk to patient safety. For example, a Swiss study of 1,425 nurses and physicians working in ICUs found that emotional exhaustion—a precursor to compassion fatigue—among ICU staff was associated with higher ICU mortality.[240] So it's not just a higher error rate… it's a higher *death* rate.

> A lack of compassion among health care providers can be a serious patient safety risk.

An anonymous survey study of 681 emergency physicians in the U.K. found that compassion fatigue among emergency physicians was also associated with reducing their quality standards in the emergency department in a way that could harm patients.[241] In fact, one-third of physicians with compassion fatigue reported these behaviors at least monthly. Taking all of the available data together, the evidence is clear. A lack of compassion among health care providers can be a serious patient safety risk.

What Compassion Fatigue Looks Like in Practice

Recently, a cardiologist shared an experience about a favorite patient of hers, Gina, an elderly woman who came to an appointment very anxious about an imminent surgical procedure that she needed. Normally, Gina was very energetic and outspoken. She was full of life.

But at this appointment, Gina was a wreck. Her family explained that she wasn't sleeping at night—she had not had a good night sleep in weeks, actually—because she was so worried she might not survive the surgery. They asked the cardiologist if she could possibly prescribe a medication to help her sleep.

Normally, a cardiologist doesn't prescribe these sorts of medications. When needed, they are usually handled by the patient's primary care physician (PCP). But when the cardiologist looked through Gina's electronic medical record, she noted that Gina had already communicated with her PCP about it.

She saw notes about telephone communications between that PCP and his staff in the office. Essentially, that doctor blew off the request. He instructed his staff, "If surgery is the reason why she can't sleep, tell her to ask the surgeon to prescribe it."

Why couldn't he help his patient?

The cardiologist made the diagnosis just from reading the notes in the computer. The PCP was burned out. It was obvious. His failure to appropriately care about his patient's well-being was depersonalization in action. Gina's PCP wasn't thinking about her as a *person*...a person who was in need of his help. To the PCP, Gina was just one more task to get through in an overflowing inbox of tasks at the end of a long day. It was easier to just "pass the buck."

The cardiologist cared deeply about Gina, and of course she helped her. Not just with a sleep aid, but she also treated Gina with compassion. She took the time to talk with Gina, to find out *why* she was so afraid of surgery and why she thought she was not going to survive it.

She reassured Gina and helped her to understand that she was not going to die. She told her that she would not go through this experience alone. And, just as we saw the scientific evidence for the power of compassion in the treatment of anxiety (Chapter 4), that compassionate connection with her cardiologist made all the difference for Gina. It made her much less anxious, helped to quell her fears, and helped her get through the surgery with peace of mind.

Emotional Harms: Invisible but Real

So far in this chapter, we have examined how a lack of compassion can reduce the quality of care leading to physical harms, such as major medical or surgical errors or other adverse outcomes. But are those really the only outcomes that matter? What about the harms to patients that do not leave a mark on the outside, but rather leave a mark on the *inside?*

Recently, *The New England Journal of Medicine* asked health care providers to imagine scenarios such as these:[242]

- A patient with a recent diagnosis of cancer goes to the emergency department, due to a complication of chemotherapy. The emergency department physician reads through his medical records from the oncology clinic and says bluntly, very matter-of-fact, "Since your cancer is incurable…" Wait, incurable? The patient's oncologist had not yet used those words with him. This is the *first time* the patient has heard this.
- A physician has to notify her patient about test results. They're not good. The physician has to give her the bad news. No one thought to ask the patient ahead of time how she wants to receive the information or who she wants to be around for support when she receives it. The phone call from the physician comes when she is away from home. All alone. And she is driving sixty-five miles an hour on the interstate.

- A morbidly obese woman is admitted to the hospital. Speaking to a colleague, a resident physician makes a judgmental, derogatory statement about her obesity after he steps outside the patient's room. What the resident physician does not realize is that the patient is still within earshot. She heard everything and is humiliated. It's not the first time in her life she has been humiliated by someone because of her weight, but this time it's different. It's her *doctor.*
- A son receives a 3 a.m. phone call from an ICU resident physician asking for his consent to do an emergency procedure on his elderly father. "Wait, ICU?" he asks. "My father is not in the ICU." But actually, he is. He's dying. Hours earlier on the cardiology floor, the patient suddenly and unexpectedly went into cardiac arrest and, with all the various caregivers' efforts to keep him alive, no one remembered to call his family.
- A woman comes to the emergency department because of abdominal pain and, ultimately, she needs to be evaluated by a specialist. Unannounced, the consulting physician barges into the patient's room while she is sitting on the bedpan. Clearly in a hurry, after barely explaining who he was or why he was there, the physician does exactly what he came to do: he begins to examine the patient's abdomen.

  Without asking permission or any forewarning, the physician lifts up the patient's gown, but does not pull the bedsheet up to maintain her privacy. The physician does not even remember to close the curtain around her bed. Family members from the next room over can see her. She is mortified—totally *exposed.*
- A patient complains on a hospital's Facebook page that the pre-operative paperwork for his surgery instructs him to check in at 5 a.m. He makes sure he's up by 3:30 a.m. because he has over an hour drive to get to the hospital, only to arrive and learn that patients can't actually check in until 6 a.m. When he expresses frustration, the staff tells him, "The 5 a.m. thing is a little 'trick' we use to make sure patients don't arrive late." The whole experience makes him wonder what other little "tricks or surprises" they might have in store for him during his surgery later that morning.[241]

These are all true stories…very real *emotional harms* that occur in hospitals and other types of health care facilities daily. In the constant quest to keep to a schedule and deliver quality clinical care, health care providers frequently overlook things like these that they don't deem important.

Dr. Lauge Sokol-Hessner, a professor at Harvard Medical School and the associate director of inpatient quality at Beth Israel Deaconess Medical Center in Boston, and his colleagues are studying just this problem. They define an emotional harm as harm to a patient's *dignity* caused by a failure to demonstrate adequate *respect* for the patient as a person.

Further, they define dignity as the intrinsic, unconditional value of all human beings that makes them worthy of respect. They see respect as the sum of the actions we take to protect, preserve, and enhance the dignity of our patients.[243] But most importantly, they believe that emotional harms are just as important as physical harms to patients and should be treated accordingly.

A few pages back, you were introduced to health care systems' gargantuan efforts to track medical errors, bad outcomes, and the process of care measures that may lead to physical harms. Quality reporting is a multi-*billion*-dollar industry in health care today. In fact, a research study examining just four specialties found that U.S. physician practices spend more than $15.4 billion annually to track, analyze and report quality measures.[244]

There are dozens of consulting companies—Healthgrades, Advisory Board, Huron Consulting Group, and so many more—all dedicated to helping hospitals improve their reporting on metrics that CMS wants data on. It makes sense, as the government is the largest health care payer in the U.S.

But there's something missing: Despite all of these efforts to reduce physical harm (and all of the spending on these efforts), *emotional harms* are not tracked at all. None of the vignettes about emotional harms you just read would show up on a health care system's quality dashboard. They are not systematically identified or addressed in hospital quality improvement programs.

That's why the unconventional—and probably long overdue—approach by Sokol-Hessner and his colleagues is so welcome.[242, 243] At Beth Israel Deaconess Medical Center, they are not only capturing and tracking emotional harms, but they've reconfigured their safety reporting tool to include a category for emotional harms.

Emotional harms are a big, big problem in health care today. Research shows that when asked about the impact of adverse events in health care, patients emphasize emotional harms more than physical harms.[243, 245, 246, 247] And emotional harms may be more common than physical harms; some research indicates *three times* more common.[246] Plus, they may "hurt" more than physical harms and can have lasting effects.

Think back for a moment to the bus crash study shared at the beginning of Chapter 1, the one about what the survivors remembered most five years after their harrowing experience.[18] What they said was that in addition to the physical pain they experienced, what was seared in their brain—five years after the accident—was a lack of compassion from caregivers at the hospital. They suffered an emotional harm that day, and they cannot forget it, even now.

Let's consider the six vignettes at the beginning of this section one more time. Five years from now, if you asked the patients or family in each of those scenarios what they remembered most of their experience, guess what they would most likely remember? They likely would not remember the specifics of the technical care. They might have very little recollection of those details. But they would definitely remember exactly how the caregivers made them *feel.* They would remember the indignity. Emotional wounds can run deep. And, unfortunately, they are sometimes never forgotten.

Maria's Story

Here is a true story of emotional harm, one that persists even today:

Maria thought she was dying. She felt like she was coming apart at the seams. She had trouble walking and trouble speaking. Her body was stiff. Her face was changing. Sometimes she would just have a blank stare, expressionless. Emotionally, she was withdrawing. She wondered if these were just the effects of aging, but she was only 65 years old.

When her primary care doctor put her arm around Maria and said the words, "I think you have Parkinson's disease," Maria's whole world changed in an instant. She was terrified. What did that mean? What would happen to her?

But, thankfully, things started to get better that day as Maria's primary care doctor also started her on a low dose of medication to treat Parkinson's disease. Almost immediately, Maria's movement got better. Her speech improved.

She was more herself, engaged, and able to connect with people. Her smile came back and her family was thankful. They had their "Nonna" back.

But then Maria's primary care doctor referred her to a specialist, a neurologist, to confirm the diagnosis was correct. On the day Maria and Peter, her husband of more than forty years, went to see the neurologist, they were quite anxious, but also hopeful that a good quality of life was possible. They were encouraged by the progress Maria had made on medications. But in that neurologist's office, everything changed.

The neurologist confirmed for Maria that it was Parkinson's disease and that she was started on the right medication already. But then, Maria asked him, "What can I expect with this diagnosis? What will happen over time?" She wanted to know what would happen to her, long term. What would the rest of her life *look like*?

The neurologist could have told her that although there is no cure for Parkinson's disease, there are effective treatments to slow the progression, and that a good quality of life is still possible for quite some time. He could have said, "Although there is no way to make this disease go away, Maria, we can treat it, and we will go through this *together*."

Instead, this is what he told her she had to look forward to. These are the actual words he used:

> *"There are two common patterns 'in the end.' The first is that, because you will have trouble walking, you will fall down and break your hip. That usually triggers a downward spiral of progressive weakness that you won't be able to get out of that will lead to your death. The second is that you will have trouble swallowing and you will choke on (aspirate) your food and you will die from that."*

Not only was there no compassion, there was no sensitivity—actually no *humanity*—in the words he spoke. Maria crumbled. She was shaking, unable to speak. She couldn't stop envisioning a horrible end to her life. Maria doesn't remember anything about the appointment beyond that point. She was unable to hear anything further that the neurologist said.

But Peter remembers every word. *Every* word. To this day when he thinks of that neurologist, he replays those words in his head and remembers how that doctor deeply wounded his wife, the love of his life. It is an emotional wound that to this day Maria keeps reliving. It cannot be undone. How could someone be so callous?

As soon as the appointment was over, Maria actually regressed *physically*. The medicines stopped working. Parkinson's disease causes rigidity of the body, an inability to move. Maria was frozen. The emotional harm triggered a physical harm. In the days and weeks that followed the neurologist visit, Maria fell into a deep depression which just exacerbated her physical symptoms.

Over time, after a rocky course, Maria started to respond to treatment again, but the experience still haunts her today. Anytime she is reminded of it, she breaks down in tears. All the feelings she felt back in that neurologist's office come rushing back all over again. And every time this happens, she slides backward with her physical symptoms as well. She crumbles again.

Everyone who knows her husband Peter would say, without question, that he is an extremely gentle man. But to this day, any time he thinks back to the words that the neurologist said, and how those words cut his precious wife to the core and stole a piece of her spirit, his jaw clenches, and so do his fists. He fights back tears. This typically gentle man shakes with anger at the memory—even now, many years later. Don't tell Peter that emotional harms aren't real.

If you are a health care worker of any kind, there are three key take-home messages in this regrettable story. First, always remember that being a patient means being *vulnerable*, and often extremely vulnerable. Second, compassion protects the vulnerable. Failing to practice compassion means that emotional harms are more likely to occur.

Emotional harms are usually *preventable*, and when we fail to prevent them we should consider that unacceptable. When a physician graduates from medical school and takes the oath that we often translate as "Do no harm," that includes the kind of harm that is *invisible* also...the emotional wounds.

And third, know this: *every word* out of your mouth *matters.*

Emotional Harms Can Be Expensive for Health Care Systems

What about when health care providers don't take their responsibility to prevent emotional harms seriously? In one especially egregious case in the news recently, a jury ordered two physicians to pay a patient $500,000 after they made disparaging comments about him while he was under anesthesia.[248]

Here's what happened: A patient was preparing to undergo a colonoscopy. He knew that he got very groggy with sedative drugs, and he wanted to accurately capture any post-procedure instructions that his physician would give him. So right before the procedure started, he pressed "record" on his smartphone.

Imagine his surprise when he pressed play on the way home from the hospital and realized that he captured the chatter of his doctors during the whole procedure. As soon as he was asleep, the insults began. "After five minutes of talking to you in pre-op, I wanted to punch you in the face and 'man you up' a little bit," the anesthesiologist said to her colleagues.

But it didn't stop there. When the medical assistant pointed out a rash on the man's penis, the anesthesiologist joked that the medical assistant should not touch it because he might get "some syphilis on your arm or something," and then added, "It's probably tuberculosis in the penis." It went on and on and on. The doctors even talked about how to avoid the patient after the procedure and asked an assistant to lie to him![248]

As a result, the jury awarded the man $100,000 for defamation, $200,000 in punitive damages, and another $200,000 for medical malpractice.[248] Later in Chapter 7, we will do a deep dive on the evidence for the effects of compassion on health care costs but, for now, this story is an example of how an extraordinary lack of compassion for a patient leading to an emotional harm can also be extraordinarily expensive.

Rethinking Quality and Safety Measures

As you've seen, Sokol-Hessner and his colleagues at Beth Israel Deaconess are convinced not only that emotional harms are real but also that we need to treat them very seriously, just like all other avoidable harms that are tracked in health care systems. We should track them just like other adverse events.[242]

Just as hospital-acquired infections, surgical complications, and the most serious adverse events are preventable (sometimes called "never events" in hospitals), health systems also need to have a method to report, track, and investigate cases of emotional harm. Of course, if we can't measure it, we can't improve it. Sokol-Hessner reminds us that dignity and respect for patients are, in fact, legitimate quality measures. Period.

Perhaps most important to remember, emotional harms often can be prevented through compassion and maintaining dignity and respect for patients. Therefore, unlike many adverse events that are tracked in health systems, the occurrence of which may be mostly (or in some cases totally) unavoidable, emotional harms are almost always preventable.

Now, following the lead of Dr. Sokol-Hessner and colleagues, it is health care's responsibility to prevent them. Research from the University of California Berkeley found that physicians are often reluctant to respond to disrespectful or uncaring behaviors toward patients by members of their medical team.[249] These researchers also found that physicians often avoid or rationalize these behaviors by colleagues, respond in ways that avoid moral judgment, do not actually address underlying attitudes towards patients, and leave room for face-saving reinterpretations of the behavior.

This is a problem. This failure to hold people accountable for bad behavior that results in emotional harms for patients could be passed on to the next generation of health care providers. (Think back to our discussion of the "hidden curriculum" for physicians-in-training from Chapter 1). We must begin to hold our colleagues (and ourselves) accountable—across all health care worker roles—and do our very best to prevent emotional harms for patients and families every day.

But let's be clear, we are not talking about eliminating heartbreak for patients and families. That's not possible. Every day in every health care system, people will grieve over devastating unavoidable loss, such as the death of a loved one or receiving bad news about a diagnosis or prognosis.

These are the outcomes that are largely unavoidable. What we are talking about is the avoidable, preventable heartbreak that comes from a patient's loss of dignity and respect, the preventable emotional harm that adds the insult to injury. That is what must be prevented.

Compassion in Times of Heartbreak

Going back to the story of Kenneth B. Schwartz from the end of Chapter 4, the inspiration behind Schwartz Rounds, he said that compassion can make the unbearable, *bearable*. So for patients and families who are dealing with unavoidable loss and grief, compassion from their health care providers can help lessen the emotional pain people are experiencing, at least to some extent. Schwartz was convinced of this; he experienced it himself firsthand.

Some health care providers just understand this intuitively. Like the entire care team did recently one night at Cooper University Hospital when a 60-year-old man was admitted to the ICU due to a spontaneous brain hemorrhage. Sadly, the bleeding was so severe that there was nothing the neurosurgeons could do to save him. He was dying, and rapidly declining with only hours to live.

But that was not the only tragedy: His grief-stricken wife relayed the story that the patient's daughter, who was on her way to the hospital with her fiancée, was to be married in just two weeks. She said it was going to be the highlight of the patient's life. She begged the ICU team to do whatever they could to keep him alive until the daughter arrived.

His daughter—who was, of course, devastated by the news that her dad was so gravely ill—was praying there was some way that he could be there when she got married. It was a heartbreaking scene when the daughter and her fiancée arrived in the ICU, saw his life slipping away, and realized that their dream wedding day would not include him.

That was when the ICU nurses and technicians on duty that night—moved by deep compassion for this patient and his family in their moment of tragedy—sprang into action…as wedding planners!

It was 2 a.m., and they did not have much time. An ICU nurse crafted two rings out of IV tubing and medical tape. Two ICU technicians quickly scoured the hospital for the rest of the essentials. The cancer unit had a beautiful bouquet of flowers that they gladly donated. There was a frozen pound cake in the back of the freezer of the staff break room that was fashioned into a wedding cake. Something blue? They borrowed a blue ribbon from some Easter decorations on another floor.

But who was going to marry them? They called the clergy on-call, but since it was 2 a.m. and Dad was fading fast, it looked like the chaplain would not make it in time. Just then, one of the other ICU nurses stepped forward. He was an ordained minister and able to perform weddings.

Imagine the scene: With wedding music playing from a nurse's cell phone, and the family (including the bride's sister who was on speaker phone from California) plus the entire ICU staff gathered around Dad's bedside, there was a wedding. It was not the wedding that was planned, but it was nonetheless beautiful.

In her father's presence (and holding his hand), the bride and groom said their vows. Minutes later, he died. The patient and family went through unspeakable pain in the ICU that night. But the compassion that the ICU staff showed them is something that no one will ever forget.

Weeks later, the bride wrote a very touching letter to the ICU staff, thanking them for all their compassion and for going the extra mile to allow her to be married in her father's presence. It meant the world to her. She concluded the letter with this:

"Thank you from the bottom of my heart. Although my heart is broken, at the same time, because of you, it is very full."

Emotional Harm Can Be Heartbreaking...Literally

Now let's look at an entirely different type of experience that happened in a different ICU in a different hospital and with a different broken heart.

Do you recall (from Chapter 1 on the compassion crisis) the NIH-funded University of Washington study where researchers found that fully one-third of end-of-life discussions with patients or families in the ICU included *zero* statements of compassion from physicians?[54] That study was especially striking, because if there ever was a time when people need compassion, it is when facing the end of life.

Remember also the description of Takotsubo cardiomyopathy from Chapter 3? That is the condition where, following an extreme emotional stressor or other triggering event, a patient goes into sudden heart failure and can suffer fatal cardiovascular collapse.[96] A patient can actually *die* from a broken heart.

One especially dramatic case highlights—and brings together—both of these scientific facts. A 72-year-old man was in the ICU with progressive multiple organ failure. As his critical illness continued to deteriorate, it was clear to the ICU team that his condition was not survivable.

The next step was to talk with his family. The plan was to meet with them and explain how grave the situation was and then to recommend withdrawal of life sustaining therapy, to allow the patient to pass away peacefully. As sad as that situation is, if you practice intensive care medicine you encounter these matters on a regular basis. It is, of course, imperative to approach the family with all the care and compassion that one can muster.

But that's not exactly what happened when meeting with the wife of this particular patient. It was quite the opposite. When the patient's wife of almost fifty years came to the patient's room in the ICU, she had absolutely no idea what was in store for that meeting. She knew he was sick, but she did not yet have an understanding of how grave the situation was.

The first error the team made was to fail to ask the wife who else in the family should be present (for multiple reasons, not the least of which is emotional support). The second error was to fail to ask her what her current understanding of the situation was, in order to predict how shocking the information may be to her.

The third error was to fail to ask her to sit down. The wife and the ICU team were standing up next to the patient's bed for that heavy talk. (Note: Always ask somebody to sit down before you give them the news that delivers the worst day of their life.) The fourth—and most egregious—error was a striking lack of compassion. Just like the University of Washington study: there was *zero*.

In the first thirty seconds of the meeting, the physician just blurted it out in a way that was not only matter-of-fact and insensitive (like it was nothing), but also downright cold: "He is dying. He won't survive the day. There is nothing we can do." Full stop.

Mind you, all of those statements were true. He was dying, and there was no way to change that. And the physician had a responsibility to communicate those facts to the wife so that she had a full understanding. It wasn't the message. It was *how* the message was delivered. While a physician needs to be honest with the facts, communicating such sensitive information in such a thoughtless way is clearly an avoidable emotional harm.

BAM! It happened so fast that no one could catch her. His wife, who was more than 70 years old herself, collapsed and hit the floor…face first. There was blood everywhere, pouring out of her nose onto the floor of the patient's room.

But as soon as the doctors flipped her over onto her back, they realized she did not just faint following the bad news. Something very different was happening to her. There was barely a pulse, and she was barely breathing.

The trauma of the fall was not the primary problem; it was a catastrophic heart problem that caused her to collapse. It was a full-on resuscitation situation, but not for the patient...for his wife.

The ICU team worked valiantly to try to revive her. When the cardiologist did an echocardiogram to look at the heart, it had the characteristic signs of Takotsubo cardiomyopathy. Sadly, she could not be saved. She and her husband both passed away within 24 hours of each other. A striking lack of compassion from a caregiver appears to be the trigger for the event that culminated in her dying from a broken heart.

Health care providers should think of this story the next time they have to give a patient or his family bad news. A caregiver's responsibility often extends *beyond* the patient.

Compassion Elevates the Quality of Care

Now that we have seen a myriad of ways in which a lack of compassion can lower the quality of health care, let's look at the flip side: how having compassion for patients can lead to higher quality of care.

There are multiple potential mechanisms by which this can occur, including:[14]

- a higher level of health care provider commitment (i.e., going the extra mile)—to ensure optimal clinical outcomes;
- higher quality standards—more diligence and meticulousness around technical quality of care—among health care providers;
- a higher level of patient trust in health care providers, creating a better therapeutic alliance; and
- more patient self-disclosure in medical interviews, resulting in better information gathering by health care providers and better diagnostic accuracy.

But what is the *evidence?*

In the Johns Hopkins study in HIV patients that you saw in Chapter 5, you may remember that researchers asked patients if their physician knew them as a person.[201] They found that knowing the patient as a person was associated with better patient adherence to antiretroviral therapy and, accordingly, better clearance of HIV virus from the blood.

Well, there was another finding in that study that matters here. The researchers also found that knowing the patient as a person was associated with *41 percent higher* odds that the antiretroviral medication regimen prescribed by the physician matched up with experts' best practice recommendations for treating HIV. In other words, there were 41 percent higher odds that the physician was prescribing the *right* medications.

Why? This seems unlikely to be causation, right? Knowing the patient as a person probably does not cause a physician to rethink what they are prescribing. More likely, it's correlation.

Perhaps physicians who are the type of people who get to know their patients as a person also happen to be the type of people who make sure they are prescribing the right medications. Maybe physicians who care enough to get to know their patients as a person are also more careful in what they are prescribing.

Or perhaps knowing the patient as a person is just a sign of *competence* for a physician. That is, physicians who are more competent know that building a relationship with the patient is an essential part of care.

So, are there data on compassion and competence? Yes, multiple studies support this link, especially the assessment of competence from the patient perspective. If a patient heard a surgeon say "oops" during their operation or observed a physician Googling their disease during an office visit, the patient's confidence in the physician obviously would take a nosedive. It's no different with compassion.

For example, a study of physicians in training found that compassion communicates competence.[250] One way that medical schools evaluate the competence of physicians-in-training is through an objective structured clinical examination (OSCE).

In an OSCE, an experienced independent physician evaluator (e.g., a professor in the medical school) watches a physician-in-training perform a "history and physical" on a patient and scores the physician-in-training on the competence of his or her clinical skills using a pre-defined and validated scoring system. Sometimes they videotape the OSCE and then show the video to lay people and patients who grade the physicians-in-training on their communication skills. This methodology has been shown to be a valid and reliable method of assessing the quality of physician communication in numerous studies.[251]

Likewise, in a study of 57 physicians-in-training, researchers found that observed behaviors—both verbal and non-verbal—that were expressions of compassion were strongly associated with perception of clinical competence, as rated by both the physician evaluator and by patients.[250] In fact, the mean score for clinical competence among high compassion individuals was *15 percent higher* than it was for those with low compassion.

In a unique study from Harvard Medical School and the Department of Psychology at Yale University, researchers tested the association between compassionate non-verbal behavior by physicians and patient perception of physicians' clinical competence using an online crowdsourcing platform to recruit more than 1,300 people to evaluate the physicians.[252] (As mentioned earlier, using lay person observers to evaluate physician communication is recognized as a sound methodology for physician communication research).[251]

In this study, all of the participants read an identical passage of text that was a scripted communication from a physician to a patient. But the participants were provided different visual images to accompany the text. Some of them were shown photographs of a physician with compassionate non-verbal communication like eye-contact, being at eye level, no physical barriers, having an open posture, leaning in, and showing a concerned facial expression.

The other participants were shown photographs of a physician with the opposite non-verbal behavior, such as no eye contact, looking down at the patient from a standing position, sitting behind a physical barrier, crossing his arms, and looking rather annoyed with their facial expressions.

After adjusting the analyses for potential confounders (like the participants' mood at the time of the evaluation), they found that participants rated physicians with compassionate non-verbal behavior as being not only more compassionate but also more competent. Similar to the prior study we just discussed, the mean competence scores for the high compassion physicians were almost *15 percent higher* than the competence scores for the low compassion physicians.

> Research shows if health care providers consistently demonstrate compassion, patients are more likely to believe they know what they are doing.

So what's the take-home message for health care providers? If you consistently demonstrate compassionate behaviors (both verbal and non-verbal communications) for your patients, they are more likely to believe that you know what you are doing. These data support that compassion and competence—at least perception of competence—just go together, naturally. But is it just perception, or is the quality of care *actually* better?

Compassion Inspires Quality Communication with Patients

If health care providers do not care enough to find out what is worrying their patients the most, they might never know. In an interesting study from the University of Colorado School of Medicine, researchers distributed cards to patients seeking care in the emergency department asking, "What worries you the most?"[253]

The patients wrote in their answers. Then the researchers compared the patients' greatest worries to what was listed as their chief complaint on their medical chart by the emergency department triage nurse. (Chief complaint, in emergency medicine speak, is the main reason someone has come to the emergency department in the first place.)

Here's what they learned: Patients' most pressing worries were often unrelated to their chief complaints. In fact, only *26 percent* of people's worries actually matched their chief complaint.[254] For example, for a 68-year-old man who presented with a chief complaint of neck pain and stiffness, his greatest worry was actually, *"Dying and not seeing my children and grandchildren again."*

One 45-year-old man had a chief complaint of chest pain on his chart, but his greatest worry told a different story. He wrote, *"I worry about dying too young to see my kids grow up—they're 14, 15, and 8. I've got trouble with my heart because of the drugs. I don't want to be here again, but I can't stay away."*

A 27-year-old pregnant female had a chief complaint of vaginal bleeding, but her greatest worry was actually depression. She wrote, *"I don't want to go into depression again. A miscarriage is hard."*

This qualitative data shows quite clearly: if health care providers do not care enough to *ask* patients what their greatest worry is, they may never know. How can health care providers possibly give their patients the highest quality, patient-centered care if they do not even know their patients' greatest worry related to their health?

Compassion for patients not only makes a health care provider more likely to ask their patients what their greatest worry is, but it also makes them more willing to *listen*. Part of caring deeply about patients is letting them tell their story.

Sir William Osler, who is one of the most famous physician scientists in the history of medicine, once said, "Listen to your patient; he is telling you the diagnosis." Health care providers who listen intently to what patients are saying are likely to get the necessary information. Those who do not listen intently to patients are prone to errors, both in making the diagnosis and in making clinical judgments.

And this appears to be a two-way street. When physicians have high compassion for patients, not only are they more willing to listen to patients, but patients are also more willing to listen to the physicians. Research shows that compassionate care from a physician is associated with more accurate patient recall of the medical information communicated by the physician.[174, 175] This is an important part of clinical quality because it promotes adherence to treatment recommendations.

When patients stop talking, the real trouble begins. A health care provider's diagnostic accuracy is based largely on having all of the right information, and the completeness of information gathering is essential. Let's face it: sometimes seeking medical care is downright embarrassing. Patients often have to share some of the most personal information imaginable. They are often reluctant to disclose information if it is of a sensitive, intensely personal nature. Patients frequently shut down and do not disclose everything fully if they think their doctor doesn't care and doesn't want to hear it. That's a serious threat to patient safety.

In Chapters 3 and 4, we reviewed data demonstrating that compassion enhances patient trust in health care providers, and that this can affect patient outcomes. But compassion also enhances patient trust in a way that facilitates patient disclosure in the medical interview. Patients don't place their trust in physicians and nurses because of the number of diplomas they have on the wall or the reputation of the school that they graduated from. Rather, research shows that patient trust is about the relationship that they have with their providers.[43]

In Chapter 5, you heard about a University of Virginia study of patients with HIV where physician compassion was associated with a patient's belief that therapy would be effective.[202] Well, they also measured patient disclosure in that study and found that patients of highly compassionate physicians disclosed more information during the visit.

Importantly, it was not just more information that was important from a psychosocial and human connection standpoint, but also information that was important from a biomedical standpoint (i.e., relevant to the treatment of HIV disease).

Rigorous research from Columbia University backs up this finding. Researchers found that compassion for others is a very strong predictor that another person will confide secrets in us, while mere politeness is not.[205] So science shows that for others to trust us with their most closely held secrets, we need to go deeper than just common courtesy, and just having the formal role of one's health care provider is not enough. Here too, science shows that compassion matters.

Earlier we shared a study published in *Annals of Internal Medicine*, where more than three-quarters of physicians interrupted patients before they completed their opening statement of concerns.[34] This is a real problem; the inability to listen attentively signals a lack of compassion and caring about the patient. That will shut down a patient quickly, making it more difficult to elicit all the necessary information for diagnosis and treatment. Here's a more in-depth (and true) story that really illustrates the impact that compassion can have on the quality of communication, and even save a life.

John's Story

It was a night shift in the emergency department of a busy academic medical center. At 1 a.m., a 45-year-old male, John, arrived complaining of a headache.

It was clear from the moment that he arrived that John didn't want to be there. He sat up on the gurney in the exam room of the emergency department, arms crossed, looking only slightly uncomfortable, but mostly just annoyed. He was only there because his wife made him come in. She made him come because he almost never gets headaches, and so it concerned her. He didn't like hospitals.

The resident physician talked with John, examined him, and did not find anything unusual to suggest something serious. But he decided to order a CT scan of John's brain, just to be sure that everything was okay.

It took a long time to complete John's evaluation that night. *Hours* really, mostly because of how busy the rest of the emergency department was. Everything was backed up, including the CT scanner and the radiologist who had to read the CT scan. Once the test results were available, it took time for the attending emergency physician to get freed up from caring for other patients in order to review them. That annoyed John even more. Remember, he did not want to be there in the first place.

But during that time delay, there was actually a bonding opportunity for John…not with his physician, but with his nurse, Jackie. She sensed his frustration and did all she could to make him more comfortable during his time there.

Jackie closed the door of his exam room so that the noise from the rest of the emergency department would not exacerbate his headache. She brought him a warm blanket and turned down the lights in his room so that he could try to close his eyes and get a little rest while waiting.

And she talked with him. She talked in soft, soothing tones. Clearly, Jackie was the type of person who really cared. She did not just talk with him about the formalities (like chief complaint, history of present illness, review of systems, and all that), but she *really* talked with him.

She sensed that there was more to the story. There must have been a reason why he did not want to come to the hospital when his wife insisted. John was notably more relaxed after the care Jackie provided. (By the way, Jackie is a nurse who is known for exceptional care and compassion for patients, so this extra care was nothing out of the ordinary for her on a busy night shift in the emergency department. That's just who she is. Also, you might think that it takes Jackie extra time for this kind of extra care. In Chapter 8, you will see that is not necessarily the case.)

After the CT scan was read by the radiologist as normal, John still had a bad headache. But by that time, he'd had it with being in the emergency department. He was ready to get out of there. So the attending physician, seeing that the CT scan was normal, discharged him home. It was 4 a.m. John went home to bed.

End of story? Not by a long shot.

Toward the end of his night shift, the attending physician was catching up on completing his charts for all the patients he treated overnight. He reviewed the resident physician's note for John's care: it looked okay; nothing unusual. But when he reviewed Jackie's nursing notes, he noted something peculiar. She jotted down: "+BM".

"+BM"? What did that mean? He went and found Jackie and asked her.

She explained: in her time talking to John, and showing him extra care, she learned that the patient was annoyed about being there because he was actually completely *embarrassed* to be there.

"Embarrassed?" the physician asked. "What do you mean?"

She went on, "He's a really stoic and private guy, you know. Well, there was something he hadn't said...and he was really embarrassed about it. I could tell that he didn't want to talk about it at first, but over the night he warmed up to me.

So here's the real story: Over the past couple of days, he had been really constipated. He tried fiber, prune juice, you name it. It was not providing relief. He went to the bathroom right before bed and decided: 'This was it.' He was going to have a bowel movement, no matter what. He strained and strained and strained. And finally, he had a huge bowel movement (actually a 'blowout,' is what he said) and he instantly felt better in his stomach. But that was when his headache came on."

"When I was talking with him, he admitted that he was so embarrassed to be there. I remember him saying, 'I feel so stupid—here as a patient in a trauma center in the middle of the night, surrounded by people who have real problems like car crashes and heart attacks—only because I overdid it in the bathroom. I'm an idiot.'"

So when Jackie made the note "+BM," that meant that the headache started when the patient was straining to have a bowel movement. As Jackie was speaking, she noted that the face of the attending physician was becoming more and more pale.

"What's the matter?" Jackie asked.

"Oh my God...*I missed it,*" said the doc.

"Does it matter?" asked Jackie.

Before Jackie could even get an answer, the physician was off like a shot. This attending physician, who was a veteran of more than ten years in the emergency department and was known for being exceptionally calm—even in the most dire, life-and-death situations—was right now on fire. His body language made it clear: this was a red alert, all hands on deck moment.

The attending physician grabbed the resident physician by the arm (which no one had ever seen him do before) and commanded, "Find that patient right now and get him back here immediately. Call the police to go to his house if you have to." Just in case there was any grey area, he added, "This is no joke."

But the resident demurred. "It's 5 a.m.," he said. "This guy had to wait three hours, only to be told nothing was wrong and be discharged. He probably just fell asleep. He's going to kill me if I wake him up and tell him to come back!" (By the way, this is the same resident physician who saw the "+BM" in the nursing notes and did not think to ask Jackie what it meant.) The resident thought his attending physician was crazy. The CT scan was fine; it was time to move on.

The attending physician had enough of the eye rolling from his junior colleague. He was going to call the patient himself. He needed to make sure the patient would come back and could not entrust the communication to anyone else.

Here's the deal: There are many warning signs in patients with headache that can signal a potential catastrophic diagnosis, even if a CT scan of the brain is normal. A headache that starts when someone is straining—like having a bowel movement or lifting an exceptionally heavy weight—can signal that it is a brain aneurysm that has popped (i.e., ruptured, bleeding).

An aneurysm is an abnormality—actually, an enlargement—of a blood vessel caused by a weakening of the blood vessel wall. A brain aneurysm can be difficult to diagnose in the emergency department, and it doesn't get any more high stakes than this.

A bleeding brain aneurysm, if not diagnosed and treated promptly, can result in devastating brain damage and is often fatal. In the earliest stages of a bleeding brain aneurysm, a conventional CT scan of the brain can appear normal. In that case, other imaging is needed, or the physicians need to insert a needle into the spinal canal to sample some of the spinal fluid (also called a spinal tap) to look for evidence of bleeding.

It's important to point out that it wasn't Jackie's job to know the significance of "+BM." It was the emergency physician's job. But it was Jackie's expertise and extra care that got the patient to open up. It was her extra care that got him to disclose it.

Imagine how that phone call went: calling John and requesting that he return immediately. If the patient was a 9 out of 10 on the annoyance scale when he was in the emergency department, he was an 11 when the attending physician woke him out of a deep sleep with a phone call and asked him to come back.

Keep in mind, the physician was also saying that they might need to stick a long needle into his spine! But the physician was insisting. Actually, he was *begging* John to come back. Of course, the physician had to acknowledge to the patient that there was also a very high likelihood that a bleeding aneurysm was not present, but with something potentially devastating you just can't take any chances.

Still groggy from being awakened, John muttered "okay," and then hung up. But the physician, who was about to turn the emergency department over to the oncoming day shift attending physician was not convinced he would actually come back. He felt sick to his stomach. He told the day shift physician the whole story and prepared to go home. In the back of his mind, he was thinking he might do something he had never done before…drive to a patient's house on the way home from the hospital!

But then, on his way out the door, the physician passed John walking back in to the emergency department. He was so happy to see John, the physician nearly hugged him. The doc went home and went to sleep. And then, when he woke up that afternoon, he called his colleague in the emergency department to see what happened with John.

"Are you sitting down?" she asked. "He's in the operating room right now." Further testing showed a brain aneurysm that had just started leaking, a very early stage of rupture. But when the neurovascular surgeon tried to stop the bleeding by threading a catheter up into the blood vessels in the brain, he could not stop the bleeding.

The shape of the aneurysm was such that they could not get control of the bleeding with a catheter. They had to rush him to the operating room for brain surgery—a craniotomy (surgical opening in the skull)—to clip the aneurysm, in order to get the bleeding to stop. Thankfully, the surgery went exactly as planned, and John made a rapid and complete recovery. He is 100 percent back to normal today.

So what does this story have to do with compassionomics? Yes, the physician was tenacious in following up once he realized the warning sign but, let's be honest, he was also one of the people who missed it. In reality, it was Jackie that saved John's life.

Earlier, we reviewed the scientific data showing that a compassionate human connection is what makes people confide their secrets in others. Specifically, in health care, we saw that compassion leads to greater disclosure by patients.

In John's case, he was totally embarrassed about the details of how his headache started. He thought his headache was nothing serious—just a byproduct of his constipation—and he did not really need to be in the emergency department among people with obvious life or death conditions. His wife made him come. He felt stupid.

He did not tell the triage nurse the "+BM" part. He did not tell the resident physician. He did not tell the attending physician. He did not even tell his wife. But he told Jackie.

Jackie could tell there was more to the story, and that he was embarrassed about something. She cared enough to ask. Like we said earlier, that's what Jackie was known for: exceptional caring and compassion. And because the patient could tell that she truly cared, he confided in her the critical piece of information that no one else could get…the only piece of information that actually mattered.

Jackie knows that compassion matters. Although she helped to save victims of car crashes and heart attacks on that same busy night in the emergency department, nothing was more heroic than the way she cared enough to inspire this man to open up and confide in her. And this is an important reminder of how compassion can actually *save a life.*

Going the Extra Mile

If you are a resident physician on duty at Cooper University Hospital, these words from the unit secretary might make you cringe: "Dr. Viner is on the phone and he wants to speak to you."

"Oh no," you might mutter under your breath. "Not *another* Dr. Viner patient."

You see, Dr. Viner's patients are special. At the end of Chapter 3, you were introduced to Dr. Viner. He was the chair of the Department of Medicine at Cooper for two decades, and he was also the patient in the story of the "angel" nurses who helped him get off the ventilator in the ICU.

As a young man, Dr. Viner experienced the power of compassion firsthand, as a patient himself. From then on, he dedicated his life to showing the same level of care for others. That's also why he founded the Center for Humanism at Cooper Medical School of Rowan University.

If you are a resident physician and one of Dr. Viner's patients is admitted to your service in the hospital, it's a special experience. Most of Dr. Viner's patients have been his patients for years, and often for decades.

Dr. Viner will first make sure you know the whole story, every detail about the patient, all the way back to the beginning. Even if the patient is only being admitted to the hospital for a very discrete issue, you will get to hear his or her life story. You might also get the life story for everyone in the patient's family. (Dr. Viner takes knowing the patient as a person to a whole new level.)

You will also get Dr. Viner's mobile phone number. And you will get the opportunity to use it…frequently. You will get to call Dr. Viner to update him about every little detail in the patient's care. If you don't call him at the expected time interval to give him the update, you can expect to be paged in the hospital. It's Dr. Viner calling to check in with you.

If something important and unexpected happens to one of his patients, good luck to you, if Dr. Viner hears it first from anyone other than you. Also, he "cyber stalks" the electronic medical record from home, so he likely knows the test results before you do. He knows every detail.

One summer night while Dr. Viner was on vacation at the Jersey Shore, he got a phone call from the wife of a man who had been his patient for nearly forty years. The man had been admitted to the hospital and needed a consultation from a specialist.

After spending much of the night on the phone discussing his care with the various caregivers involved, Dr. Viner decided that it was taking too long for the specialist to come and see his patient. He got in his car late at night (leaving his vacation, mind you) and drove all the way from Ocean City, New Jersey to Cooper in Camden, New Jersey which is more than sixty miles away, arriving close to midnight, just to stand by his patient's bedside and make sure that he got everything he needed as quickly as possible.

That's Dr. Viner. So, if you are a resident physician on duty when one of Dr. Viner's patients is admitted, you can expect he will be all over you to make sure that you provide the best care to his patient that you possibly can. Not acceptable care, but *exceptional* care.

Why? Compassionomics. Research shows that compassion for others makes people more likely to exhibit altruistic behavior and "go the extra mile."[234, 235] Dr. Viner cares deeply about his patients. He doesn't just know them as patients, he knows each patient as a whole person. He has celebrated with them life's wonderful blessings—when their kids got married and their grandchildren were born—and he has stood by them through unspeakable pain, such as suffering and loss.

When his patients are sick, he walks with them. He meets them in their pain and suffering with an authentic desire to help. You will remember from Chapter 2, that's actually the *definition* of compassion. And the manifestation of Dr. Viner's compassion for patients? Going the extra mile.

Going the extra mile for his patients ensures that the care they receive has a characteristic kind of meticulousness, the highest standard. On a Dr. Viner patient, nothing falls through the cracks. He makes certain of it. Every little detail goes under the microscope and is attended to diligently. And quality of care is all about the *details*.

His compassion elevates the quality of care by elevating the expectations for everyone's care of his patients, the whole team. He is legendary for this, and it has left an indelible mark on trainees at Cooper for decades. Essentially, Dr. Viner has taught physicians-in-training a whole new level of what it means to care.

But, you do not have to know a patient for decades in order to care enough to go the extra mile and make a difference. Sometimes, those bonds can be built in just a matter of minutes, and in the back of an ambulance of all places.

Consider this story:

A previously healthy young man in his mid-thirties, Joe, was brought to the emergency department by ambulance because he passed out cold while at work. He just collapsed with no warning. When paramedics arrived, Joe's vital signs were okay, but he was out of it. They put him on a stretcher, slapped an oxygen mask on his face, and loaded him in the ambulance.

When the ambulance began to pull away from the scene, Joe was now fully awake with normal mental status. He sat up and asked, "What happened?" He recalled having a dull headache during his shift, but that was all he remembered. Then he woke up in the back of an ambulance.

But then Joe went into panic mode. He wanted out of the ambulance immediately, saying that he had to get back to work. But Layla, the paramedic in the back of the ambulance, was able to calm him down and recognize that he needed medical attention. That's when a much unexpected compassion connection happened.

Joe explained the reason for his panic to Layla: He had been out of work for a number of months, almost a year, until this current job came around just two weeks ago. Through a very fortunate set of circumstances—a friend of a friend—he landed a job as a forklift operator, and (thankfully) it was the best paying job he ever had.

He needed the money desperately. He and his wife had a two-year-old at home and, unexpectedly, they had just learned she was pregnant again. They were almost evicted from their apartment the prior month, until a family member floated them a last-minute loan to pay the rent.

His wife was in school full-time, so Joe *had* to find work. He said he had been so stressed out. And then he got the call about this job—it was a godsend and just in the nick of time. He broke down in tears in the back of that ambulance, terrified that his boss who barely knew him yet would think he was flaky if he missed work so soon after starting the job and would want to let him go.

Layla knew *exactly* how he felt. She had been there before—living paycheck to paycheck, barely making ends meet. Before landing this steady (not to mention rewarding) paramedic job two years ago, she was unemployed herself…a single mom with two kids to care for. She had felt his stress and fear.

But healthy people in their mid-thirties don't just pass out for no reason, so she tried to convince Joe that he had to let her take him to the hospital. What finally convinced him was when she said, "You won't be of any use to your family if you end up dead." Layla smiled at him warmly and held his hand so he would not be afraid as she said, "C'mon, let's get you checked out." He agreed, so off to the hospital they went.

On arrival to the emergency department, Layla said her goodbyes, took his hand once more, and let him know that she wished the best for him. Then she left on another ambulance call. The emergency department team put him in an exam room and the evaluation began:

Vital signs: normal
Chief complaint: None (He was asymptomatic now…"I feel fine.")
History: "I think I blacked out." (That's what Layla told him.)
Past medical history: None
Physical exam: Normal
Electrocardiogram (heart tracing): Normal
Chest x-ray: Normal
CT scan of the brain: Normal

The emergency physician was perplexed. Totally stumped. What would make this young man suddenly collapse and go unconscious? Everything in his history was unrevealing and all of his tests were coming back normal so far.

That's when Joe started back with the panic. He *had* to get released, to get back to work. "Please tell my boss everything is totally fine if he calls," Joe urged. That's when Layla showed up…again. She was out on another ambulance call and could not get Joe out of her head. She knew the fear and anxiety he was going through, and even though she just met him, she was very worried about him.

Why did she come back? One thing was bugging her. In thinking about his case some more, she thought it was sort of striking that Joe started to recover his mental status as soon as they put him in the back of the ambulance...like immediately. It was as if getting him out of the warehouse where they found him had made a huge difference. He had been operating a forklift in there.

Layla said to the emergency physician, "I think you should check the carbon monoxide level in his blood."

The nurses gasped and almost started laughing; did the paramedic really just say that to our doc? Now, there are a few things you should know about the emergency department in this story: It's a very busy urban academic trauma center that has an impressive reputation. Their emergency team knows exactly what they are doing, and they don't like being told their business...by anyone.

Let's just say that it is unusual in this emergency department for a paramedic to talk with the attending physicians, let alone tell them what to do. And let's just say that in this emergency department if that did happen it would be unusual for the attending physicians to listen.

But this physician decided to take a different approach. After all, he did not have a good explanation for the patient's blackout, so he was willing to listen to suggestions. And he had not considered carbon monoxide. Also, in his more than ten years of working in that emergency department, he had never seen a paramedic care so much about a patient's well-being that she would come back specifically for the purpose of checking on a patient. That was special care. So, the physician agreed to do the test.

There was definitely some eye rolling from the nurses when the physician ordered the test. And then the result came in...

The nurse and the physician just stared at each other in disbelief. They repeated the blood test, thinking it must be a lab error, and got the same result. His carbon monoxide level was through the roof. It was more than *ten times* higher than the upper limit of the normal range for carbon monoxide level in the blood. It was a wonder that Joe was alive at all, let alone awake and talking.

A level that high is such an emergency that they immediately started a special treatment called hyperbaric oxygen therapy to drive down the carbon monoxide level. Even though Joe survived the initial event in the workplace, he still could have suffered severe long-term side effects of a carbon monoxide level that high. The special care from the paramedic—going the extra mile for a patient—made all the difference.

The physician went to thank Layla, but she was gone. But the story does not end here. Since the accident happened at work, the hospital toxicologist immediately called local authorities to check the warehouse to determine if others were at risk. When they arrived, the carbon monoxide meter read "error." They could not even get a reading. That's because the number—the carbon monoxide level in the air—was too high. They had to open up all the windows and doors to ventilate the area for quite some time before the meter would actually register a number. It was off the charts.

Somehow, carbon monoxide was spilling unchecked throughout the warehouse. But here's the most striking part: at the time that the authorities arrived to measure the carbon monoxide level, there were actually several people working in the warehouse who did not (yet) start to show symptoms.

If it hadn't been for Layla, a paramedic that cared enough to go the extra mile for a patient and come back to the emergency department with her revelation, *many people* could have died in that warehouse that night. And, in some sense, Layla's special care had a major impact on the physician, too. How, you ask?

Imagine being that physician at home later that night after he completed his shift and was sitting down to catch the local news headlines on television. What if he heard then that multiple people died from carbon monoxide exposure in a warehouse?

The news reporter would have discovered that one of the employees was rushed to the emergency department earlier in the day, but that no one at the hospital put "two and two together" to identify that the employee was suffering from carbon monoxide poisoning and then check everyone else who was working in the warehouse that day.

To this day, that physician swears that if they had missed that in the emergency department, and people died because of it, he would have been so devastated by his failure that he would have had to quit practicing medicine. He would have felt responsible, and there would be no way to recover from that kind of guilt.

Never underestimate the power of going the extra mile for a patient. The ripple effects from this one act of compassionate care by Layla truly changed multiple lives.

CHAPTER 7:
Compassion Drives Revenue and Cuts Costs

"Show me the money."

—Rod Tidwell

You've seen the evidence that compassion can dramatically improve the quality of clinical outcomes. And yet, some may still be skeptical that compassionate care will ever truly become the new standard of care. After all, it's really finance that drives change within the health care industry, right?

Anything that is to become widely adopted needs to make good financial sense. No matter how strongly one might feel about the value of compassion from a moral standpoint, the health care industry will only see impetus for meaningful change if the dollars also add up.

So, the next question is: Does the evidence show that compassion can make a difference when it comes to financial outcomes? The answer is an unequivocal *yes*. Compassion actually drives higher revenue and reduces cost for health systems and providers. The potential benefit is huge, when you consider the scope of the cost problem.

We're Drowning in Health Care Costs

While it's no surprise to any of us that health care is expensive, let's take a quick look at some of the specific financial challenges the industry faces so we can fully grasp what we're up against here. Then you'll understand why the potential for compassionate care to "move the needle" on health care costs is such an important topic.

If you were a person who had lived your whole life in a single town—someone who still took your kids to the very same pediatrician's office you visited as a child—you would likely be struck by two things on a visit today, if you could compare it side-by-side to your visits as a child.

First, you might feel comforted by how some things have remained the same. The office where your pediatrician practiced over the last twenty or thirty years might look very much the same, with the very same art on the wall and those slightly uncomfortable seats in the waiting room. You might smile as you watched children reading those familiar issues of *Highlights* magazine in the waiting room, just as you once did.

But you know what would seem quite different? You wouldn't see a lot of people writing personal checks and exchanging money as they checked in or out of the doctor's office. Nope.

You would also see a lot more staff behind the front desk than you remember from back in the day. What do all those new people do? They manage the huge tangle of insurance pre-authorizations and the bureaucracy of reimbursement that defines the U.S. health care system today.

The practice of caring for patients has not changed much over the years, but the *business* of caring for patients has changed dramatically. And that business is incredibly complex and growing.

Typically, something that's growing means it's becoming more profitable, but that is not necessarily true in health care. There are so many stakeholders and so many aspects of practice administration that, while overall spending is increasing at an alarming rate, some parts of the health care system are doing better, and others are not.[255, 256]

Just as in the case of the pediatrician's office described above, when physician offices—particularly in primary care—add more staff, they are responding to an increased administrative burden in order to collect revenue that does not always bring in more profit.

The administrative costs of physician practices have grown sharply over time.[257] A study from ten years ago showed how—even then—efforts around billing and insurance were eating away at 14 percent of physician office revenue. That same study also showed that 27 percent of office operating revenue was already going towards other administrative overhead.[258] Again, that was more than ten years ago. Things have not improved since then.

In reality, all those new people in that pediatrician's office are just hemorrhage control. Their goal is just to stop the bleeding of lost revenue. And the end result of their efforts is that the practice will likely be stagnant or declining in profitability, compared to the previous year.

It's not just outpatient offices that have been forced to add administrative costs to deal with the complexity of the health care system either. It's all across the healthcare industry. According to a Kaiser Family Foundation analysis of national health expenditure data from the Centers for Medicare & Medicaid Services, between 1970 and 2016, the percentage of health care costs attributable to administration more than *doubled*.[259]

That can be difficult to appreciate, though—what "doubling" means for a problem of this scope. So, let's bring a little perspective to the size of the U.S. health care system in terms of cost and money, courtesy of Steven Brill.

Brill is a lawyer, journalist, and founder of the television channel CourtTV, the monthly law magazine *The American Lawyer*, and the news reliability service *NewsGuard.*[260] In their March 4, 2013 issue, *Time* magazine, for the first time in its history, dedicated an entire feature section to a single article: Brill's piece entitled "Bitter Pill: Why Medical Bills Are Killing Us."[261]

In the report, Brill tackles the complex, and often absurd, pricing schema that has developed within the U.S. health care system. However, it is his overview of the scale of the U.S. health care system that serves our purpose here:

> *"According to one of a series of exhaustive studies done by the McKinsey & Co. consulting firm, we spend more on health care than the next 10 biggest spenders combined: Japan, Germany, France, China, the U.K., Italy, Canada, Brazil, Spain, and Australia. We may be shocked at the $60 billion price tag for cleaning up after Hurricane Sandy. We spent almost that much last week on health care. We spend more every year on artificial knees and hips than what Hollywood collects at the box office. We spend two or three times that much on durable medical devices like canes and wheelchairs, in part because a heavily lobbied Congress forces Medicare to pay 25% to 75% more for this equipment than it would cost at Walmart."*[261]

So yes, costs are seriously high…and still getting higher.

The U.S. spent 17.9 percent of the gross domestic product (GDP) on health care in 2016—that is $3.3 trillion, or $10,348 per person. It is projected to grow to $5.7 trillion by 2026 and, since health spending is expected to grow faster than GDP per year, the health share of GDP is expected to grow from 17.9 to 19.7 percent by 2026.[262]

This growth in spending is driven by a number of factors, but an interesting one to note that is a change from prior decades is the so-called "Silver Tsunami." That refers to the ten thousand baby boomers that turn 65 years old every day and, therefore, move from private insurance to government insurance (Medicare).[263] That's why Medicare is expected to grow in spending 7.4 percent each year until 2026.[262]

> **Medicare is expected to grow in spending 7.4 percent each year until 2026.**

There is a similar situation that is also challenging state Medicaid programs as it struggles to limit the growth of costs. While Medicare covers those over age 65 (as well as the disabled), Medicaid covers individuals below a designated poverty level. Medicaid is expected to grow at 5.8 percent per year through 2026. The primary driver here is spending per enrollee (rather than enrollee growth).[262]

As you might imagine, the politics surrounding Medicare and Medicaid are intense. Meaningful efforts for change—those that would impact the elderly, the disabled, and the poor—make major overhauls of these programs somewhat unlikely. Therefore, program costs will continue to gallop upward.

Spending is rising throughout the health care system, and since so much of the private health insurance in the U.S. is tied to employment, it is causing employers—and consumers, too—to buckle under the pressure of being asked to absorb more and more of the health care tab. Measures that can help control costs, without cutting access or hurting quality, would likely be welcomed by all stakeholders.

Health care costs have been growing for decades. While we are used to inflation as we look at costs over a timeline, the cost curve for health care is much steeper than it is for other items.[256]

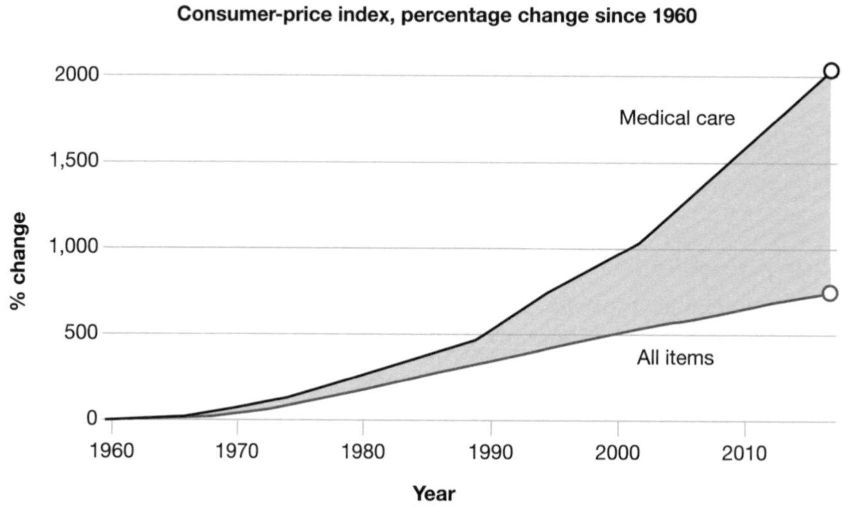

Figure 7.1: Rise in Health Care Costs Relative to Other Goods and Services (1960-2017). Health care costs are not only growing faster than all other costs in the economy, but they are outpacing them at an alarming rate.
Source Labor Department
(Walker 2018)

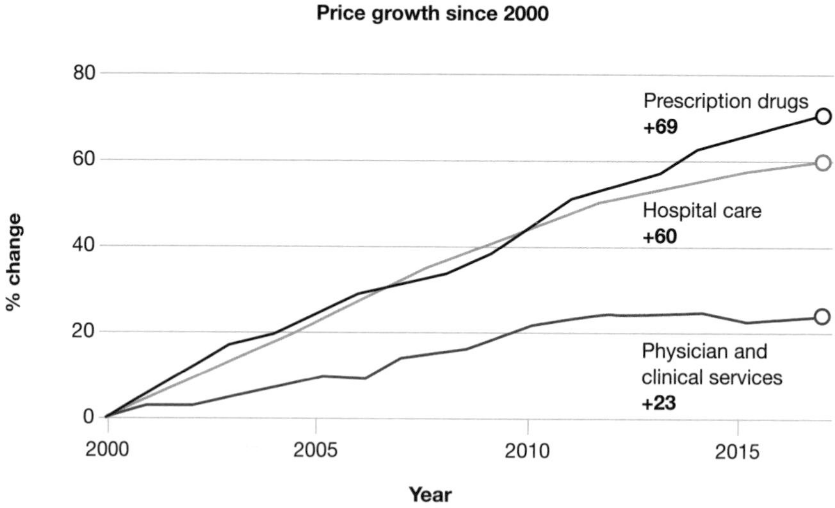

Figure 7.2: Components of Rising Health Care Costs (2000-2016). The sharpest rise in health care costs is seen in prescription drugs and hospital care.
Source Centers for Medicare and Medicaid Services
(Walker 2018)

Let's put this into perspective. If the costs of all other goods had grown as quickly as health care costs since 1945, a gallon of milk today would cost $48! If that doesn't make the point clear enough, let's complete the breakfast analogy: You would need to shell out (no pun intended) $55 for a dozen eggs and $134 for a dozen oranges.[264] That's a pretty crazy cost escalation.

So why has there not been more public outcry or outrage? The answer is that, even though we each feel our own medical pain acutely, very few of us actually feel much of our own pain from medical bills. We may pay co-pays or fill out paperwork, but several factors insulate us from feeling the full force of the rising costs.

First, according to the Congressional Budget Office, as of 2016, almost 92 percent of Americans have some form of health insurance. So, while there may be a rise in premiums, the insurance model helps absorb and redistribute a portion of the cost burden. Secondly, and perhaps more importantly, health insurance does not pass on rising costs to individuals in the same way that individuals feel rising costs with consumer goods and services.

The government regulates what individuals actually pay, when it comes to the 45 percent of Americans that have some form of government insurance (i.e., Medicare, Medicaid, or military). The 48 percent of Americans that have employer-sponsored insurance do see some costs passed along, but often employers absorb the majority of a rise in premiums to remain competitive for workers in the marketplace.[265, 266]

Even the 6 percent of Americans that get insurance through the individual exchanges mandated by the Affordable Care Act are eligible for subsidies relative to their ability to pay. So they, too, are insulated from portions of rising costs.

However, this pattern of accelerating costs (and subsequent insulation from them) cannot be sustained indefinitely. Between 1999 and 2009, the average

American saw a 38 percent increase in salary, as health care premiums increased by a whopping 131 percent![267]

That means that either employers are absorbing those costs, they are being passed on to employees, or some combination of the two. Of course, if employers are absorbing the rising costs, this affects their ability to raise wages and salaries, so workers are being negatively impacted in an important way, whether they realize it or not.

Health Care Costs Are Rising Faster than Revenue

If the above scenario isn't worrisome enough, consider this: Expense growth is outpacing revenue growth for most American health systems (and many health care providers) today. That's the reason why Moody's Investor Service, the bond credit rating agency, downgraded the whole health care sector from stable to negative in 2018.

> Expense growth is outpacing revenue growth for most American health systems.

When analysts looked at the combination of the industry's rising pharmaceutical, medical supply, and labor costs (the steep curve in Figure 7.1) next to lackluster volumes, the future for the health care industry just didn't inspire confidence (despite overall growth in spending).[256]

Why is revenue for organizations that provide health care diminishing? For one thing, people are putting off expensive procedures. For another, payers—who are looking to cut costs—are increasingly cutting their reimbursement to health systems for services rendered.

At the same time, there is currently a shift in medical care from more costly settings (such as in the hospital) to less costly settings (such as an outpatient site) as technology and the advancement of medical knowledge about the safe practice in outpatient settings continues to improve.

It's also worth noting that 60 percent of Moody's downgrades went to smaller hospitals and health systems.[268] That's because analysts know it's easier for larger systems to absorb losses from a lower performing facility through a more profitable one. They can better offset any losses without a threat to the whole enterprise.

Small rural hospitals obviously don't have that advantage, and they're in serious trouble. In fact, in 2016, 50 percent of Pennsylvania's rural hospitals operated at a net loss (compared to 29 percent of hospitals overall).[268] These are also hospitals that have disproportionately large Medicare and Medicaid patient populations, so they get reimbursed at a lower rate than they would through commercial payers.

> When it comes to cost, the health care industry is teetering dangerously at the edge of a precipice. You might even call it a *tipping point*.

Here's why: In 2016, for the first time, costs eclipsed revenues in a major way. Sure, in the past, there were some lean years for the industry. There were even a few years when costs were a bit higher than revenue for the industry as a whole. But now the gap is widening like never before.[269] There's no sign of the cost escalation slowing down anytime soon.

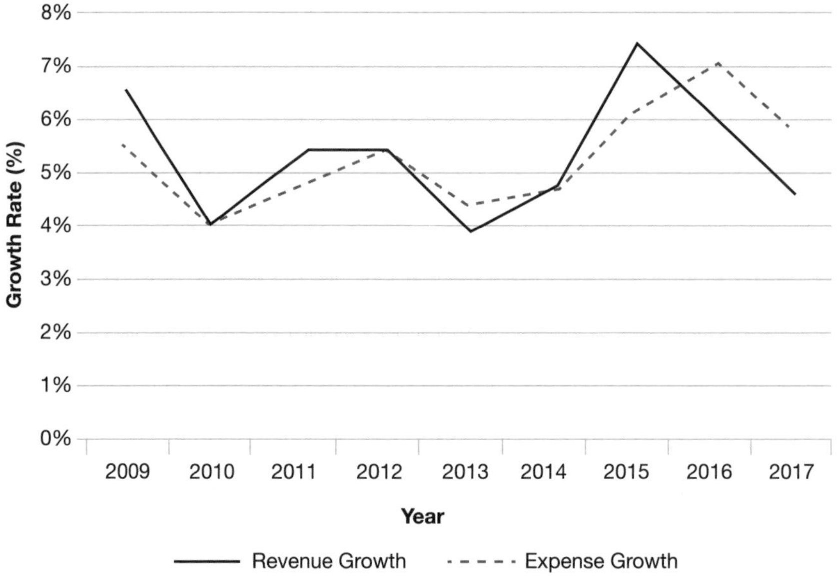

Figure 7.3: Revenue and Expense Growth Rates (Median) For Non-Profit Hospitals in the U.S. (2009-2017). Between 2015 and 2016 costs for non-profit hospitals began to rise faster than revenue, and eclipsed the growth in revenue in 2016 for the first time. The growth in expenses was a full 1% higher than growth in revenue in both 2016 and 2017. This means that the gap between cost and revenue in the health care industry is increasing. Figure prepared by Kevin O'Leary, Cooper University Health Care.

In health care, there is a saying that is repeated quite often: "No margin, no mission." It refers to the noble intent of many health systems to serve patients, particularly underserved populations, and the importance of money to succeed at it. Put simply, the only way to keep the doors open to serve patients is for revenue to outpace costs. The math is unavoidable. Otherwise, there is no way to pay the bills and keep the lights on.

So the healthcare financial situation is dire and, frankly, depressing. But do you know what can make a meaningful difference in reversing this situation for health systems? Take a guess.

That's right. *Compassion*. How? Because it actually drives revenue *and* reduces costs.

Let's first take a look at revenue. Compassion not only improves clinical quality, motivates better patient self-care, and confers all the other benefits discussed so far, but it actually drives revenue in health care organizations that excel in compassionate care.

It won't make the total revenue "pie" for the industry any larger. Rather, it will increase the piece of the pie for organizations that consistently use it. And why would that be?

Patient Experience Drives Business

The term "patient experience" (also sometimes called "patient satisfaction") encompasses the range of interactions that patients have with the health care system, as rated by the patient. It includes several aspects of health care delivery that patients value highly when they seek and receive care, such as good communication with health care providers.[270] In recent decades, hospitals and other types of health care organizations have conducted surveys to assess this. Quite frankly, the surveys have not been that popular among those that deliver care.

Physicians—and staff, too—have sometimes balked at being rated on things like how responsive or timely they were. When patients ding them for poor performance, they can sometimes feel resentful because they don't always see those things as under their control or related to the quality of the clinical care they have provided.

For example, a surgeon doesn't just want to be judged on how well they explained instructions at the time of a patient's discharge from the hospital; the surgeon would rather be judged on the complex factors that were carefully navigated in the operating room to save the patient's life…while the person filing out the survey was unconscious. Some physicians and nurses also worry that patients will rate them poorly if they refuse unreasonable requests (such as pain medications or antibiotics when they're not clinically warranted).

Dr. Zubin Damania, also known as "ZDoggMD" within the medical community for his viral comedy sketches and parodies, captures this conflict adeptly in one of his videos.[271] In the video, his character, Doc Vader, who often models poor behavior, suggests that the survey should only have one question: "Did you die?" Because if the patient is still alive, the doctor should receive a perfect score on the survey.[272] (Along the same lines, you may have seen a nurse, during non-work hours, wearing a t-shirt that proudly proclaims, "I'm a nurse. My job is to save your butt, not kiss it.")

But think about this a moment. Isn't it sort of crazy that medicine hasn't always taken an interest in asking patients what they think about the care we provide? In most other aspects of our lives, we expect to be asked for customer service feedback on purchases we make and services we use. But *not* when it comes to health care, arguably one of the most critical services we will ever purchase?

ZDoggMD's Doc Vader suggests that if the patient isn't happy, he can just go somewhere else.[272] And that, in fact, is exactly what patients do.

So while critical feedback from patient surveys may upset some health care providers, and may not be a true proxy of quality, it is insight into how patients feel about the care that is provided. No matter how physicians and nurses feel about it, patients will make decisions based on how they are treated, and the payers—including the federal government—want to know that the care they are paying for includes valuable aspects of customer service.

In any case, back in 2006, the federal government rolled out a mandated and standardized patient experience survey for hospitals, the Hospital Consumer Assessment of Healthcare Providers and Systems (HCAHPS). Its 32 questions ask patients about everything from how well nurses and doctors communicated, to how clean the room was, and how well staff explained medications and discharge instructions.

Since then, the HCAHPS survey has also been adapted so patients can rate a whole range of health care organizations—everything from outpatient office practices and emergency departments to dialysis centers and hospice care. The results on those surveys are an important determinant of how well a health care organization is reimbursed for the care they provide.

> **Hospitals that are rated highly on their patient experience scores are also higher performing hospitals financially.**

But let's stick with the hospital example specifically in our examination of patient experience here. It turns out that hospitals that are rated highly on their patient experience scores are also higher performing hospitals financially. That's probably not surprising when you lay it out. It's kind of a "duh" moment, isn't it?

Happy customers drive business in all industries, and health care is no different. That's why we get so many requests to rate the businesses we use—so that other potential customers can read about how happy we were (or not) with the service.

So yes, happy customers drive business and revenue in health care. In fact, a Deloitte study showed that hospitals rated by patients as "excellent" on the survey earned (average net patient revenue, per adjusted patient day) 127 percent of what hospitals that were rated as "low" earned.[273]

The costs were also higher for high-performing hospitals, but this was outpaced by the revenue increase. Another way of explaining the higher associated costs might be that hospitals whose patients rate them highly also tend to have more revenue to invest back into the patient experience.

In a similar vein, hospitals with higher reported patient experience are also more profitable; their revenue exceeds their costs by a higher amount. Those that were rated "excellent" outperformed low performers with a margin of 4.7 percent, on average, compared to just 1.8 percent.[273]

To people who don't study health care financials for a living, that 2.9 percent difference might not sound like much money. But for many U.S. hospitals, it could be the difference between seeing patients or shuttering the place.

So how does compassion for patients factor in? One Virginia Commonwealth University study of 269 hospitals found a direct link to compassion with respect to profitability: It was all about the employees.[274] Researchers found that hospitals with a "compassion culture"—they rewarded employees who practiced compassion and even supported struggling employees with pastoral care—were more likely to be rated higher by patients, and patients were more likely to recommend the hospital to others. These compassion practices translated directly to top ratings by patients on the federal HCAHPS survey mentioned above.

Compassion creates "patient-centeredness."

One of the reasons why a compassion culture translates into delivering top patient ratings is because compassion creates "patient-centeredness."[274] When an organization encourages its employees to detect and respond to suffering, they put the patient at the very center of everyone's care, and patients can sense it. Rather than feeling that they are just one more body being shuttled into and out of the system, they feel "seen as a person" and valued.

Hospitals that recognize the value of this approach are intentional in creating a workplace culture of compassion. They understand that health care workers experience suffering, too, and actively work to address and heal those effects. For instance, Cleveland Clinic has employed a practice called "Code Lavender."[275] They deploy a team to support employees who need emotional support after a tragic event occurs (like an unexpected patient death) or a series of especially stressful events in the workplace.[276] By demonstrating compassion for employees, they prime them to care for patients with the same sensitivity because they are more engaged and invested in the organization.[274]

This all has important implications for an organization's financial health because a positive patient experience gets rewarded by payments from the federal government. One reason that hospitals delivering a better patient experience are more profitable is because CMS actually reimburses hospitals that perform better on the survey at a higher rate through its Medicare value-based purchasing (VBP) structure.[277]

But the Deloitte survey also suggests that this tendency to perform better financially goes deeper than just the bump in reimbursement or increase in volume. In fact, when the researchers looked at the correlation between hospital financial performance and a variety of factors, they found that Medicare VBP incentives accounted for just seven percent of the association between patient experience and strong financial performance.[273]

Hospitals and health systems can increase their margin, the difference between their revenue and expenses, if they are able to reduce costs. In a study that analyzed cost data for three thousand U.S. hospitals, researchers found that better patient experience in the hospital was associated with lower health care spending per episode of care.[278] In fact, there was a 5.6 percent difference in spending between the hospitals with the lowest and highest patient experience ratings. The research adjusted the analysis for complexity of care and socioeconomic status of those hospital patient populations, so we can be confident in these results.

But let's consider the results from the Deloitte study again for a moment. Do you know what they found mattered most, when they considered all the factors that could account for stronger financial performance based on patient experience survey ratings? It was the nurse-patient relationship.[273] Communication with nurses is one of the things measured on the HCAHPS survey instrument. That matters to patients. Again, the results are not surprising, right?

One of the key ingredients to communicating effectively with patients is, of course, the ability to genuinely express compassion. Health care providers are frequently surprised that when patients are surveyed, time and again, they say that they value their doctors' interpersonal skills even more than any of the items on their résumé.

Patients Want Compassionate Care

In one Harris Poll, published in *The Wall Street Journal*, that asked people what they believed were the most important qualities in a physician, 85 percent of people said "treating me with dignity and respect," 84 percent said "listening carefully and being easy to talk to," and 81 percent said "truly caring about me." In comparison, the proportion of patients who said that the physician being trained at one of the best medical schools was important was just 27 percent.[279] So *three times* the number of patients value human connection and caring from their physician more than the prestige of the institution where the physician was trained.

> Three times the number of patients value human connection and caring from their physician more than the prestige of the institution where the physician was trained.

Just a little over *half*—58 percent—agreed that having "a lot of experience treating patients with your medical condition" was extremely important![279]

Moreover, 14 percent of respondents who said they had changed doctors in the past five years said that was because the doctor "didn't listen carefully."[279]

That's because what people really want from health care goes to the very core of the doctor-patient relationship. Compassion is at the very top of that list.

Consider the results from one "man on the street" study. Researchers from George Washington University asked random adults—people in coffee shops, senior centers, community centers, and transportation stops—what they most wanted from health care and also what they thought could be done to most improve health care.[280] They asked them to recall a positive and negative experience with health care and to explain the factors that made it such.

Just like in *The Wall Street Journal* report, the top three suggestions for improving health care were: more doctors who listen (85 percent), doctors who are caring and compassionate (71 percent), and doctors who explain well (69 percent). The doctor-patient relationship was at the very heart of their answers.

Conversely, only 22 percent of people indicated "ensuring doctors disclose financial conflicts of interest." And only four percent said, "having a doctor of the same language" is important. Not just that, it's also 17 to 20 times more important to patients in this study that their doctor listens and is compassionate than that their doctor even speaks their native language.

> People's perceptions of health care are all about relationships.

Patients clearly value a doctor who listens, who is caring and compassionate, and who explains well. Note that when people are asked about their health care experiences, they speak about the *interaction* between themselves and their doctors. People's perceptions of health care are all about relationships.

Just listen to some of the things that patients in this study shared about their experiences below.[280] Take a moment to notice the difference between negative and positive experiences:

On having a doctor who listens:

"I have a problem with my M.D. He sends me off to lots of specialists and to get tests before he even listens to everything I have to say. It seems like he doesn't even listen to what my whole problem is. He could maybe solve it himself."

"My doctor listens to everything about me—how my medical problem affects me as a person, daily life, emotions, my family, etc."

On having a doctor who is caring and compassionate:

"I really didn't like this one doctor. He didn't even look at my face. He kept walking. I felt discriminated against. Maybe he didn't talk to me because my English isn't so fluent and I'm old. He didn't care."

"I want doctors to have compassion and show my loved one that they care about them as a human being, not just another case to solve."

On having a doctor who explains well:

"I don't like my own doctor. I go in for a sore throat and she tells me I'm fine. She trivialized my complaints. She doesn't share her thought process."

"I love my doctor...She translates things so that a normal person like me and you can understand them."

The results of online consumer research studies corroborate the results of this "man on the street" study. When the ratings companies Healthgrades and Medical Group Management Association partnered to study seven million online patient reviews of their health care providers, they found that more than half of patients wanted compassion and bedside manner from their doctors.[281]

That's a big deal since one online marketing company's survey showed that 84 percent of patients said they consult online reviews before selecting a provider.[281] Several online review sites, such as Healthgrades, are now partnering with health systems to allow patients to schedule appointments with a physician—right from the review website. Think about it like this: It's just like how you can call a retail store or restaurant from Yelp or Google on a smartphone without having to go to the official website for the business you wish to call.

The report even pointed out that "...health care consumers view health care first and foremost as a personal interaction and not just a medical transaction." Actually 52 percent of respondents' online comments mention words like "compassion," "comfort," "patience," "personality" or "bedside manner."[281]

> **Health care consumers view health care first and foremost as a personal interaction and not just a medical transaction.**

Online reviews from patients consistently focus on—in both negative and positive terms—how their doctor made them feel, if the doctor listened, and if the doctor and the staff were friendly. Perhaps most importantly, the study authors noted, "this new analysis reflects a patient population that doesn't just want to *see* a doctor; they want to be *seen*."[281]

Compassion is a vital driver of patient experience. In one study from Harvard Medical School that examined patient satisfaction with providers, researchers asked 112 new patients to complete a survey that examined everything from outcomes and functional recovery to wait times and visit duration.[282]

There was no difference between the satisfied and the dissatisfied patients when it came to waiting time in the office or lag time from calling to getting an appointment date. However, after controlling for potential cofounding effects, they found that it was compassion that accounted for fully 65 percent of the variation in how patients rated their satisfaction with their health care provider.[282]

> **Compassion accounted for 65 percent of the variation in how patients rated their satisfaction with their health care provider.**

Numerous other studies have linked compassion to patient experience. In one of these studies, researchers surveyed primary care patients and found that patients who said they were more satisfied on the survey were highly likely to rate their physicians as more compassionate, and those patients were also very likely to recommend that physician to family and friends.[283]

Another way to find out what qualities patients want in a physician is to ask them which physicians they like best and then watch those patients' interactions with the well-liked physicians. What if researchers could review these interactions—just like professional football coaches review game day tapes—to figure out how to get better? What would that show?

That's just what they did in a University of New Mexico study in the late 1970s: Researchers observed the behavior of internal medicine resident physicians with their patients through a one-way mirror. Afterwards, patients were asked to rate their satisfaction with their physician on an eight-item survey.[284]

The findings: The patients who said their physicians were especially courteous and better communicators were more satisfied. Researchers also found that when physicians were perceived as compassionate, patients were more likely to rate that physician as enjoying his or her work. On a side note, they found no correlation between how a physician looked and patient satisfaction—even among physicians that researchers identified as dressing "counter culture."[284]

For a study done in the 1970s, this means that even if physicians dressed with wide bell bottoms and flowered, wide lapel shirts/blouses, it didn't matter to patients of any age…as long as the doctor was compassionate. (This is perhaps notable because in health care organizations there is likely more time spent in new employee orientations on the dress code policy then there is on treating patients with compassion!)

Patients Would Pay More for Compassion

In 2013, Dignity Health, one of the top five largest health systems in the U.S., released findings from a survey that showed when choosing a health care provider, 87 percent of Americans feel kindness is more important than any other consideration…even wait time, how far the provider is from their home, or cost.[20] This nationwide email and online survey study included responses from 1,400 U.S. adults. We can have confidence in the reliability and accuracy of these findings because the survey included a rigorous methodology (including quotas for demographics of respondent) to ensure a nationally representative sample.

64 percent of people in the survey said they had experienced unkindness in a health care setting where caregivers failed to connect personally, were rude, or didn't listen.

Fully 64 percent of people in the survey said they had experienced unkindness in a health care setting where caregivers failed to connect personally, were rude, or didn't listen.[20] Caring is the most important thing to patients and yet, the majority of people have not consistently received it during their interactions with physicians, nurses, and staff.

Nearly three-quarters of patients in the survey said they would pay more for a physician who placed an emphasis on kindness. Nine out of ten said they would feel like switching health care providers if they were unkind.[20]

This idea that patients would actually pay for compassion is also supported by a survey that specifically studied the role of compassion in medicine.[285] The research shows that patients would pay more for compassionate care.

Eighty-five percent of patients said compassion was very important to them for their satisfaction with health care providers and that they would choose compassion over pricing when choosing a doctor. For the purpose of comparison, just 48 percent of patients said wait time was very important, and only 31 percent said cost was very important.[285]

Patients Perceive Compassionate Physicians to Be More Competent

Patients may be willing to pay more for compassion, and they may rate compassion as more important than other factors, but they still want to know that their physician is skilled. Does compassion play a role in how patients view the competency of a provider?

The data say *yes*.

You've already seen some of this data back in Chapter 6, in our discussion of the link between compassion and clinical competence. For example, you saw a study of medical students that found both verbal and non-verbal expressions of compassion contributed to the perception of clinical competence by the supervising physician evaluators as well as the patients.[250]

In that study, researchers asked independent observers to rate the compassion of students participating in the study. Then, they asked independent observers to judge their clinical competence.

When they compared these ratings, they found that more compassionate students were also perceived to be more clinically skilled. It's important to note that the student ratings of their own compassion were *not* associated with the judgments of clinical competence by the physician evaluators or the independent observer ratings of compassion.

And yet, the more compassionate group outperformed the less compassionate group in ratings of clinical competence by 15 percent.[250] Other studies have confirmed this finding that patients treated with compassionate care are more likely to believe their health care provider knows what they are doing.[252, 284]

> Multiple studies show compassion communicates competence.

Why is this important in our discussion of money? One way to beat a rival for market share and increase an organization's revenue in health care is to grow its reputation as more competent than its competitors. Compassion might just be the tool to use.

As you've seen with other studies on expressions of compassion, it's not just what providers say, but their non-verbal actions that matter as well. In Chapter 6, for example, you learned about a collaborative Harvard-Yale study that tested this relationship between physicians' compassionate non-verbal behavior and patients' perception of their clinical competence.[252] It identified a positive correlation.

To put it bluntly, you are going to have trouble building your practice and generating revenue if your patients do not think you are a competent doctor. How can you make them understand you are more competent? Treat them with more compassion. This is not our opinion; it's what the data show.

Medical Errors Erode Revenue

One of the things threatening the already razor-thin operating margins of many health care organizations is medical errors. Aside from the obvious damage to reputation that can occur from medical errors that become known to the marketplace, medical errors also have direct financial consequences to health systems and providers.

> Increased errors will decrease value-based purchasing and pay-for-performance revenue.

That's a problem: These funding sources are an increasing portion of reimbursement to hospitals and physicians, not only by Medicare, but also by many commercial insurance companies.

Earlier, you saw how the case for compassion falls into two categories: a lack of compassion causes problems and the presence of compassion confers benefits. So let's look next at both cases with respect to medical errors and clinical competence.

Provider burnout, as you may recall, is characterized as emotional exhaustion and the tendency to depersonalize patients (having no personal connection). Burnout has contributed in a big way to the compassion crisis in health care today, so you'll learn more about how to specifically counteract this unfortunate phenomenon soon (Chapter 10).

But for now, take a moment to think about the earlier link we established between depersonalization/emotional exhaustion and a greater incidence of medical errors (Chapter 6). There's a strong correlation between the two. Unfortunately, those errors have direct and widespread financial consequences that extend far beyond the walls of the organizations where those providers practice. They adversely affect the whole U.S. health care system.

According to a 2010 study sponsored by the Society for Actuaries, medical errors cost the U.S. $19.5 billion dollars annually, with $17 billion due to avoidable medical costs attributable to the errors, $1.4 billion due to increased mortality rates, and $1.1 billion due to lost productivity from missed work.[286, 287] But according to recent research, that may actually be a gross *underestimate.*

In a study in the *Journal of Health Care Finance*, researchers consider more recent data that suggest a much higher rate of medical errors. They are also more granular in their calculations, such as accounting for the lost productivity of those that lose their life due to medical errors for up to ten years, rather than just one year (depending on life expectancy)—something that was not done in the earlier study. The new annual U.S. estimate: between $735 billion and $980 billion.[288]

As you've learned, compassionate care means more meticulous care for better clinical outcomes. If an increase in compassionate care could reduce medical errors in such a way that recaptures even a small fraction of that lost revenue, it would be an enormous windfall indeed.

> If compassion moves the needle just a little bit on medical errors, the economic impact could be substantial.

And, as you'll soon see, there are effective ways to counteract burnout to achieve this goal. The take-home point here is that if compassion moves the needle just a little bit, the economic impact could be substantial because of the massive costs that are involved.

Compassionate Physicians Refer Less and Order Fewer Tests

One of the reasons that compassion can make such a meaningful difference to cost cutting is because connecting with patients is associated with lower medical expenditures. That's because it's part of patient-centered care. Compassion is "other-focused."

It's not about the needs of the physician or the nurse or the organization; it's all about the needs of the patient. Patient-centered care is not some vague concept. Studies have determined that the impact of patient-centeredness on quality outcomes can be reliably measured.[289]

So why do compassionate physicians order fewer tests? Let's start with some myth-busting. There is a misperception that the best doctors order lots of tests and refer patients to every possible specialist. The myth goes like this: "My doctor is the best. He orders every test under the sun."

But it's just not true that this is what patients want. A few pages back you read that when patients are asked what they want from doctors, they ask for more caring and personal connection, not necessarily more tests.

But let's see what happens in practice.

In one study from University of California Davis that considered the practice styles of nearly a thousand primary care physicians and the outcomes of their patients, researchers concluded that patients who felt their primary care doctors practiced patient-centered care were less likely to utilize excessive health care services.[290] They also had lower medical bill charges. Median charges per patient were *51% lower* with patient-centered care.

One big reason why was fewer referrals to specialists. That makes good sense, right? If your doctor takes time to listen to your concerns and shows compassion for your suffering, you are more likely to trust the doctor's recommendations. Conversely, if your physician seems distracted, doesn't make eye contact, or generally seems burned out, your confidence in those recommendations might wane. You might be thinking, "Better to get another opinion," as you request a referral to see a specialist.

Or maybe you don't actually verbally ask for a referral, but you transmit your anxiety and uncertainty about what your physician is recommending with lots of non-verbal cues. The physician gets the sense through your fidgeting and hand-wringing that you're not on board with the plan.

So, to pacify you, extra tests or referrals are ordered. Or if the physician does not really care enough to spend time talking with you, he might find it easier to just order the extra tests or refer you to someone else.

> Patients who do not feel a strong personal connection with their physician receive more referrals to specialists and undergo more diagnostic tests.

And that's exactly what researchers in this study concluded. When these primary care patients didn't feel a strong personal connection, they ended up with higher referrals to specialists and more diagnostic tests. They measured specific communication behaviors like eliciting understanding, validating the patient's perspective, and coming to a mutually shared understanding of the problem.[290]

Patient-centered physicians in this study also made an effort to understand what the study authors called the "psychosocial" context of the patients: the combined factors that come together to "know them as a person," as we've discussed. They wanted to understand the things in patients' lives that might derail their recovery or motivate them to work hard to regain their health.[290]

Recall our earlier discussion from Chapter 5—the chapter about patient self-care—on patient "activation." That was the concept where a health care provider successfully engages patients in independently managing their own care when they're not in the doctor's office. Well, this study also measured the ability of the physicians to create just this sort of partnership where patients took ownership and responsibility for their health.

The researchers believe the reason that the patients who received compassionate, patient-centered care had lower health care resource utilization was because the patients trusted their physician, believed he or she had a good understanding of them, and the physician was able to effectively manage both their anxiety and expectations. That's because physicians who demonstrated compassionate, patient-centered care took time to ensure good information exchange, manage uncertainty, and ultimately, better understand the patient.

That's the power of compassion at work.

The patients in the study above who had lower resource use didn't need lots of extra tests to feel confident in their provider's diagnosis and treatment plan. And that's an important benefit of compassion. Unnecessary testing and specialist referrals are expensive for health care organizations and payers.

Another primary care study from the University of Rochester found similar results. First, researchers collected data in two ways: through patient surveys and audio recordings of clinical encounters. Based on those, they scored each physician on his or her patient-centeredness using a validated methodology. Just as in the earlier study, they concluded that those who scored the worst also had patients with higher costs due to higher use of diagnostic tests.[291]

A U.K. study on compassionate, patient-centered primary care published in *BMJ* (formerly known as *The British Medical Journal*) went even further in its conclusion.[292] The authors found that when patients perceive their physician to be patient-centered, they use this as a "marker" for quality care.

> **Primary care patients who had unmet expectations for a personal connection with the physician had 41 percent higher odds of referral to a specialist.**

So when they don't experience compassion, patients tend to be less satisfied and are more likely to be referred to a specialist. In fact, primary care patients who had unmet expectations for a personal connection with the primary care physician had *41 percent higher odds* of referral to a specialist after controlling for patient factors such as anxiety and the type of diagnosis.

In a unique Canadian primary care study, researchers tested the hypothesis that patients who received compassionate, patient-centered care recover more quickly from the symptom that brought them to the doctor, report better health, and have fewer visits, tests, and referrals.[289] They audiotaped each of the office encounters to score them for patient-centered communication, and then the research assistant interviewed the patient in person right after the visit. Finally, they reviewed the patient's chart to assess the amount of follow-up care for the next two months, and conducted a follow-up assessment by telephone.

The results? Compared to patients who did not perceive their care as patient-centered, the patients who perceived their care as patient-centered had significantly lower referrals to specialists. Specifically, the proportion of patients referred to a specialist was 51 percent lower (only 7.9 percent of patients who said their care was patient-centered versus 16.2 percent who said it was not).

Similarly, patients who perceived their care as patient-centered had significantly less diagnostic testing performed. The proportion of patients who underwent diagnostic testing was 40 percent lower (only 14.6 percent in the patient-centered group versus 24.3 percent in the non-patient-centered group).

Upon further testing, the researchers found that the associations between the patient perception of patient-centeredness and fewer referrals and diagnostic tests was mainly driven by the patient's perception that "common ground had been attained." In the subgroup that specifically expressed this perception, the results were even more impressive: The proportion of patients who were referred to specialists was 59 percent lower, while those who underwent diagnostic testing was 84 percent lower.[289]

Some may worry that if physicians seem too attentive to a patient's every worry that they might be unnecessarily racking up costs through more tests and referrals as a result. This study proved just the opposite: Compassionate patient-centered care *reduces* costs!

Compassionate Care Drives Lower Costs through Better Adherence

Earlier, you read about the importance of patient adherence to therapy (Chapter 5), the extent to which patients follow the treatment recommendations from their health care providers. That includes taking medication as prescribed, behavior modification (like losing weight), and following through with scheduled treatments.

Nonadherence—when a patient doesn't do those things—is a huge threat to public health, as discussed. That's because disease proceeds unchecked when patients don't take their medicine as directed or follow through on best practices their doctors recommend. Non-adherence is a complex and multidimensional problem.

But you know what else? This preventable epidemic of unchecked disease results in a massive number of deaths and hospitalizations that have very real and staggering economic costs. As noted earlier, one estimate puts the cost between $100 billion and $300 billion per year in the U.S. alone.[194, 196]

And as you learned, compassion effectively promotes and improves patient adherence. Therefore, some of the $100 to $300 billion is up for grabs as a way to reduce overall costs in healthcare.

There's no need to spend massive amounts of money to develop and bring new drugs to market if patients don't take them. What about using compassion to convince people to take the drugs we already have instead? This simple shift in care has the potential to save billions of dollars.

A Compassion Culture Cuts Employee Absences

Now that you understand how compassion can cut the expense associated with medical errors, overutilization of health care resources, and non-adherence by patients, let's look at another place compassion makes an important difference: with the well-being of those that take care of patients. Earlier, we looked at how a compassionate culture in a hospital translates into more compassion for patients, but what about compassion for everyone who provides that care?

You know how airlines advise that, in the event of an in-flight emergency, parents should put on their own oxygen masks first—before attempting to put on a child's oxygen mask? It's the same kind of phenomenon at work here. If health care organizations want their health care providers and staff to show compassion to patients, the organizations must first demonstrate compassion to the employees.

It's no secret that working in health care can be emotionally exhausting and even sometimes traumatic. If those negative effects are not addressed proactively, people tend to take more sick time and medical leave. Or look for another job that's not so taxing.

In a University of Pennsylvania study of health care workers in 13 long-term care facilities (i.e., "nursing homes"), researchers tested this very hypothesis. They asked everyone—including certified nursing assistants, nurses, social workers, physicians, food service personnel and others—to complete a survey that assessed their perception of the workplace culture in their facility.[293]

Specifically, they used a validated measurement scale to determine if a compassionate culture was present. It's important to understand that they were not asking workers to assess their own compassionate behavior, but rather the behaviors of their coworkers all around them.

What is a compassionate culture exactly? These researchers described it as the way that coworkers helped each other and expressed care for each other... how they were thoughtful about the feelings of their co-workers and shared compassion when things didn't go well for someone, either at work or in their personal lives.

But they weren't only interested in how compassion flowed between two coworkers. They wanted to understand how it flowed in group situations and between supervisors and their direct reports (as well as the degree to which it flowed back to those supervisors).

Here's what they found: The emotional culture of the health care facility had a strong association with how employees treated their patients, the patients' experience, and even patient outcomes. As you might anticipate, employees were not able to effectively show compassion to their patients if they didn't experience it in their work environment themselves.

The emotional culture of the health care facility had a strong association with how employees treated their patients, the patients' experience, and even patient outcomes.

However, in health care facilities where a more compassionate culture was established, there were better employee outcomes: better experience and teamwork, lower emotional exhaustion, and less absenteeism from work. The improved workplace culture for employees even had a positive impact on the nursing home residents: better quality of life, fewer emergency department visits, and better patient and family experience.[293]

This association between a compassionate culture and lower emotional exhaustion among employees is an important finding. One important aspect of emotional exhaustion is when a health care provider loses the ability to feel "compassion satisfaction." Compassion satisfaction is the degree to which a person feels pleasure from efforts to relieve others' suffering.

Doctors who are unable to feel compassion satisfaction due to emotional exhaustion tend to take more sick days and medical leaves of absence. Consider, for example, the findings from a 2013 study of 7,584 physicians.[294] It was a survey study to elicit information about both their professional satisfaction and emotional exhaustion.

Here's what they found: Among physicians who said they had no compassion satisfaction and were experiencing compassion fatigue (emotional exhaustion, depersonalization, and, in this case, also taking on stress from taking care of those that are stressed from being sick) *68 percent* of the physicians had taken a leave of absence due to medical reasons. They also had taken the greatest number of sick days among all the physicians in the study.

It would be easy to blame the pressures of the health care environment for why a culture with a lack of compassion leads to increased workforce issues. However, there are studies across multiple other industries showing similar results:[295]

- 74 percent of employees reported that work is a significant source of stress and one in five has missed work as a result of stress.[296]
- 55 percent of employees reported they were less productive at work as a result of stress.[296]

- 52 percent of employees reported that they have considered or made a decision about their career such as looking for a new job, declining a promotion, or leaving a job, based on workplace stress.[296]
- In 2001, the median number of days away from work as a result of anxiety, stress, and related disorders was 25 days, substantially greater than the median of six days attributable to nonfatal injury and illness.[297]
- Job stress is estimated to cost U.S. industries more than $300 billion a year in absenteeism, turnover, diminished productivity, and medical, legal and insurance costs.[298]

Dr. Emma Seppälä is the science director of Stanford University's Center for Compassion and Altruism Research and Education (CCARE) and the author of the book *The Happiness Track*.[299] She often writes about the benefits of compassion in the business setting.

In an article entitled "Why Compassion in Business Makes Sense," she sums up the most current data in the field in this way:

> *A new field of research is suggesting that when organizations promote an ethic of compassion rather than a culture of stress, they may not only see a happier workplace but also an improved bottom line. Consider the important—but often overlooked—issue of workplace culture...Employees in positive moods are more willing to help peers and to provide customer service on their own accord... In doing so, they boost coworkers' productivity levels and increase coworkers' feeling of social connection, as well as their commitment to the workplace and their levels of engagement with their job. Given the costs of health care, employee turnover, and poor customer service, we can understand how compassion might very well have a positive impact not only on employee health and well-being but also on the overall financial success of a workplace.*[300]

When the work of researchers, such as Dr. Seppälä and her colleagues, on compassion in the workplace is applied to health care—where the intensity of the work and the amount of stress is so high—the results are likely even more dramatic. As a result, the expected economic benefits will likely be magnified as well.

Investing in Physician Well-Being Pays Off

Turnover of staff in any organization is costly, when you consider the direct exit costs as well as the additional costs to recruit and train new hires. There is also the decreased productivity of being short-staffed while seeking a replacement and the loss of morale that goes along with people leaving. Then there are other intangibles, such as the loss of institutional knowledge that is missing in new employees when a veteran employee leaves.

These costs are magnified even further for employees who earn higher salaries, like physicians and nurses. These may include lost revenue (i.e., losing people who bring in revenue) or the recruitment costs of using a professional search firm.

Let's take a closer look where there is the most data on this phenomenon in healthcare: physicians. By now, you understand that physician burnout is expensive. It compromises clinical quality and adds significant costs—through medical leave and sick days—for organizations that employ physicians.

It's a widespread problem. Burnout affects approximately a half million physicians in the U.S. alone.[301, 302] While it's difficult to calculate with precision, a conservative estimate is that the increase in physician turnover that is produced by burnout costs the U.S. health care system approximately *$12 billion* annually.[303] And this is just for physicians.

So it's not just that we have a moral responsibility to care for our physicians in the best interest of patients, but we also have a compelling economic imperative to care for those who provide care.

To that end, some forward-thinking health care organizations are formalizing their efforts to do just that. For example, in a first for an academic medical center, Stanford University hired its first "chief physician wellness officer" in 2017.[304] Dr. Tait Shanafelt, who was hired for the job, is a recognized thought leader and researcher on the topic of physician wellness, having led pioneering work on physician burnout and resiliency at Mayo Clinic.

Later in the same year that Stanford hired him, Shanafelt made a compelling business case for investing in physician well-being in a paper published in *JAMA Internal Medicine*. In it, he detailed the financial toll that burned out physicians take on a health care system. In addition to factoring in hard recruiting costs and lost revenue during onboarding and lost efficiencies, the cost to a health care organization to replace a physician is *two to three times* a physician's annual salary.[305]

Plus, when one member of a care team leaves, that physician puts other members of the care team at higher risk for burnout as they work to pick up the slack due to his or her absence.[305] So there's a potential domino effect to worry about in case other team members also decide to leave.

What makes this even more troublesome is the fact that it's getting harder and harder to replace physicians who leave, since we're already facing a shortage of physicians in many specialties today. The burnout epidemic is dangerous, indeed. In one study led by Shanafelt at the Mayo Clinic, they found that the smallest measureable increase in burnout (i.e., just a one point increase on the burnout scale) increased the likelihood—by *30 to 50 percent*—that a physician would reduce his professional work effort over the next two years.[306]

Cutting back on work seems like a reasonable thing to do when faced with burnout, right? The problem, however, is that the health care system can ill afford fewer physicians. While it's tempting to think you may just need a little extra time to meditate in the woods—to get your groove back—stay tuned for our upcoming discussion of what really works to create resiliency in Chapter 10.

Importantly, it's not just U.S. physicians who are thinking about cutting back because of burnout either. It's everywhere.

For example, in a survey study of emergency physicians in the U.K. National Health Service, researchers found that physicians with less compassion satisfaction (i.e., not experiencing pleasure or satisfaction from relieving patients' suffering) were more likely to complain about patients or colleagues, reduce their quality standards, and even more likely to retire early. (In fact, *59 percent* of physicians with low compassion satisfaction were contemplating early retirement).[241]

Compassion Lowers Malpractice Costs

According to an article published in *Health Affairs*, the annual cost of the U.S. medical liability system, including the cost of defensive medicine, is $56 billion. That doesn't even include the cost of insurance premiums.[307] While it's a hefty price tag, those costs might be worth it if the system is achieving its goals. And yet, there is scant evidence that's true. In fact, it is just the opposite.

In order for malpractice to have occurred, there needs to be a breach of duty to a patient, a deviation from the standard of care, and harm or damage to the patient that has been caused due to that deviation.[308] A poor outcome or damage alone does not equate to malpractice.

Despite how it feels to health care providers, the purpose of the legal system with respect to medicine is not to punish those that commit malpractice. Rather, the purpose of a malpractice lawsuit is to make the patient whole (as if the interaction had not happened) and to incentivize providers to take appropriate precautions against accidental harm.

Does the U.S. system do either of these things well? *No.*

According to a landmark study, the Harvard Medical Practice Study, only 1 in 15 patients who are actually injured due to medical malpractice ever receive any compensation. On the contrary, five out of every six cases that *do* receive compensation have no evidence of malpractice.[309]

These same findings were even reproduced in a second, more recent study looking at the same thing.[310] In other words, the overwhelming majority of acts of negligence never become malpractice claims and, at the same time, the overwhelming majority of malpractice claims have no actual occurrence of malpractice.

This means that patients that are wronged are not getting compensated, and the messages that are being sent to providers about taking precautions are not being heard. As one team of Harvard researchers described it, the malpractice system is "sending as confusing a signal as would our traffic laws if the police regularly gave out more tickets to drivers who go through green lights than to those who go through red lights."[311]

Even with perfect technical expertise or with strict adherence to the standard of care, poor outcomes can occur; that is always a risk in medicine. Poor outcomes alone should not create a malpractice claim that leads to a court case, a settlement or the need to defend anything at all.

However, patients often ask lawyers to file lawsuits based on poor outcomes. This often leads to malpractice claims despite the absence of the very elements that define such a case. That leads to "tickets for green lights," using the traffic analogy from the Harvard study.

So why do patients sue? And what can be done to avoid these lawsuits?

That's right…it's *compassion*. Yet again.

A perceived lack of caring – rather than negligence – is frequently what gets a doctor sued. In one study of plaintiff depositions for malpractice lawsuits that were settled against a large metropolitan medical center, researchers found that, in general, patients and families decided to litigate because they perceived their doctors didn't care.[312]

Specifically, they complained that doctors weren't available, they discounted their concerns, they weren't good at conveying information, and they just didn't seem to understand the patient's or family's perspective. It wasn't the technical part of the medical care; it was the caring part of the medical care.

> A perceived lack of caring – rather than negligence – is frequently what gets a doctor sued.

A study of new mothers' experiences with their obstetricians by researchers from Vanderbilt University uncovered the same finding.[313] They interviewed nearly a thousand new mothers and analyzed the data based on the malpractice history of their obstetricians. They separated the physicians into those that had a large number of malpractice cases in the past (i.e., the "high malpractice" group) and those that had low to no malpractice history in the past.

They wanted to learn about the relationship between malpractice history and the doctor-patient relationship with the obstetrician. Would physicians that got sued more often reveal a different pattern in the way they treated their current patients?

Although none of the women in the study had an active malpractice claim against their obstetrician, researchers were nonetheless struck by the emergence of a clear pattern. Compared to patients of obstetricians with low or no malpractice history, the patients of obstetricians in the high malpractice group complained they felt rushed, didn't receive good explanations about recommended tests, and were often ignored.

In fact, when the patients were asked to share which part of their care had been the least satisfying, the patients of high malpractice obstetricians had a list of complaints twice as long as the patients of obstetricians with low/no malpractice history. At the top of the list of these moms' complaints was poor physician communication.

Remember our earlier discussion about the relationship between compassion and trust? When a health care provider authentically expresses compassion, it's likely that he or she is also making eye contact and giving lots of verbal and non-verbal cues that he cares about the patient. That's what confers trust. The absence of that type of communication creates *distrust*...and those are the patients who sue.

Several studies have suggested that the doctor-patient relationship—or lack of it—is a major determinant, if not the *deciding* determinant, of a patients' overall assessment of their treatment, and, therefore, a major factor in the decision to pursue a malpractice claim.[314, 315, 316, 317, 318, 319]

None of these studies, however, used an experimental design—like a randomized controlled trial, for example—which is the more definitive way to show cause-and-effect in research. But researchers at the University of California San Francisco designed just such a study with obstetric patients (the population of patients most likely to file a lawsuit in the event of an adverse outcome).[320]

Women who had delivered babies within the last six to 12 months were enrolled in the study and were randomly assigned to consider one of four hypothetical scenarios describing interactions between a patient and an obstetrician throughout a patient's pregnancy, labor, and delivery. Essentially, they were asked to imagine themselves in the scenario described, where there were ultimately complications with childbirth, and explain how they would feel.

Multiple different communication behaviors of the physician were described in these scenarios as well as different severities of complications for the baby, some of them quite disabling. One of the questions asked was

"Given what happened in the pregnancy described earlier, I would be likely to file a malpractice claim against the physician (yes/no)."

The findings? In scenarios describing a strong doctor-patient relationship, the participants were more likely to believe that the obstetrician was competent and not at fault for the occurrence of the complications of childbirth. As a result, these women were less likely to express intentions to file a malpractice claim, even in cases where the outcomes for the baby were more severe.

In summary, a take-home message for health care providers: When patients suffer bad outcomes, whether or not you get sued may not be based on how you treated patients (i.e., the technical aspects) but rather how you *took care* of them.

Could Compassion *Increase* Costs?

As stated at the very outset of this book, being both data-driven and open-minded are prerequisites for good science. So in addition to a willingness to accept the hypothesis that compassion might *not* make a difference, there must be a similar willingness to examine the possibility that compassion might cause harm in certain circumstances.

This was a particular possibility when it came to examining the effect of compassion on costs. Would a more compassionate physician with a stronger doctor-patient relationship understand the patient's situation more and, as a result, order more tests and referrals? You've seen that the evidence shows that just the opposite is true.

But then an emergency medicine colleague of ours pointed out a very common scenario—one in which emergency department staff almost universally believe that compassion drives up costs: the homeless patient. It's frequently an individual who comes to the emergency department with no identifiable diagnosis. It's presumed he is there just looking for a warm place to sleep for a while.

This is a very common scenario. In fact, these patients typically return to the emergency department repeatedly, sometimes several times per month. The logic of the emergency department staff is that since federal law mandates that every patient must be seen, these patients know that they will have some amount of time sheltered.[321]

Sometimes nurses and staff are actually reluctant to be kind to these patients. They may be slow in calling them from the waiting room in a timely manner or hesitant to offer them some small amount of hospital food. Their fear is that such kindnesses might send the wrong message…making them more likely to return, even though they do not actually need medical care.

It's not that these nurses and staff are cold, heartless individuals, of course. They're just doing their best to make sure there are beds available in the emergency department when truly sick patients arrive and urgently need them. They don't want anyone to be gaming the system.

The logic is sound here, but the science tells a different story.

In a fascinating randomized controlled trial from the University of Toronto that appeared in the *The Lancet*—one of the most prestigious clinical journals in the world—researchers tested if especially compassionate care for homeless patients in the emergency department would affect their subsequent use of emergency services.[322]

They randomized 133 homeless patients arriving in the emergency department with no identifiable diagnosis into two groups: one group was assigned to receive extra compassionate care from a trained volunteer (a person whose only job was to treat the homeless patients with extra compassion) in addition to usual care from the emergency department staff. The other group was assigned to usual care only. They tested the association between extra compassion and return visits to the emergency department over the next thirty days.

> Extra compassion reduced subsequent emergency department visits by homeless patients by 33 percent.

And what did they find out? *Compared to usual care, randomization to extra compassion reduced subsequent emergency department visits by homeless patients by 33 percent.* These results are based on a randomized trial with a rigorous experimental design. So they are based on science; not a set of beliefs or opinions.

What could be the explanation then for why the homeless patients did not return to the emergency department as often after receiving extra compassion? The authors postulate that perhaps the patients just finally got what they wanted: someone to care.[322]

Shouldn't compassion be the default—rather than the exception—when interacting with patients? When interacting with *anyone*?

There's simply no reason—neither moral nor scientific—whether you're considering the art or the science of compassion, to ignore the profound benefits it confers.

CHAPTER 8:
The Power of 40 Seconds

"Be kind whenever possible. It is always possible."

—Dalai Lama

One reason health care providers don't show compassion is because they're concerned it's going to take time they just don't have. After all, time is money in health care, right?

Time is clearly a crucial factor in the efficiency and the economics of health care. So does it really take a lot more time to show patients compassion?

> Researchers found that 56 percent of physicians believe they do not have time to treat patients with compassion.

As you saw earlier, health care providers frequently feel they're just too busy for compassion. More than half of physicians feel this way, according to one Harvard Medical School study: 56 percent of them, specifically, believed that they *do not have enough time* to treat patients with compassion.[323]

But why are health care providers so frenetically busy these days? For one reason, there is a continuous push for them to see more patients in less time.

This is often a financial pressure, because payments from insurers to health care organizations are generally going down, and the costs of running a health care enterprise keep going up.

Another reason for health care provider "busyness" is what many consider to be the "red tape" of health care. There's been a sharp increase in the demands for documentation of the care that physicians provide.

To avoid fines or losses in revenue, health care organizations must comply with an ever-increasing list of rules and regulations that document compliance. That burden lands squarely on the shoulders of the people providing care to patients. In fact, many health care quality metrics tracked by the federal government rely solely on this documentation.

Another time suck is the increased demand for administrative tasks to satisfy payers. There's always one more process required to get patients the care they need. Lots of time is spent on obtaining prior authorization for services or appealing denied services. This ever-increasing administrative burden makes it particularly challenging to see more patients in shorter time intervals.

But seriously? No time for compassion? Compassion for others is supposed to be one of the main reasons that providers choose to go into the health care profession in the first place!

This begs the very important question: How much time does it really take? So let's consider the scientific data for how much time is really required to make a compassionate connection with a patient.

Spoiler alert: The evidence may surprise you.

It's Time to Take the Time

To address the question of time, researchers from Johns Hopkins University performed a randomized controlled trial in cancer patients during a consultation with an oncologist.[97] The main outcome measure for this study was a well-validated measurement scale for patient anxiety. If you understand what it's like to receive a cancer diagnosis, then you already know that reducing anxiety is a critically important outcome for cancer patients.

The researchers found that, compared to a standard consultation from an oncologist, patients randomized to an enhanced compassion intervention from an oncologist had significantly *less* anxiety at the end of the consultation.

So what was the enhanced compassion intervention? It was a few words offered at both the beginning and the end of the consultation.

Here was the message from the oncologist, at the beginning of the consultation:

> *"I know this is a tough experience to go through and I want you to know that I am here with you. Some of the things that I say to you today may be difficult to understand, so I want you to feel comfortable in stopping me if something I say is confusing or doesn't make sense. We are here together, and we will go through this together."*

And then at the end of the consultation, the oncologist said:

> *"I know this is a tough time for you and I want to emphasize again that we are in this together. I will be with you each step along the way."*

So how long did it take? They timed it: just *forty seconds.*

Patients that were randomized to this enhanced compassion intervention and heard these messages from the oncologist rated the oncologist as warmer and more caring, as well as sensitive and compassionate. Patients in the enhanced compassion group also rated the oncologist higher in terms of wanting what was best for the patient. But what was most striking was that, using a validated scientific scale to precisely measure patients' level of anxiety, patients randomized to the enhanced compassion intervention actually had measurably lower anxiety.

This randomized controlled trial demonstrates two important things: First, in accordance with what you already learned in Chapter 4, compassion for patients can effectively reduce the anxiety they are experiencing, thereby improving their psychological health. Second, and perhaps most importantly, forty seconds of compassion is all you need to make a meaningful difference for a patient.

> Forty seconds of compassion is all you need to make a meaningful difference for a patient.

But are these results from Johns Hopkins—that it only takes forty seconds—the exception or the rule? Let's take a look at more data:

In two studies from the Netherlands Institute for Health Services Research, researchers tested the effects of compassionate communication on patient anxiety among patients receiving "bad news" about their diagnosis and prognosis (e.g., a terminal condition).[174, 175] Of note, this study had to be conducted in a sample of "analogue" patients—healthy patients who put themselves "in the shoes" of a patient receiving bad news—because, of course, it would be unethical to randomize a patient receiving such bad news to a lack of compassion.

As a reminder, numerous scientific studies have shown that use of analogue patients is not only a valid, but actually an optimal method for studying the effectiveness of health care provider communication with patients, so we can have confidence in the study results.[251]

Half of the study subjects receiving bad news were randomized to standard communication from the physician and the other half were randomized to an enhanced compassion communication from the physician.

The enhanced compassion intervention included all of the following communications from the physician:

"Whatever we do, and however that develops, we will continue to take good care of you."
"We will be with you all the way."
"We will do, and will continue to do, our very best for you."
"Whatever happens, we will never abandon you. You are not facing this on your own."
"Together, we will have a careful look at decisions you have to make and will keep a close eye on your concerns."

Similar to the Johns Hopkins study, the researchers found that participants who were randomized to the enhanced compassion communication had significantly lower anxiety following the consultation, as measured on a validated anxiety measurement scale.

But here is the most important piece of data: How long did this enhanced compassion communication take in total? Again, they timed it: just *38 seconds.* Similar to the findings of the Johns Hopkins study, 38 seconds was all it took to make a meaningful and measurable difference.

What about Endless Concerns and Questions?

A skeptic might critique these data as being one-sided, only reflecting the health care providers' part of the communication. What about the patient side of the communication? When you factor that in, doesn't compassion take a lot longer?

Health care providers sometimes express concerns that if they start regularly exploring their patients' emotions, it might open up "Pandora's box" of endless concerns, where it seems like the patient will never stop talking, and so the provider won't be able to get his or her work done efficiently. As we saw in the Harvard Medical School study at the beginning of this chapter,

56 percent of physicians believe that they do not have time to go down this path of exploring emotions with their patients.[323]

But the available data in the biomedical literature do not support this thinking. In fact, when precisely measured, the scientific data support that a compassionate exchange with a patient actually takes far less time than one might think.

For example, researchers from Northwestern University studied real-world patients in a general internal medicine practice, using a validated methodology to measure compassion opportunities from patients and the corresponding responses by physicians.[324]

They identified these as "opportunity-response" communication sequences. They found that compassionate opportunity-response communication sequences took, on average...*31.5 seconds.*

> **Compassionate opportunity-response communication sequences take about 30 seconds.**

This 31.5 seconds included hearing what the patient had to say that presented an opportunity for compassion, plus the health care providers' response, including "confirmation" (conveying that the patients' emotion or concern was legitimate) or "pursuit" (asking the patient a follow-up question or offering support).

So this time sequence included both the patients' part of the communication as well as the physicians'. On average, the exchanges with the most compassion—including confirmation or pursuit—took about half a minute.

Now, to be fair, if there was a long series of compassionate opportunity-response sequences between the patient and the physician, it could be longer. For example, if a patient was really struggling on a particular day and was especially in need of compassion, a back-and-forth exchange of ten compassion sequences between the patient and the physician could then take, on average, 315 seconds (31.5 seconds per sequence for 10 sequences).

But even still, let's recognize that those ten sequences add up to barely over five minutes in total. And the available evidence indicates that this level of need for compassion would be an outlier or extreme case.

The truth is that patients in some medical visits do not communicate *any* need for compassion during their visits, and so, may not even require the extra thirty seconds. In the Northwestern study, for example, many of the clinic visits had zero compassion opportunities.

But among all clinic visits with one or more compassion opportunities, the mean number of compassion opportunities per visit was 2.5. Think of it like this: If a compassion sequence takes, on average, 31.5 seconds and there are 2.5 sequences per patient, providers can expect to spend an extra 79 seconds (on average) with a patient who is in need of compassion.

So if a single sequence of communicating compassion probably takes half a minute, can health care providers spare that for compassion? How about a whole forty seconds, as in the Johns Hopkins study?

Does Compassion Lengthen Doctor Visits?

The findings in these studies are also corroborated by other rigorously conducted research that shows compassionate care does not add a significant amount of time to a health care encounter. In Chapter 4, for instance, you saw the data from a University of California San Francisco study of inpatients admitted to the hospital, where each additional compassionate statement from a hospitalist physician was associated with an incremental (or cumulative) reduction in patient anxiety.[48]

In that study, researchers also measured total encounter time—the length of time physicians spent face-to-face with patients—and found that the number of compassionate statements from the physician was *not* significantly associated with encounter length. More compassion did not equate to longer visits. So the data support that being compassionate does *not* add a significant amount of time to the total time spent with patients.

Similar results have been found in studies of patients in the primary care setting. In a study supported by the National Institutes of Health (NIH), researchers from Johns Hopkins University conducted a randomized controlled trial of compassionate communication training (including "emotion handling" skills) for physicians.[185]

They found that, compared to a control group of primary care physicians who received no special training, the physicians randomly assigned to training in emotion handling had higher ratings for compassionate care from patients, and their patients were less emotionally distressed. And here's an amazing finding that probably surprised the authors of this study: In follow-up evaluations by telephone, they learned that compassionate care not only reduced patients' emotional distress, but the effects also persisted up to *six months* after the clinic visit.

But the researchers were also interested in the time during clinic visits that it took to get those kinds of benefits. So they measured the time that the physicians spent face-to-face with patients in the initial appointment. The hypothesis was that it might take more time in order to make a compassionate connection.

What they found is that the compassion-trained physicians did *not* spend significantly more time. It was slightly longer, but the difference was so small that it was not statistically significant. Compared to a control group of physicians who did not get any special training, the clinic visits with the compassion-trained physicians were, on average, only *54 seconds* longer.

Lower emotional distress for six whole months from just 54 seconds of extra care? That's a lot of mileage from less than one minute of compassion!

More data on the time required to make a compassionate connection with patients is available from the experience of Christy Dempsey, chief nursing officer at Press Ganey, Inc. A patient experience thought leader, Dempsey is the author of the book *The Antidote to Suffering: How Compassionate Connected Care Can Improve Safety, Quality, and Experience.*[325]

In Dempsey's thirty years of personal experience in health care, both at the bedside as well as working with groups of health care providers to improve their ability to connect compassionately with their patients, she has found that a meaningful compassion connection takes, on average, *56 seconds* (and she reports that it almost never exceeds two minutes).

The Perception Problem

Given a plethora of data that the time required to show meaningful compassion to a patient is, on average, less than a minute, could it be that health care providers' belief that they do not have time for compassion is all "in their heads"?

Compassion Takes Less than 60 Seconds

Bylund et al[324]	32 seconds
Bensing et al[174,175]	38 seconds
Fogarty et al[97]	40 seconds
Roter et al[185]	54 seconds
Dempsey[325]	56 seconds

Studies show that demonstrating compassion to patients takes less than one minute. The median value based off these five studies is 40 seconds.

Perhaps it's not really about actual time, but rather about their *perception* of time.

Think back to the "good Samaritan" study from Princeton University that you learned about in Chapter 1.[24] That was the research on seminarians (i.e., students studying to be pastors of a church) where just 40 percent of the seminarians stopped to help a person in obvious distress...someone disheveled, moaning, and lying in an alley.

You will recall that the person in distress was a "confederate" (i.e., an actor who was part of the research study). You will also recall that hearing a lecture about the Good Samaritan parable from the Bible right before encountering the person in distress had no effect on whether or not the seminarian stopped to help.

But you haven't heard the rest of the story yet. We explained that half the seminarians were randomly assigned to hear a lecture on the Good Samaritan parable, to see if that would make a difference in helping behavior. And that it did not.

But the seminarians were also randomized in one other way. All of the seminarians were instructed to go to another nearby building on campus for their next assignment. In doing so, they would have to walk right past the person in distress lying in the alley.

But here was the next level of experimental randomization: Half of the seminarians were randomly told that they did not need to rush. In this experimental study, the researchers called this the "no hurry condition." The other half of the seminarians were given the exact same instructions about which building to go to next, but with a twist.

Instead of being told not to rush, these seminarians were told that they were already late for their next assignment, and they needed to hurry. The researchers called this the "hurry condition." (Of course, the seminarians were not really late for anything at all; they were just made to believe they were in a hurry.)

What the researchers found was that seminarians who believed they were in a hurry to reach their destination were significantly more likely to pass by the person in distress without stopping. Compared to seminarians who believed they were in a hurry, the proportion of seminarians in the "no hurry" group that stopped to offer meaningful help was *six times* higher. Specifically, 63 percent of the "no hurry" group stopped to help, but just 10 percent stopped to help among those in a hurry.

Further analyses even took into account multiple other factors beyond whether or not they heard the lecture on the Good Samaritan parable. Researchers considered the seminarians' personal attributes—including their degree of "religiosity"—and found that believing to be in a hurry was the only factor that predicted whether or not they stopped to help a person in need. And the seminarians weren't really even late for anything...they just thought they were.

> Researchers found that believing to be in a hurry was the only factor that predicted whether or not participants stopped to help a person in need.

So you've seen that 56 percent of physicians believe they don't have enough time for compassion. And that it really only takes forty seconds or so. Is it possible that this disconnect—a perception problem by health care providers—is a major contributor to the compassion crisis that we have in health care today?

A Virtuous Cycle

In a fascinating series of experiments from The Wharton School at the University of Pennsylvania published in the journal *Psychological Science*, researchers examined a person's perception of "time affluence." Time affluence is the perception of having plenty of time, not being in a rush, and thus a willingness to donate more time to others.[326] This research sought to examine the determinants of time affluence, and specifically how the ways that people use their time makes them feel about the time that they have.

What the researchers found was surprising, and perhaps counterintuitive. Although the objective amount of time people have cannot be increased—after all, there are only 24 hours in a day—this research demonstrated that people's subjective sense of time affluence (i.e., the perception that that they have plenty of time) can actually be increased. Their solution to the common problem of feeling that one does not have enough time? Give some of it away!

In a series of experiments, these researchers compared the effects of four things on people's perception of their time affluence: (1) spending time helping other people, (2) spending time on oneself, (3) wasting time, and (4) gaining an unexpected windfall of "free" time. What they found was that spending time helping others actually *increases* one's perception of time affluence.

In fact, spending time helping others had a statistically significant larger boost in perception of time affluence compared to self-focused time, wasting time, or gaining more free time. The researchers concluded that the mechanism by which giving time to others raises one's perception of time affluence is driven by an elevated sense of purpose and self-efficacy in helping others. That is, the positive emotions associated with making a difference for others changes how people feel about the time that they have.

So what does this have to do with compassionomics?

The answer: *Everything.*

> The research is quite clear that giving time actually gives you time.

Given that research shows 56 percent of health care providers believe that they do not have enough time for compassion, it is quite possible (based on this rigorous research from the University of Pennsylvania) that spending a little more time on compassion for patients will change health care providers' experience in a way that makes them feel like they actually have more time for compassion.[323, 326]

It's a *virtuous* cycle. The data are quite clear here...giving time away actually gives you time!

Maybe when we consider how much time we have to show others compassion, we should make the next leap in our thinking: Compassion doesn't necessarily take any extra time at all.

Dr. Robin Youngson, co-founder of the Australian organization Hearts in Healthcare and author of the book *Time to Care: How to Love Your Patients and Your Job*, relates a story of a patient admitted to the hospital due to a serious illness who is awakened in the wee hours of the morning by a nurse coming in to his hospital room to administer his next dose of intravenous medication.[327, 328]

The nurse loudly opens the door with a bang, abruptly turns on the lights, and roughly pulls back the sheets of the patient's bed to check his wrist band identification. After she finishes giving the dose of medication, she marches out the room...leaving the lights on.

"There is no possibility of rest in this place," mutters the patient.

Contrast this experience with the next night, when a different nurse is on duty and takes a totally different approach to the same task with the same patient. She tiptoes quietly into the room and uses a flashlight so that she doesn't have to turn on the overhead room lights. She gently checks his wrist band identification, and quietly administers his medication before tiptoeing out of the room. The patient never wakes up.

Which nurse was compassionate? How much extra time did it take?

The point of Youngson's story is that when health care providers are doing their necessary clinical tasks, they can do so with an approach of compassion or with what he calls "brusque efficiency." They can either greet patients with warmth and engage them in conversations about their needs, or alternatively, they can ensure their patients know just how busy they are (or how busy they *think* they are). [328]

Each option actually takes exactly the same amount of time.

CHAPTER 9:
Nature versus Nurture: Can We Learn Compassion?

"One of the most powerful forces in human nature is our belief that change is possible."

—Shawn Achor

It is likely that your junior high school biology teacher once asked you—between teaching you how to dissect a frog and mount a glass slide onto a microscope—whether you could roll your tongue. Tongue rolling is the ability to roll the lateral edges of the tongue upwards into a tube.

Then you likely learned that some people have the genetic ability to roll their tongue while others do not. Ever since the prominent geneticist Alfred Sturtevant published the article "A New Inherited Character in Man" in 1940, biology teachers have used this example to demonstrate basic genetic principles as well as give a solid example of "nature" in the "nature versus nurture" explanation of human traits.[329, 330]

But what about compassion? Is that something that falls squarely in the "nature" category? Something similar to Sturtevant's description of tongue rolling: you either have it or you don't? Or is it something that can be "nurtured?" In other words, can we train people in this powerful intervention? Can compassion for others actually be *learned*?

Some people feel intuitively (and quite strongly) that the answer is "no." They believe that compassion for others cannot be learned. They scoff at the suggestion that one can be taught to be compassionate.

In fact, they would probably tell you that some people are just "wired" for compassion, while others simply are not. Or that compassion is something intrinsic that one is born with—it's in the fabric of who you are—and you cannot pick it up along the way. They might also believe that people without compassion cannot change their character—the old idea that "a leopard never changes its spots."

In fact, some people believe this about *themselves*. You will recall from Chapter 1 that an important reason why health care providers sometimes fail to treat patients with compassion is a belief that it is not in their nature (e.g., "I'm not a 'touchy-feely' person").

The problem with this kind of thinking is that it is *not* supported by the available evidence. Science tells a different story. The preponderance of data in the scientific literature shows quite clearly that compassionate behaviors can, in fact, be learned. This includes compassionate behaviors towards patients by health care providers.

> The scientific literature clearly shows that compassionate behaviors can be learned.

Therein lies a key distinction: It's all about *behaviors*. Whether or not a health care provider can be taught to care more for others in his or her own mind is a separate (perhaps more philosophical) question. But what matters from the patient perspective is what a patient experiences. That is shaped almost entirely by the behaviors that health care providers display toward them. So, for our purposes, the main question is: Can a health care provider learn compassionate behaviors?

The answer, you will see, is a resounding *yes*.

Be Intentional

Implicit in the idea of behaving in a compassionate way is the concept of "emotional labor," which we briefly touched on in Chapter 1. Emotional labor is the management of one's emotions (both one's experienced emotions as well as one's displayed emotions) to present a certain image.[56]

For decades, researchers in management and organizational behavior have been studying emotional labor by service workers across all types of service industries. For health care providers, emotional labor includes the expectation of compassionate behaviors toward patients, even if those providers aren't actually feeling an emotional connection with the patient in that particular moment. (A word of caution here: Please resist the temptation to trivialize emotional labor as "faking it." It goes much deeper than that, as you'll see in a moment.)

> Compassion makes you a better healer. Period.

If you are a health care provider, implicit in emotional labor is the recognition that your patients are counting on you. In earlier chapters, you saw a tidal wave of data that demonstrated that compassion is an essential ingredient for optimal health outcomes and quality of care. Compassion makes you a better healer. Period.

Therefore, you have a responsibility. Everyone has bad days, of course. Maybe your own life circumstances at the present time are not what you intended, or ever expected. But when there are patients in front of you who need your compassion, it is your responsibility to find a way to show it to them.

Renowned University of Houston researcher Dr. Brené Brown reminds us that "Compassion…is a commitment. It's not something we have or we don't have—it's something we *choose* to practice."[331]

So it's a conscious decision. Being intentional about compassion is not only allowable; it's necessary. Without question, people in health care (and all helping professions, for that matter) will not always feel like being compassionate. In those instances, it's not only okay to "dig deep" and force oneself to muster compassionate behaviors, it's essential.

What does that look like exactly? A classic paper published in *JAMA* explains the different types—or layers, really—of emotional labor as they pertain to health care providers.[56] For example, one is called "deep acting." This is when health care providers intentionally generate compassionate emotional and cognitive reactions in themselves before and during interactions with patients who are in need of compassion. You can think of it as analogous to the famous "method acting" tradition used by some stage and screen actors.

But let's be clear: There is no "faking it" here. The compassionate feelings are 100 percent genuine and sincere; they are just the product of being intentional. They are feelings generated by health care providers within themselves… explicitly for patients' benefit.

Anyone who has small children at home does this quite frequently. No matter how stressed, tired, overworked or overwhelmed caring parents become, they almost always summon up the necessary energy with their children. They offer a consistent message of love, understanding, and hope when speaking to them, especially when their kids are frightened or upset.

People intentionally put on a different face with their children to connect with them in those moments. It's because parents take the responsibility of how their kids respond to their words and behaviors very seriously. Parents understand that their interactions make an imprint on them.

The energy it takes for a parent to push worries—work stress, paying the bills, etc.—to the back of the mind in favor of a positive, nurturing message about why doing your homework or being kind to others is important sometimes requires emotional labor. It's not always easy if you're feeling completely stressed in the moment. But you do it anyway, because that's what parents do.

It's a form of "deep acting," really. And yet, the sentiments and caring that those parents summon up within them are 100 percent genuine and sincere.

The other type of emotional labor in health care described in the *JAMA* paper is called "surface acting."[56] This is when a health care provider shows compassionate behaviors toward the patient, but without consistent emotional and cognitive reactions. When it comes to surface acting, the outward compassionate behaviors are there, but the health care provider is not actually feeling it on the inside. So this *is* kind of like faking it.

> **Compassionate behaviors are a health care provider's responsibility.**

The *JAMA* authors suggest that although deep acting is preferred, it is okay for health care providers to rely on surface acting in those situations when an emotional understanding and connection are impossible. What's key to remember is that, in either case, compassionate behaviors are a health care provider's responsibility.

Engaging in emotional labor, in a meaningful way, can also begin to transform how a health care provider feels about his or her patients. In other words, treating patients with compassion by being very intentional—through emotional labor—may result in a health care provider actually *feeling* more compassion for patients.

Some might consider this to be a "fake it 'til you make it" approach. But remember that many prominent thinkers throughout history have attested to the fact that making a habit of altruistic behaviors can transform oneself from the inside.

The literary giant and theologian C.S. Lewis observed that: "When you are behaving as if you loved someone, you will presently come to love him." Mahatma Gandhi taught that "Compassion is a muscle that gets stronger with use." In *Nicomachean Ethics*, Aristotle wrote: "Virtues are formed in man by his doing the actions."

Emotional labor—and specifically compassionate behaviors towards others—can, in fact, make one more compassionate which, in turn, yields more compassionate behaviors. So giving patients *your* forty seconds of compassion will not only make you feel like you have more time to give (see the section on time affluence in Chapter 8) but also it will make you feel more compassion.

It's a *virtuous* cycle...born from intentionality.

Can You Really Change Your Mind?

Shortly, you will see the data for how compassion training can change health care providers' behaviors towards patients. But can this change in compassionate behavior begin to change who they really *are*?

We do not mean this to be an existential question, but rather a scientific one. To answer it, we need to dive into some rigorous neuroscience data…to see what immersing oneself in compassion can actually do to one's *brain*.

Let's begin with the concept of "neuroplasticity." Essentially, that's the brain's ability to adapt over time. Traditionally, neuroplasticity used to refer to the brain's ability to adapt in response to a brain injury. The brain can, to some extent, reorganize itself by forming new connections between neurons (brain cells) in order to compensate for damage or disease. Neuroplasticity explains why some patients are able to recover from brain injury and regain functional status over time.

But there is another very important aspect to neuroplasticity, one that has become more widely appreciated in recent years. The brain can adapt to far more than just a physical injury; it also adapts to new situations and challenges, new environments, and new demands for performance. Over time, brain "wiring" can actually change to allow people to do things they could not do before.

This specific aspect of neuroplasticity actually represents a monumental shift from historical thinking about neuroscience. In decades past, most neuroscientists believed in a "fixed brain" paradigm which assumed that once a person reached adulthood, his or her brain could not change anymore.

This is the belief that the brain could no longer reorganize itself—that people "are who they are" once they reach adulthood. Put plainly, neuroscientists were true believers that you could not teach an old dog new tricks.

But emerging data on neuroplasticity have shattered that thinking and resulted in a paradigm shift. Neuroscientists now recognize that the human brain is actually malleable, at least to some extent.

Take taxi cab drivers, for instance. Researchers from University College London used MRI scans to study the brains of experienced taxi cab drivers in London and then published their results in *Proceedings of the National Academy of Sciences*, one of the most prestigious scientific journals in the world.[332] The evidence for neuroplasticity was eye-opening indeed.

If you have ever driven in London, you know that it is a maze of streets; the layout is anything but predictable. In London, the streets were not designed like a grid. The map looks more like a spaghetti diagram, actually.

But the most experienced cabbies in London know this maze like the back of their hands. They seem to have a "sixth sense" about where they are going and how to navigate around town. They have navigated the maze so many times, day after day, they just know—by second nature—where to turn and what shortcuts to take. Based on the demands of their job, they utilize their navigation skills all day, every day. Could this experience actually change their brains?

What the researchers found was downright amazing. By examining brain MRI scans they found that compared to control subjects (people who were not cab drivers), the London taxi cab drivers had significantly *larger* posterior hippocampi. The posterior hippocampus is a brain structure involved in spatial relations and spatial memory. This is an area of the brain vital to navigation and remembering how to navigate a challenging environment.

So what is the explanation? Is it possible that people born with larger posterior hippocampi are intrinsically better at navigating, and therefore decide to go into the taxi cab driver business?

No way.

The only plausible explanation is that daily exposure to the demands of complex navigation actually *changed* the structure of their brains. In response to the constant use of that navigation area of the brain, it actually grew larger!

The most common evidence of neuroplasticity is an improvement in brain function, but in this unique study—with the advent of MRI scans—the researchers found scientific evidence that the brain can change its structure as well. This study, along with others that shared similar findings, has turned the idea of a "fixed brain" on its head (no pun intended). The MRI data show quite clearly: change is possible!

So, can a leopard change its spots? Can people truly change who they are? Philosophers have been asking this question throughout the ages. And the answer is in: Indeed they can. From a neuroscience perspective, and based on rigorous scientific evidence of neuroplasticity, it's increasingly clear: change *can* happen.

Of course, change does not happen from casual, fleeting, or inconsistent exposure to new challenges or environments. As in the study of taxi cab drivers, the differences found in brain structures were the result of intentional, disciplined, and sustained practice over many years.

But is this kind of neuroplasticity limited only to navigation and spatial relations? Or could it also be true for...*compassion*?

Could it be that immersing oneself in compassion and practicing compassion intentionally and consistently over time, in a disciplined way, could change who you are?

To find out, let's take a look at the most extreme example of people devoted to practicing compassion: Tibetan monks. If you study in a Buddhist monastery in Tibet, compassion is serious business. And it requires serious training.

> **Buddhist monks become "outliers" in compassion, not only in the time they spend training in compassion, but also in how this training changes their brain function.**

In their preparation to become monks, these individuals spend over ten thousand hours meditating on loving-kindness and compassion for others. They become "outliers" in every sense of the word, not only in the amount of time that they spend training in the practice of compassion, but also in how this experience changes their brain function.[333]

Want proof?

Dr. Richard Davidson and his colleagues from the Center for Healthy Minds at the University Wisconsin-Madison have studied some of the most experienced Tibetan monks—the "outliers of the outliers" in how much time they spend fully immersed in compassion. Specifically, these monks are the world's experts in a specific type of meditation technique called loving-kindness meditation (LKM) to increase one's compassion.[334]

Using 256 tiny electrodes attached to the skull and measuring brain electrical activity (i.e., "brain waves") with a test called electroencephalography (EEG), Davidson and colleagues found that compared to control subjects (regular people), these compassion adept monks had brain waves that were literally off the charts.[335]

There is a specific type of brain wave, called a gamma wave, that is seen on an EEG during moments when differing brain regions are firing in harmony, such as when you have an exhilarating "Aha!" moment of extreme insight. Typically, when gamma waves are observed they are only fleeting, found in isolated brain areas, and the amplitude of the brain waves is rather small.

What the researchers found when they studied the monks' brain waves was stunning, and particularly when the monks were meditating on compassion for others. When the monks were in "compassion mode," they generated EEG data unlike anything Davidson and colleagues had ever seen before in their lab.[335]

When the monks generated feelings of compassion during meditation, their brain activity began to fire in a rhythmic harmony. The monks' gamma waves were markedly stronger and more sustained than those of normal subjects. Plus, they were in synchrony across widespread brain regions.

But here is perhaps the most interesting finding: When the monks stopped meditating on compassion, the gamma wave activity decreased, but this activity was still markedly greater than control subjects' gamma activity, independent of any specific mental activity. This difference persisted even when the monks were sleeping![335, 336]

Davidson and colleagues were seeing, for the first time, an enduring transformation of the brain that was the result of thousands and thousands of hours of intentionality and practice in meditation on loving-kindness and compassion. It changed the monks' brains…it changed who they *are.*

Corroborating the findings from Davidson's lab are compelling data from MRI studies that look inside the brains of expert compassion meditators. Just as the London taxi cab drivers had an increase in the size of brain regions involved in navigation, researchers identified a similar phenomenon in the compassion meditators. Compared to control subjects, people who are expert practitioners of compassion meditation—those with ten thousand or more lifetime hours of meditation—have more gray matter volume in regions of the brain that are involved in affect and emotion regulation.[337, 338]

Again, it is unlikely that naturally having more developed brains in these regions drew them to become experts in compassion meditation. Rather, because they immersed themselves in compassion for thousands of hours, resulting brain changes can be seen on MRI. Again, over time, their dedication to compassion changed who they are.

So will it require ten thousand hours or a monk's life-altering commitment for compassion to change people? Fortunately, the answer is no.

And here is a crucial thing to understand: There is rigorous scientific evidence that thousands of hours of practice are *not* required in order to begin to see changes in brain function. In fact, with just a little bit of practice, one can start to see some functional changes right away.

In two studies from the Max Planck Institute for Human Cognitive and Brain Sciences in Germany, researchers found evidence of functional changes in the brain with just a little bit of compassion training.[11, 12] Using functional MRI, the researchers found increased activity in regions of the brain associated with affiliation and positive affect after study subjects took a short course (six-hours in total) in compassion meditation led by an expert practitioner.

Similar brain changes on functional MRI scans have been reported by the Davidson lab at the University of Wisconsin-Madison after a two-week compassion training course.[339] Considering the minimal time investment required to begin to see change, these data indicate that change is not only possible but also is readily available.

Now that we know that the act of practicing compassion can change our brains—our brain waves, brain structure, and brain function—let's look at the evidence that compassion training can actually change our *behavior* in meaningful ways, too…as well as the perception of compassion from the receiver's perspective.

Compassion Training Works!

A University of Oxford meta-analysis of data from 64 different clinical studies shows quite clearly that there is major variation in health care provider compassion, as assessed by patients.[55] This inconsistency is not surprising; there are both high performers and low performers when it comes to showing compassion…and a glut of health care providers that rank in between. (Some are clearly capable of compassion but perhaps inconsistent in delivering it.)

So can individuals who don't excel at compassion get better?

There is scientific evidence that certain genetic polymorphisms—for example, in the oxytocin receptor gene—are associated with a more compassionate disposition toward others.[340, 341, 342] There are also clinical studies that show that female health care providers may have greater compassion for patients compared to their male counterparts.[55, 323, 343] (Sorry, guys.)

But no health care provider should get a "pass" on the expectation of compassion, regardless of their genes or their gender.

To this point, French scientist Matthieu Ricard (who also happens to be a Buddhist monk) uses the metaphor of throwing a javelin to explain the value of compassion training.[344] Ricard teaches this: Every person can learn the basics of how to throw a javelin.

Some people will intrinsically throw it better than others from the start. But with practice, every single javelin thrower can improve. Although it is true that not all people can or will become Olympic-level javelin throwers, with effort and dedication, every person can improve their ability to throw the javelin significantly further than they initially threw it.

Similarly, every person can get better at showing compassion for others, at least a little bit. And, as we have seen throughout these pages, just a little bit more compassion may make all the difference in the world to a patient in need. Ricard's javelin throwing analogy is apt indeed.

Back in Chapter 4, you met Dr. Helen Riess, the Mass General psychiatrist and empathy researcher who discovered her patient's deep-seated and previously unrecognized need for empathy and compassion during a psychotherapy session. You may remember that she had an epiphany when she monitored her patient's electrodermal activity (skin conductance) in a research experiment and measured her off-the-charts anxiety that was otherwise undetectable.[146, 147] This realization was not only a life-altering experience for the patient, but for Dr. Riess, too.

Dr. Riess realized we need to advance the science of empathy in the scientific community…to better train health care providers to pick up on subtle non-verbal cues from patients indicating that they are in need of compassion… and to teach them optimal methods to use in patient interactions. As a result of her research, she has dedicated her career to teaching health care providers, through the development of rigorous training programs, to be more empathetic. This, in turn, inspires them to act differently towards their patients and to provide more compassionate care.[345]

Now, we know what you might be thinking: Are these training programs just "smile school?" Hardly.

There is no fluffy stuff here. Every technique that Dr. Riess and her colleagues at Empathetics, Inc., teach to health care providers in three 60-minute modules is evidence-based and rooted in *bona fide* neuroscience.[149]

In fact, they call it a "neuroscience-informed curriculum." The behaviors she and her colleagues teach reflect state-of-the-art understanding about the science of human connection.[323] The training modules include how to decode subtle facial expressions for accurate emotion recognition as well as specific verbal and non-verbal communications to express compassion for patients.

The results speak for themselves. In a randomized controlled trial, Riess and her colleagues tested their neuroscience-informed curriculum in a population of resident physicians at Mass General, and found that the physicians who were randomized to empathy training had a statistically significant rise in positive patient ratings of physician compassion.[323]

Riess' results are actually consistent with what the vast majority of studies have found. One meta-analysis addressed the question: Can people (in general) be trained to be more compassionate?[346] They examined 18 randomized controlled trials of compassion training programs in heterogeneous types of trainees (more than a thousand people in total). They found that compassion training programs are effective overall, and that the calculated effect size of all trials combined was in a range that, statistically speaking, is considered to be a substantial effect.

> In *80 percent* of the most scientifically rigorous published studies, compassion training successfully increased physician compassion.

Another meta-analysis conducted by researchers from the Children's Hospital of Philadelphia focused specifically on compassion training for physicians.[347] What they found is that in *80 percent* of the most scientifically rigorous published studies, compassion training successfully increased physician compassion.

Similar results have been found in meta-analyses of compassion training studies conducted in medical students.[348, 349] Compassion training also appears to be effective in nurses and nursing students as well.[350, 351, 352, 353]

You will also recall from Chapter 8 the description of the randomized trial from Johns Hopkins and funded by the National Institutes of Health (NIH), demonstrating that training primary care physicians in "emotion handling" skills with an eight-hour training program was effective for improving compassionate communication by physicians...and without significantly lengthening the clinic visits.[185]

But taking the effects one step further is another study from Dr. Riess and her group at Mass General.[354] Up to this point, the studies discussed above have provided evidence that compassionate behaviors can be learned by health care providers. But what are the effects of these training interventions on *patients*?

To answer this question, Riess and colleagues performed a meta-analysis of randomized controlled trials that systematically manipulated the patient-clinician relationship and tested the effects on patient outcomes. The interventions to augment relationships with patients included various methods of boosting human connection, for example, training in communication skills, recognition of emotional cues, increasing eye contact, sitting down (versus standing up), goal setting, shared decision-making, and avoiding interrupting the patient.

> **Interventions to improve the patient-clinician relationship are associated with better outcomes for patients.**

The patient-oriented outcomes were either objective measures, like blood pressure, or validated subjective measures, such as pain scores. The researchers found that interventions to improve the patient-clinician relationship were associated with better outcomes for patients.

Not only that, but after pooling the data Riess and colleagues found that the size of the effect of the interventions was greater than the effects of aspirin in reducing the incidence of heart attack over five years or the influence of statins (cholesterol-lowering medications) on the five-year risk of an adverse cardiovascular event.[354, 355]

In other words, statistically speaking, interventions to augment the patient-clinician relationship have a greater effect on patients than some of the most common and well-known advances in clinical practice across all of medicine in the last half century! Those are striking findings.

The Power of Mindset

So now you have seen the data that compassionate behaviors can, in fact, be learned and that compassion training works. But there is a key characteristic that's required for success: the learner's *mindset.*

You may be familiar with the research on "growth mindset" from Dr. Carol Dweck and her colleagues at Stanford University. In her book *Mindset: The New Psychology of Success*, Dweck explains how a vital part of learning new things is the belief that you *can*. You must believe that change is possible.[356]

According to Dweck, many people believe that successful learning is based solely on innate ability. She describes such people as having a "fixed" theory of intelligence, or a fixed mindset. Others, who believe that successful learning is based on hard work, training, and perseverance are said to have a "growth" theory of intelligence, or growth mindset.

Here's why that's so important for learning new things. "Fixed mindset" people believe their abilities are fixed traits. They dread failure because they believe that it exposes their inherent lack of ability. As a result, they do not eagerly take on new challenges because of their fear of failure and looking or feeling stupid.

On the contrary, "growth mindset" people understand that their abilities grow through good teaching, effort, and persistence. They do not fear failure because they recognize that is how learning happens. You need to work at it.

As a result, such individuals are inherently more eager to take on new challenges and grow in their abilities. Dweck's research has shown that, over time, these types of people are more likely to be successful in whatever they are trying to accomplish.

Most of Dweck's work has been on learning and education in the broad sense. But could these principles also apply to learning to be compassionate to others? The answer is *yes*.

Growth mindset is crucial for becoming a more compassionate health care provider, or more broadly, a more compassionate person. Not just one, but a whole series, of studies from Dweck and colleagues found that in contexts where being compassionate is challenging, people who hold a growth mindset about compassion (believing that compassion can be developed) put significantly more effort into being compassionate, compared to people who hold a fixed mindset (believing compassion cannot be developed).[357]

> A person's mindset powerfully affects whether they exert effort to be compassionate when it is needed most.

The researchers found that people with a growth mindset worked harder at being compassionate because they had a stronger interest in improving their compassionate behavior. These studies indicate that a person's mindset powerfully affects whether they exert effort to be compassionate when it is needed most.

The data you've reviewed here have demonstrated quite clearly that one can learn to treat others with compassion; however, one must have a growth mindset to realize this change. You must first believe in your mind that *change is possible*!

You Gotta Want It

So if health care providers understand that change is possible, can't health care organizations and administrators just mandate that their providers participate in compassion training programs and work hard at being more compassionate to patients?

Nope. And this part is critically important for administrators of health care organizations to understand.

> **Science shows that health care providers have to want to get better at compassion. Compassion cannot be mandated.**

Health care providers have to *want* to get better at compassion. They have to have intrinsic motivation for improving, rather than extrinsic motivation, like being forced to do it. That's what the science shows.

In a series of studies that were designed to test the importance of intrinsic motivation in helping others, researchers from the University of Rochester found that the degree to which helping others is "autonomous" (i.e., voluntary), rather than "controlled" (i.e., mandated or forced), predicts the effectiveness of help—as perceived by the receiver.[358] In other words, receivers of help perceive the help to be more effective when the helper is doing it because they want to. Maybe that's because people do a better job of helping when they intrinsically want to help, rather than it being forced upon them.

This is why health care administrators can't just mandate health care providers to be compassionate to patients. That's not how compassion works. For patients to really benefit from compassion, the health care provider behaviors need to be self-initiated (or self-endorsed).

But here is an even more interesting part of what the University of Rochester researchers found: The degree to which help was autonomous (versus controlled) predicted the effects of helping on the well-being and self-esteem of the helper.[358] So helpers that intrinsically want to help are not only more effective at it, when they offer it freely (versus being forced), they feel better about the experience of helping.

In the next chapter, you will see more about how compassion for others powerfully impacts health care provider well-being and resilience. But for now, just remember that compassion can't and shouldn't be forced upon health care providers. Rather, help them to understand the "why" behind compassionate care so that they *want* to use compassion in every opportunity that they have.

Understanding that "why" is what this book is all about.

Learning to Care When Caring is Hard

During busy shifts or challenging days, it can be easy for health care providers to lose sight of the *people* they're caring for…not just a person's clinical diagnosis or symptoms, but all of the things that make them unique, important, and beloved to the people in their lives. Sometimes disease can ravage a body and make that harder for health care providers to see.

Nicki was a perfect example of that.

She was beautiful. Long brown hair. Kind eyes. A radiant smile that could light up the room. Her high school graduation portrait was picture perfect: a girl happy and full of life who brought happiness to those around her. It was a picture of a girl ready to take on the world…with her whole life ahead of her.

Things are much different today. That graduation photo sits on the windowsill in her room in the ICU, a poignant reminder to those caring for her of what her life used to be. Nicki's mom, Susan, brought the picture in, along with some baby pictures. The beautiful smile of that toddler was the same one as in the graduation photo. It was unmistakable.

It's hard for Nicki's caregivers to see her distinctive smile in the ICU today, with all the tubes and medical equipment. She has been unconscious on a ventilator for days with no sign of improvement. The reality of today is light years away from that graduation photo. She is almost unrecognizable.

Nicki has also withered away to less than 100 pounds. She is so emaciated that the beautiful face from the graduation photo is now sunken and sallow. The dirt on her feet was so deep-seated that despite repeated scrubbing by the ICU staff, her feet still tell a story of homelessness and being on the streets for way too long.

Covering her arms is the evidence of what caused her to abandon her home after high school. Years of injecting drugs into her veins have left awful scars on her body.

Nicki may never wake up. And if she does, she may never be able to communicate... to tell her mom how sorry she is for all the pain and anguish she's caused or how much she loves her, despite all the battles they've been through during all the times Nicki bounced from rehab to home and then, inevitably, back out on the streets again.

Susan knew she would get that dreaded phone call one day. She had been called to the hospital many times for Nicki's overdoses, and the repeated bloodstream infections that came from her heroin injections. She knew that one day she would get the call that would change everything.

She received that call one week ago. Since then, Nicki has not opened her eyes. Twenty five year-olds are not supposed to have strokes...let alone massive strokes. But when infections in the bloodstream collect on the valves of the heart, those big chunks of bacteria can break off and quickly migrate into the brain to cause a massive stroke, as they did for Nicki—changing the trajectory of her life instantly and forever.

As the reality of it all begins to sink in, Susan shares the story of another heartbreak in this very same ICU: when her older brother died several years ago from liver failure. She describes him as kind, gentle and outgoing, the kind of guy who would do anything for anybody. But privately, he battled demons. He could not stop drinking.

Jared spent a month in the ICU before he died. Susan recalls that whenever the doctors would do hospital rounds and discuss his case, the resident physician's opening sentence always described him as "a 53-year-old alcoholic with liver failure." To them, that was who Jared was. That hurt her a lot.

She knew him very differently. She knew him as a loving brother who was with her always as they were growing up, in good times and bad. He was her rock. Susan misses him desperately, especially now when she has to face saying goodbye to Nicki. She has no one left to lean on.

Just as she did during Nicki's hospitalization, Susan recalls also propping up Jared's graduation photo and baby picture on the ICU windowsill in a desperate attempt to help the nurses glimpse her brother the way she still sees him in her mind's eye… before addiction ravaged his body and made him unrecognizable, too.

She mentions overhearing doctors and nurses sometimes refer to Jared's condition as "self-inflicted"—just as they have with Nicki's. As if they both deserved the suffering they were experiencing.

This, too, hurt her a lot.

Stories like Nicki's and Jared's play out in hospitals around the country daily. While these kinds of statements from staff aren't very compassionate, perhaps we shouldn't be surprised.

There is extensive data in the psychology scientific literature to show that people's compassion for others often drops—sometimes rather sharply—when they believe that poor choices played a major role in the condition an individual is in; they believe they did it to themselves.

And in its simplest form, it's true. When a person's body is ravaged by the effects of addiction, that individual has clearly made some poor decisions—perhaps repeatedly—and especially in the beginning.

But today there is simply no longer a debate about whether addiction is a disease or a choice. Medicine has firmly concluded that addiction is a disease.[359]

It is critically important to recognize that, in the history of the world, no one has ever awakened in the morning and said to themselves, "Hey, I've got a great idea! Today I'm going to go out and get addicted to heroin." Or alcohol. Or anything else for that matter. That's just *never* happened.

If you've ever witnessed someone's body destroyed by the effects of addiction, you know how ugly it is. At the very end, they are unrecognizable. They suffer unspeakable pain. *No one* would ever willfully intend to be in that horrifying place. And thinking that they would makes it that much harder to summon the compassion needed to provide compassionate care.

But this idea that patients "do it to themselves" also extends far beyond patients who struggle with addiction. What about morbid obesity, for example? Some providers might be judgmental toward a morbidly obese person—because they believe such a condition results from bad personal choices and a lack of willpower.

It's not. It is far, far more complex than that.

Morbid obesity destroys a person's health. And when he is lying there in the hospital bed, with his life slipping away due to the cumulative effects of obesity on his body over many years, he too suffers unspeakable pain. *No one* would ever willfully intend to be in that horrifying place.

And what about people who don't take their medicine? Or follow doctors' orders? The so-called "non-compliant" patients. These patients are repeatedly readmitted to the hospital because they do not (or cannot) adhere to treatment recommendations. Do they "deserve it," too?

Maybe the reason why a patient doesn't refill his medication prescriptions to maintain better health is because he's used every dollar he has to make sure his kids don't go hungry. Poverty brings difficult decisions.

Or maybe it's because of mental illness. Or maybe health care providers have never really done a good job of explaining things in a way he can understand.

No one would ever willfully intend to be admitted to the hospital over and over again.

So let's be clear about one thing: When a person's health is failing and he or she is suffering terribly, remember this:

> *No one* "deserves it." Ever.

You've seen the scientific data that people can, in fact, learn to be compassionate to others. But it's not enough to simply learn compassionate behaviors. Or to have a growth mindset. Or to believe that change is possible.

Before one can learn to be more compassionate, there is a vital first step. First, one must believe that *every* patient deserves compassion.

Every single one.

A Final Few Thoughts: If We're Being Honest...

In case you're thinking that we must be the most compassionate doctors in the world, wonder no longer.

Just because we're sharing revolutionary scientific truths about the power of compassion here doesn't mean that we never slip ourselves. The truth is: We are both very much "works in progress." But we *see it* now. And what you focus on always grows stronger.

We used to believe that people were either wired for compassion or they were not. But the data in the scientific literature don't lie. The data—for both in the general population and in health care workers specifically—show that compassionate behaviors can most definitely be learned. And that is good news.

So we are working hard to get better at compassion—every day.

And last, a final note on tongue rolling: It's time for some more myth busting. It turns out that Dr. Sturtevant, and hence your junior high school science teacher, was actually wrong. Not only have rigorous scientific studies (conducted in twins and families) shown quite clearly that tongue rolling is *not* an inherited trait, but they have also found that tongue rolling can actually be *learned!*[360, 361, 362, 363, 364]

CHAPTER 10:
Compassion as an Antidote to Burnout

"If you want others to be happy, practice compassion. If you want to be happy, practice compassion."

—Dalai Lama

It's true. Compassion is not only a powerful therapy for the person receiving compassion, but it is a powerful therapy for the person giving compassion, too. That's what the latest science shows. And that's why compassion can be such a powerful treatment for burnout among health care providers.

Burnout: A Public Health Crisis

Earlier, you learned that two cornerstones of the burnout syndrome are depersonalization—the inability to make a personal connection—and emotional exhaustion, which is an important precursor to compassion fatigue.

When depersonalization and emotional exhaustion are present, it's no wonder that patients experience a lack of compassion. In fact, depersonalization and emotional exhaustion act as important surrogate markers for an *absence of compassion* when researchers study the effects of the compassion crisis on patients and patient care.

You've also read about the link between burnout among health care providers and lower quality of care (Chapter 6), including major medical and surgical errors as well as how health care providers "cut corners" in the care of patients.[365] In fact, new research from the Mayo Clinic demonstrates that burned out physicians have *two times higher odds* of making major medical errors.[366]

This is true cause for alarm because medical errors have been identified as a leading cause of death in the U.S. In short, health care provider burnout takes a toll not just on the people providing care, but the human toll also includes devastating effects on patients as well.[367]

You've also learned about the dire financial implications of burnout (Chapter 7), including the billions of dollars in direct costs and lost productivity for those that are harmed through medical errors and the ways in which burnout is associated with higher costs of care, especially with respect to physician and employee turnover. (The latter is estimated at $12 billion annually for physicians alone).[288, 301, 302, 303]

We also described the link between burnout and lost revenue to health care organizations that results from the effect of burnout on patient experience. (That's key because patient experience is one of the main drivers of the "business" of health care.) So you already understand the economic toll of health care provider burnout on the financial sustainability of organizations and our health care system overall.

> Research shows that approximately *50 percent* of U.S. physicians are suffering from burnout.

Through your own experience, you may also be aware that the prevalence of burnout symptoms among health care providers is enormous and growing rapidly. The medical literature supports this. For example, based on rigorous research using validated measures of burnout, multiple independent researchers have found that approximately *50 percent* of U.S. physicians are suffering burnout symptoms.[30, 301]

The National Academy of Medicine (NAM) concurs.[368] The NAM is a branch of the National Academies of Sciences whose aim is to provide unbiased, evidence-based, and authoritative guidance on health policy to policymakers and leaders in every sector of society and the public at large. The NAM sees burnout for what it is: a crucial problem for public health.

When you consider all of this evidence together—the effects on patients and patient care plus the effects on costs of care—and then add in the enormous prevalence of the problem, it becomes clear that burnout among health care providers is a major and growing public health *emergency*. It's no secret in health care circles.

But you know what else? The general public knows about it, too. The epidemic of burnout in medicine has been widely covered in the press, from *The Atlantic* and *The New York Times Magazine* to *The Wall Street Journal* and scores of other media outlets.[369, 370, 371]

Burnout among health care providers is serious business. What you may not yet appreciate, however, is the full effect of burnout on health care providers *themselves*—the effects on the individual caregiver. This is the other side of the human toll, and these effects can be staggering.

In Chapter 7, you learned that health care providers are leaving the profession in droves. But what are they actually experiencing before they "pull the rip cord" on the career for which they have been training their whole lives?

The Personal Toll of Burnout

Did you know that approximately *four hundred* physicians die by suicide every year? Research going back more than fifty years demonstrates that physicians die by suicide at a rate that significantly exceeds that of the general population.[372] In fact, recent research reports that physicians experience the highest suicide rate of *any* profession.[373]

> **Physicians die by suicide at a rate that significantly exceeds that of the general population.**

A systematic review of the medical literature reported that the suicide rate among physicians is 28 to 40 per 100,000, which is more than *double* the rate in the general population (12 per 100,000).[373] Research from the Mayo Clinic found that almost 40 percent of U.S. physicians have some symptoms of depression, and an astonishing 6 percent of those are depressed enough to think about suicide.[30]

What about nurses? Nobody knows precisely. According to researchers at the University of California San Diego, there is an alarming paucity of data on the nurse suicide rate. Considering the extreme occupational pressures on nurses, the National Academy of Medicine is concerned that nurse suicide is a hidden tragedy: *"Until such data are available, silence and the preventable loss of life will prevail."*[374]

So burnout is not just a serious concern for patient care, or for the costs of care, but also for those who care for patients. It's a multi-dimensional syndrome that stems from a combination of factors.[375] Certainly, fatigue—being overworked—is one component. Cynicism is another.

Cynicism can arise when a person feels a loss of autonomy, insufficient support or unattainable goals. It might be due to a feeling of being surrounded by impediments with no way out.

Frustration is another component of burnout. It can show up as a negative response to self and dissatisfaction with one's own performance (i.e., "beating yourself up"). Ultimately, all of these aspects of burnout combine into a downward spiral, culminating in the most dangerous manifestation of all: withdrawal. A person gives up and loses his or her motivation to make things better. A burned out physician starts to depersonalize relationships and becomes detached.

Here's another important consideration: Burnout isn't just about being overworked; it's also about the absence of meaningful human connection in one's work. You saw the data (way back in Chapter 1) that, in the era of electronic medical records, health care providers now spend more time looking into a computer screen than looking into the faces of their patients.

According to Dr. Atul Gawande, a surgeon, prolific writer, acclaimed public health researcher, and author of *The New Yorker* article "Why Doctors Hate Their Computers," this is fuel to the fire for the burnout epidemic.[376] Gawande asserts that doctors' computer screens are increasingly coming between them and their patients. He sees this as directly eroding what is supposed to be a fulfilling experience…the human connection of caring for patients.

Most applicants to medical school say that they are going into medicine to help people. And yet, a valuable piece of that rewarding experience is being lost through a required attention to computer screens in lieu of the patient in the room.

So burnout isn't just about exhaustion. It's about much more than that. According to Stanford's Dr. Emma Seppälä, whom you met earlier, burnout is also about loneliness. In a *Harvard Business Review* article, she reported that our professional relationships with colleagues (and specifically our compassion for each other during difficult times) are a key protective factor against the development of burnout.[377]

Seppälä warns that without meaningful relationships in the workplace, the risk of developing burnout skyrockets. Accordingly, it's vitally important for colleagues to take good care of each other.

The symptoms of burnout are numerous and include physical complaints (illness or other somatic manifestations), insomnia, irritability, negative attitude, being hypercritical of others, desensitization, apathy, feeling empty, disengagement, hopelessness, and pulling away emotionally. Sometimes burnout manifests with unprofessional behavior, and possibly outbursts in the workplace ("acting out").[375]

Another common manifestation of burnout is dread of going to work. Recently, an emergency physician from a large, very busy community hospital in suburban Boston relayed the story of his experience struggling with burnout. It was, quite frankly, a shocking example of what it means to dread going to work.

After experiencing the stages and symptoms of burnout described above, he had one event that pushed him past the breaking point. During one of his shifts in the emergency department, a patient came in who was at the end-stage of a serious illness.

That is not uncommon in emergency medicine. What was uncommon was that the patient was just a teenager. A short time after arrival in the emergency department, the patient took a sudden turn for the worse and went into cardiac arrest. The physician had to perform cardiopulmonary resuscitation (CPR) on the boy for almost an *hour*. Ultimately, the physician could not bring him back. The boy was gone.

The physician went to tell the family. It is not uncommon for an emergency physician to have to pronounce someone dead and notify next of kin, but it is uncommon to pronounce a teenager dead. It is especially uncommon to pronounce a teenager dead when he is the son of the physician's best friend. The physician knew this boy like he was part of his family...a child this physician had, in fact, watched grow up.

No one would question how traumatic this must have been. The physician was already suffering from burnout, and then this intensely personal tragedy happened right before his eyes. It culminated in such severe dread of going to work that after this tragic event, just before starting his shifts in the emergency department, he frequently found himself sitting in his car in the hospital parking lot, violently *throwing up*.

Thankfully, this physician got help. And thankfully, he never became one of the suicide statistics that are alarmingly prevalent in medicine today.

Certainly, this is a shocking example of a physical manifestation of burnout. But it is also important to recognize that many of the health care providers in the grips of burnout do not demonstrate such overt signs of it.

> Health care providers going through burnout may not show overt signs. They often suffer in silence.

Often, they suffer in silence, and you may never know they are suffering. But make no mistake: Burnout is real even if you cannot see it. The human toll on a personal level can be immense.

Treating Health Care Provider Burnout

So what are the most effective, proven treatments for burnout among health care providers? There is no shortage of lectures, webinars, and conferences claiming to hold the solutions to the burnout epidemic. There is plenty of conversation. Many people say they have answers. However, at the present time, burnout still remains an unconquered challenge in medicine.

Recently, two independent groups of researchers published rigorous meta-analyses in *The Lancet* and *JAMA Internal Medicine*, reporting on the effectiveness of interventions to combat burnout. Some interventions have been targeted at the individual physician level, and some interventions have been targeted at the organizational (health system) level.[378, 379] In other words, the interventions that have been tested are very heterogeneous. But what is striking about the vast majority of them is that, collectively, they represent what could be labeled "escapism."

Essentially, escapism is the act of getting away from patient care as much as possible to achieve a better "work-life balance." Strategies include minimizing stress by working less with patients (in order to spend more time on restorative activities like nature hikes, yoga, meditation, etc.). Another approach is to cut down on working altogether by going part-time.

The mantra goes like this: "Detach...Pull back...Get away more." Escapism is built upon the belief that if health care providers just spent less time caring for patients in favor of more self-care ("*me* time") that burnout would no longer be a problem.

Without question, maintaining a healthy work-life balance is critically important; it's vital for good health and well-being among health care providers. That's intuitive. But is detaching and pulling back from patients an effective treatment for burnout? It sounds like a plausible solution. But what is the evidence?

Research shows that many interventions based in escapism do reduce burnout... to some extent.[378, 379] But the effects are only modest at best. Accordingly, at the present time, there is no magic bullet for treating health care provider burnout.

> Escapism interventions do reduce burnout, but the effects are only modest at best.

Perhaps that is because escapism alone is an inadequate approach to solving the problem. Or perhaps it is because better work-life balance is just part of the story and does not solve the fundamental problem: A paucity of meaningful (and fulfilling) human connection in one's work.

Perhaps it is because a vital ingredient of treating burnout can only be found at *the point of care* with the patient. And perhaps the real antidote to burnout is *leaning in* rather than pulling back.

Rethinking Dogma

Historically, physicians-in-training have been taught: "Don't get *too close* to patients." The thinking was that keeping a safe distance from patients—at least emotionally—would protect the caregiver by preventing emotional overextension and thus reduce the risk of getting burned out.

Accordingly, physicians may be taught not to cross what Kenneth B. Schwartz—the lung cancer patient who inspired Schwartz Rounds—called the "professional rubicon" in caring for patients. Really connecting with patients in their times of suffering could be psychologically costly, according to this teaching. Essentially, the belief was that too much compassion would burn you out.

But you won't find this teaching in any medical textbook. Rather, it's part of the "hidden curriculum" of medical training that you learned about earlier. This teaching has been passed down, albeit informally, to generations of physicians.

But here's the problem with that historical thinking: It's actually *not* evidence-based. In fact, the available scientific evidence tells a very different story.

Of course, it is intuitive to some extent that there could be risk of burnout with repeated or excessive exposure to human suffering. However, the preponderance of data in the scientific literature supports a different view: It shows that human connection can transform the experience for the *giver* of compassion, trigger positive emotion, and build *resilience*. (That's the ability to maintain one's own well-being despite stressful conditions, including witnessing suffering.)

Let's look at the data. If there were scientific studies that supported that historical thinking (i.e., "Don't get too close; too much compassion will burn you out."), we'd expect them to show a *positive* association (correlation) between compassion and burnout. That is, we'd expect that high compassion would be associated with high burnout, and that low compassion would be associated with low burnout, right? Compassion and burnout would go in the same direction.

But if you systematically analyze the available evidence in the biomedical literature, you will find that the preponderance of data among health care providers actually shows the *opposite* to be true. A recent rigorous systematic review published in *Burnout Research* reported that the vast majority of published studies testing the association between compassion and burnout in health care providers found an *inverse* correlation.[380] Inverse!

That is, high compassion was associated with low burnout, and low compassion was associated with high burnout. So when you actually dive into the published scientific data, compassion and burnout go in *opposite* directions.

So these data do *not* support the historical thinking that too much compassion will burn you out. This rigorous systematic review of the biomedical literature suggests that the historical thinking may actually be propping up a complete myth.

A quick side note: For millennia, philosophers and thinkers have intuitively understood that compassion for others could be beneficial for one's own well-being. For example, way back in the 13th century, the famed mystic and poet Rumi said, *"When we practice loving kindness and compassion, we are the first ones to profit."*

Then, in the late 1800s, American writer and philosopher Elbert Hubbard noted that, *"Human service is the highest form of self-interest for the person who serves."* Later, Dutch theologian Henri Nouwen said, *"Our greatest fulfillment lies in giving ourselves to others,"* and, *"The joy that compassion brings is one of the best-kept secrets of humanity. It is a secret known only to a very few people, a secret that has to be rediscovered over and over again."*

More recently, Buddhist teacher and compassion activist Joan Halifax explained that *"Many of us think that compassion drains us, but I promise you it is something that truly enlivens us."*[381] This is not a new idea!

Crime of (Mis)Interpretation?

Many people in health care who understand there is an inverse relationship between compassion and burnout tend to interpret the inverse relationship (that high burnout correlates with low compassion) this way: Burnout crushes one's ability to be compassionate. They believe that when health care providers get burned out this drains their compassion.

However, it is very important to recognize that one should not infer causation from the available data, only association. Inferring causation when only association is known is a really common mistake people make when interpreting scientific studies.

In academic medicine, it's considered a crime to mix up association and causation. Maybe it's not a felony, but it's a misdemeanor for sure. And it happens all the time.

Here is a famous example: People who own a washing machine are more likely to die in a car crash. Why? Do clean clothes make you a worse driver? Does using the small knobs on a washing machine make it harder to use a steering wheel?

Of course not. The two are only *correlated,* which is an association, rather than causation. People that have the economic means to own a washing machine (versus having to take their clothes to a laundromat to do laundry) are also more likely to have the economic means to own a car. Also, people who own cars are at higher risk for getting in a car crash. So, when it comes to owning a washing machine and crashing a car, the two just go together. It is not something about washing machines that *causes* car crashes or vice versa.

This mistake is so common in the interpretation of scientific data that it spurred a popular (and humorous) website that has now become a book, called *Spurious Correlations*, where the purveyor collects data on quirky correlations in which causation is ridiculously implausible.[382] (One example: There is a

99 percent correlation between the divorce rate in Maine and the per capita consumption of margarine.)[383]

While causation *might* exist with correlated data, you just can't assume it. Making the assumption of causation is considered a crime in the world of statistics, including academic medicine. But, again, it's just a misdemeanor. People make this mistake all the time.

But beware of a potential felony! An academic crime worse than mixing up association and causation is the crime of assuming causation in the *wrong direction*…mixing up which factor is the cause and which is the effect. So if you assume causation when you should not, you may get off with just a fine. But if you go beyond that to assume causation in the wrong direction, you will be thrown behind bars (academically speaking, of course).

Consider this example: Smoking is associated with lung cancer. It is also undeniable, based on decades of iron-clad research, that smoking *causes* lung cancer. Everybody knows that. But did you know that frequent alcohol consumption is also associated with lung cancer?

Mainly, it's because people who smoke are also more likely to drink alcohol. Alcohol is not the major driver of the risk of lung cancer; it's smoking that is causing lung cancer. But alcohol use and lung cancer go together, for sure, even though smoking is the main cause. It would be a crime (and an error) to attribute all of the causation that is due to smoking to the consumption of alcohol. And yet, as noted, that's just a misdemeanor.

You know what's a felony? Interpreting that data to suggest that lung cancer causes smoking or alcohol consumption. In academic circles, if you make this mistake they will throw the book at you! And it doesn't take a background in medicine to know how silly it would be to think that lung cancer causes smoking.

A Contrarian Interpretation

Now, back to compassion and burnout. As noted earlier, many in health care have fallen into the trap of assuming that the inverse relationship between compassion and burnout means that burnout causes compassion to take a nosedive.

But we can't really make that leap. Here's why: Most of the research specifically honing in on the relationship between compassion and burnout has been comprised of cross-sectional studies—testing associations at a snapshot in time—rather than longitudinal studies with an experimental design (such as randomized controlled trials).

Without experimental studies, this is not only a setup for incorrectly assuming causation when there is only association—a misdemeanor—but it is also a trap for the full-blown felony of assuming causation in the wrong direction.[384]

How so, you ask? What if burnout does not cause a drop in compassion, but rather it's *the other way around?*

> Health care providers who have low compassion are predisposed to becoming burned out.

That is, health care providers who have low compassion are *predisposed* to becoming burned out. Could it be that low compassion increases the risk of developing burnout?

It may sound like a somewhat radical (or perhaps contrarian) concept when you lay it out, that high compassion is *protective* against burnout. But after a thorough review of the scientific evidence, as you will see shortly, the preponderance of data points to this as the most likely explanation for which factor is the cause and which factor is the effect.

Here's another way to think about it: Under the same amount of stress, a determinant of who will or will not get burned out may be a person's compassion for others. And the corollary to this would be that interventions to *raise* one's compassion could prevent burnout or even counteract burnout in people who already have it. Based on the available scientific data in published research studies, this explanation for the observed inverse relationship between compassion and burnout is quite plausible.[384]

This brings us to a crucial question: Could compassion actually be an "antidote" for burnout? It's a key question to examine.

In exploring this, let's consider all of the scientific evidence that compassion for others can build resilience. In the health care environment, that's the data that connecting with patients through compassion can transform a health care provider's experience in a positive and fulfilling way that builds resistance to burnout. If you are a health care provider, it's the evidence that compassion for others is actually good for *you*.[385]

But before reviewing all of the data, let's first acknowledge something important: Without question, seeing others who are in pain can be painful. When someone sees another person suffering, and doesn't run away to escape, it hits them right in the pain center of the brain, as demonstrated in research using functional MRI scans.[10]

When we detect and resonate with another's pain, we too can experience pain by bearing witness to that individual's suffering. The recognition, feeling, and mirroring or understanding of another's emotions is empathy.

But remember that compassion is different from empathy. It's not seeing or feeling someone's pain. Rather, compassion is *action*. When taking action to relieve someone else's suffering, a distinctly different area of the brain lights up on functional MRI: a "reward" pathway that is associated with affiliation and positive emotions.[11, 12] It's a pleasurable experience for the *giver* of compassion.

But it's not just about emotions; it goes deeper than that. The personal connection aspect of compassion is vital for one's *fulfillment*. Research shows that compassion for others can be a coping strategy to overcome personal distress and strengthen one's own resilience.[11]

So how are health care providers supposed to protect themselves from the pain of bearing witness to suffering? It is intuitive that there is intrinsic risk to the psyche of caregivers that can culminate in personal distress.

One key factor identified in psychological science research is called "self-other differentiation" or "self-other distinction."[386, 387, 388] Simply stated, this is your ability to be in the presence of a person in pain or suffering and always remain cognizant that it is not your own pain and suffering.

It's the ability to experience and understand what others feel without confusion between yourself and others. It's knowing that the emotions you are resonating with are the emotions of another and not your own.

Although the pain and suffering may be terrible, it's happening to the patient and it's not actually happening to you. Be thankful for that. Blurring the self-other distinction through excessive sharing of others' negative emotions can lead to shared distress. And that could indeed be harmful.[11]

The second key way to protect oneself from a patient's pain and distress is to meet that suffering with action. Taking action to relieve another's suffering is at the very heart what it means to be compassionate and brings reward that can overcome the distress of empathy.[11, 12]

The Evidence in Neuroscience and Psychology Research

There is abundant data in neuroscience and psychology research showing how compassion for others promotes well-being for the *giver* of compassion. There's also plenty of data to support that compassion for others can promote resilience, well-being, and resistance to burnout specifically among health care providers.

Hopefully, after seeing all of the data, you'll be open to the possibility that compassion could be effective in relieving burnout. And, perhaps, if you are struggling with burnout, you'll find the data compelling enough to test the compassion hypothesis for *yourself.*

Seth Gillihan, a psychology professor at the University of Pennsylvania, once explained the symbiotic relationship between giving and receiving compassion like this: *"Coming together (in compassion) works a sort of alchemy, transforming one person's pain into a shared feeling of uplift. Indeed, compassion is the opposite of a zero-sum game in which there are winners and losers: Both giver and receiver benefit."*[389]

> Seventy percent of people experience a feel-good sensation when giving meaningful help to others in need.

For decades, scientists have been aware of a phenomenon called the "helper's high." This is the good feeling you get when you help others in a meaningful way. Research shows that approximately 70 percent of people experience this type of feel-good sensation when giving meaningful help to others in need (some scientists call it a "warm glow"), accompanied by an inner calmness and an enhanced feeling of self-worth.[390]

Research also shows that it makes people feel less depressed. That's because being focused on another's well-being can help you forget your own worries, at least temporarily.[391] When you are down, you may be uplifted by picking others up.[392] This makes sense, because extensive research published in the psychology domain has identified a similar phenomenon; people who are self-focused actually experience *more* depression and anxiety.[393]

One can definitely experience a helper's high when showing others compassion. That is, not just helping for the sake of helping, but rather helping as a response to another's pain and suffering. You will recall that compassion is defined as the emotional response to another's pain or suffering involving an authentic desire to *help*.[7]

But when your compassion for others triggers a helper's high, how does that "work" exactly? There are multiple potential mechanisms of action—some of which also apply to the effects on the receiver of compassion, as noted earlier in Chapter 3. But interestingly these same mechanisms are also in play for the giver.

One mechanism is a sharp spike in circulating endorphins, endogenous—or natural—opiates produced by the body.[390] Another mechanism is that giving meaningful help to others (and specifically, a compassionate response to suffering) activates reward pathways in the brain that produce positive affect and emotions.[394] In other words, it activates the part of the brain that gives you the experience of happiness. One more mechanism for the "helper's high" is that compassionate helping is stress-buffering.

In fact, there are two ways that compassionate helping can alleviate stress for the person giving compassion. One is a nervous system effect: Compassion for others activates the parasympathetic nervous system by increasing vagus nerve activity.[395] This results in a calming effect that counterbalances the "fight or flight" response of the sympathetic nervous system. The other is by boosting circulating neuromodulators (such as the hormone oxytocin) which not only buffers stress, but also triggers positive emotions (such as feelings of calm and closeness).[396]

All of these mechanisms are activated when we are "other-focused"—focused on service to others. A robust body of scientific evidence shows that these physiological mechanisms translate to better health and well-being for the one who serves. So serving others is actually good for *you*.

Now let's look at the data supporting that compassion for others can be stress-buffering. Psychology research shows that resonance between the giver and the receiver of compassion increases the ability of the giver to benefit from receiving compassion, through this reduced response to stress.[397] These include things like lower blood pressure reactivity, better heart rate variability, and lower cortisol (stress hormone) release.

Further, a randomized trial from Emory University tested the effects of compassion training on the response to a standardized (i.e., experimental) stressful event applied in a laboratory and found that compassion was associated with reduced blood markers of systemic inflammation, in addition to reduced psychological distress.[398]

But perhaps the most interesting data is on human *happiness*. Neuroscience research shows that the most potent activator of brain circuits involved in human happiness is actually...*compassion*.

In Chapter 9, you were introduced to French scientist (and Buddhist monk) Mathieu Ricard. In his TED Talk "The Habits of Happiness," Ricard relates the story of his experience with a scientific experiment that led him to become widely known as "the happiest man in the world."[334] Ricard is more than just an expert in compassion, he is a true outlier among outliers, having logged tens of thousands of hours over the course of his lifetime in meditation on loving-kindness and compassion.

When Ricard was studied in Richard Davidson's lab at the University of Wisconsin-Madison, they found something startling. After connecting 256 electrodes to Ricard's head and performing EEG (as described in Chapter 9), as well as functional MRI scans of the brain, they found that he was an outlier in one particular way that had never been seen before in any research.

Compared to the data for 150 control subjects—regular people—Ricard was off the charts in one very specific type of brain activity: the pattern of activity observed in the experience of human *happiness*.[335]

The data for Ricard's brain activity were not merely a couple of standard deviations away from the norm, either. His data were so far outside the bell curve (in the happiness zone) that he was in a world all his own. (Hence, his "happiest man" title.)

So when Ricard was generating brain activity for happiness unlike anything ever seen before, what was he doing? He was meditating on one thing and one thing only: *compassion for others*. Ricard considers compassion for others to be the happiest state ever. And he has the neuroscience data to prove it![335]

Other neuroscience research that has studied visual attention with precise eye-tracking methodologies has found that compassion training can help you keep your eyes focused on someone when they suffering, rather than looking away, while simultaneously *reducing* the activation in the areas of the brain associated with negative affect and emotion.[399] In other words, augmenting compassion helps you not only bear witness to human suffering, but to actually stay focused on it. Compassion does that in such a way that it does not hurt you.

Similarly, other neuroscience research showed film clips of people suffering to study subjects and then performed functional MRI scans on their brains.[400] These researchers also found that augmenting study subjects' compassion is helpful for regulating their own emotions.

> **Compassion for others can overcome the distress associated with seeing other people in distress.**

Despite being shown painful, distressing images, boosting participants' compassion activated reward centers in the brain and generated positive (rather than negative) affect and emotions. So these data support that compassion for others can overcome the distress associated with seeing other people in distress. Other neuroscience research corroborates this same finding.[11] Further, it shows that compassion can strengthen our personal resilience.

Think of it as a coping strategy: Compassion builds positive emotional resources even when confronted with the distress of others.[12] So, when it comes to caring for patients, "leaning in" with more compassion may be adaptive (rather than maladaptive) and thereby reduce the risk of burnout (rather than raising it).

Can an intense focus on compassion for others really make you feel better? That's what researchers from Stanford University investigated in one study.[401] They recruited volunteers to participate in a trial of "loving-kindness meditation" (LKM), a well-established meditation practice where one willfully and intently directs compassion and wishes for well-being toward another person in order to create changes in one's own emotion, motivation, and behavior.

They found that practicing LKM for just 1.7 hours per month (just a few minutes per day, on average) not only raised feelings of social connection but also raised feelings of positive affect. The results show that it helped people feel calm and happy.

The same Stanford University researchers then conducted a randomized controlled trial of just a single session (ten minutes) of LKM in volunteers.[402] They found that participants randomized to LKM not only had a significant boost in their compassion for others, along with a reduction in self-focus, but they also demonstrated increased positive affect and well-being.

So they felt significantly better, even after just ten minutes of intense focus on compassion for others. It may seem surprising that such a short intervention could have meaningful effects, but the data indicate that it works.

These results were corroborated by another group of Stanford University researchers who found that a compassion cultivation training program could improve emotion regulation by increasing positive affect and calmness and decreasing anxiety and worry.[403, 404] Another randomized controlled study found that augmenting the practice of compassion for others is even associated with lasting gains: up to six months in happiness and self-esteem in general and reduced depressive symptoms in people with anxiety.[405]

How? Compassion for others releases the mind from the harmful effects of negative emotions. In compelling research from the University of North Carolina at Chapel Hill, scientists found that routinely and intentionally focusing one's mind on kindness to others, as part of a disciplined practice, results in the building of positive emotions over time with an associated increase in personal resources.[406] That's to say that study participants felt an increased purpose in life, enjoyed more social support, and experienced fewer symptoms of illness.

And here's one more example of a similar finding. Dr. James Kirby, a clinical psychologist and renowned compassion researcher from the University of Queensland in Australia, recently published a meta-analysis that synthesized the world's scientific literature on compassion-based interventions for psychological conditions.[162, 407]

After collating and analyzing all the data—which included 21 randomized controlled trials and more than 1,200 total participants—Kirby and his colleagues found that interventions to generate compassion were associated with major benefits. These included significantly lower depression, lower anxiety, lower psychological distress, and enhanced well-being. The signal in the data is clear; giving compassion has tremendous psychological benefits.

Effects on Health Care Providers

Now that you know what compassion can do for one's stress, emotions, resilience, and well-being, let's revisit the relationship between compassion and burnout as it specifically relates to health care providers. Because, as Ralph Waldo Emerson once pointed out, "*It is one of the most beautiful compensations of life that no man can sincerely try to help another without helping himself.*"

As noted earlier, research shows that compassion and burnout among health care providers are inversely related: high compassion is associated with low burnout, and low compassion is associated with high burnout. The evidence for positive impact of compassion on the well-being of the giver in the neuroscience and psychology worlds certainly hints at a likely protective benefit for health care providers at risk of burnout, but that evidence was not specific to the health care context.

So what are the specific studies that show this relationship in health care providers? Numerous clinical research studies have found a link between compassion, enhanced resilience, and lower burnout among health care providers. Now that we have laid out the mechanisms by which that occurs, let's consider the evidence.

A study from Kyoto University in Japan assessed burnout in nurses, using the Maslach Burnout Inventory and performing functional MRI scans of the nurses' brains, with stunning results.[408] What they found was that burnout severity in the nurses was explained by reduced activation of areas of the brain involved in compassion.

Nurses with functional MRI evidence of low activity in compassion centers of the brain scored the highest in burnout. If the historical belief—"Too much compassion will burn you out"—were true, wouldn't you expect that researchers would find evidence to the contrary?

In a cross-sectional study of resident physicians from the Mayo Clinic, researchers measured compassion of the physicians using a validated measurement tool called the Interpersonal Reactivity Index, as well as a validated scale measuring their mental well-being.[409] They found that greater physician compassion was associated with greater well-being.

> Higher compassion is associated with lower depression symptoms, a higher sense of personal accomplishment, and enhanced quality of life.

A follow-up study from the same group of Mayo Clinic researchers, using similar methodology, examined more than a thousand medical students in a multi-center study.[410] The researchers found an inverse association with compassion; students with high compassion had low burnout and vice versa. Higher compassion was also associated with lower depression symptoms, a higher sense of personal accomplishment, and enhanced quality of life.

And this isn't true only for medical students, either. There is substantial evidence that an inverse relationship also exists between compassion and burnout among practicing physicians. A survey study of 7,500 physicians found that those who had the lowest compassion satisfaction (i.e., the least amount of pleasure from compassion for others) had the highest burnout and personal distress.[294]

These physicians with low compassion satisfaction also missed the most days of work and were more likely to take a medical leave of absence. The researchers found significantly less personal distress among physicians who had high compassion satisfaction (i.e., experienced pleasure from compassion).

In an eye-opening study of 294 primary care physicians, researchers found that in a multivariable model controlling for potential confounders, physicians' compassion was independently associated with lower physician burnout.[411] The researchers concluded that physician compassion may be *protective* against burnout.

But what about under really stressful conditions, like in the emergency department? Being an emergency nurse is unquestionably one of the hardest jobs in health care. Among emergency nurses, researchers have found that more compassion is associated with higher scores for nurse well-being.[412]

> It appears that when health care providers are under the most stress, that compassion is needed the most for their own well-being.

Similarly, researchers have found that among emergency physicians, the ability to maintain compassion for patients was a distinguishing feature of satisfaction in their professional quality of life.[241] It appears that when health care providers are under the most stress, that compassion is needed the most for their own well-being.

Most of the studies mentioned here are observational studies looking at associations between compassion and burnout. As has been mentioned multiple times in earlier chapters, the most compelling evidence comes from research with an experimental design where prescribed interventions are tested.

So are there any such studies looking at compassion and burnout? *Yes.*

One such study from the University of Rochester, published in *JAMA*, trained seventy primary care physicians in techniques to be fully present and attentive with their patients over an eight-week period.[413] The researchers found that this experience raised the physicians' belief in the importance of compassion as well as their self-ratings of their own compassion. But that's not all: They also found that the physicians' burnout symptoms decreased while their scores for well-being increased.

A recent randomized controlled trial of compassion training from Emory University holds some of the most persuasive scientific data on the power of compassion for the *giver.*[414] In a group of 132 physicians-in-training, the researchers randomized the participants to a ten-week compassion training program versus assignment to a waitlist (which was the control group).

They found that students randomized to compassion training not only developed more compassion for others, but they also experienced a decrease in any symptoms of depression that they might have had. Further, the effects on their depression symptoms were found to be the greatest among those who had the highest level of depression symptoms at baseline, suggesting that compassion training may benefit those most in need by breaking the link between low compassion and personal suffering.

Relationships Matter

When it comes to healing burnout, the Dalai Lama perhaps expressed it best when he advised: "*Cultivating a close, warm-hearted feeling for others automatically puts the mind at ease. It helps remove whatever fears or insecurities we may have and gives us the strength to cope with any obstacles we encounter.*"

So how does a culture of compassion in the workplace impact the well-being and risk of burnout among health care workers?

Think back to the University of Pennsylvania study of 13 long-term care centers (nursing homes) from Chapter 7.[293] In that study, you will recall that they surveyed the health care workers using a validated instrument to determine if there was a culture of compassion in their workplace.

Researchers also measured the health care workers' emotional exhaustion, which is a key component of burnout. They found that a compassionate culture in the workplace was associated with less emotional exhaustion among these health care workers. Clearly, relationships matter. In this study, being a part of a compassionate workplace culture transformed these workers' experience and lowered their risk of burnout.

In a similar study from Virginia Commonwealth University, researchers measured compassion practices across thirty different outpatient clinics in an academic health system, as assessed by 177 nurses who worked there.[415] They also measured emotional exhaustion and psychological vitality among the nurses, as well as patient experience.

In assessing compassion practices across the thirty clinics, the nurses were asked if employees were recognized and rewarded (through an awards program) for acts of caring shown to patients and families or for acts of caring shown to coworkers. They were also asked if there was a culture of supporting employees through difficult times or workplace stress.

What they found is that a compassionate workplace culture was associated with lower emotional exhaustion and better psychological vitality among the nurses. And there is evidence that this culture also impacted nurse behavior towards patients: Where there was a compassionate workplace culture, the patients perceived greater caring by nurses.

The evidence suggests that patients feel a compassionate culture in the health care workplace and this is associated with better well-being among the nurses providing that greater care and compassion. In summary, the data suggest that a culture of compassionate care can be a *virtuous* cycle—resulting in more compassion for those being served and better well-being for those who serve.

These data on a compassionate culture, and the meaningful relationships that flow from it, make sense if you think back to Chapter 3 and the Harvard Study of Adult Development.[416] That's the ongoing study that has been in progress for over eighty years now in which researchers have found that good relationships were a better predictor of people's health than traditional medical markers such as cholesterol levels.[86]

In fact, it was the people who were the most satisfied in their relationships with others at age 50 that were the healthiest at age 80. It appears that relationships matter in the context of health care providers as well.

In a study of physicians-in-training, researchers from Thomas Jefferson University similarly found an inverse association between compassion and burnout that was impacted by personal relationships.[417] They learned that higher compassion was associated with lower burnout and concluded that this was because compassion for others is conducive to relationship building, which builds personal resilience. Multiple other studies of physicians (and physicians-in-training) have also found an inverse association exists between compassion for others and burnout symptoms.[32, 418, 419]

So human connection and meaningful relationships may be a mediator of the association between high compassion and low burnout in trainees just beginning their careers, but what about the opposite end of the spectrum? What about for established physician leaders?

An interesting study from Dr. Kandi Wiens at the University of Pennsylvania, highlighted in *Harvard Business Review*, shines a light on the importance of practicing compassion for others among physician leaders (administrators) in health care organizations.[420, 421, 422]

Specifically, Wiens' research used structured interviews and a rigorous qualitative research methodology to study stress and burnout in 35 physicians who were chief medical officers (CMOs) of large hospitals and health systems. What Dr. Wiens and colleagues found was that 69 percent of CMOs had stress that was "severe," "very severe," or "worst possible."

And yet, despite all this stress, the majority of CMOs were actually *not* suffering from burnout. In general, burnout among CMOs was much lower than expected.

What did the researchers find was the key ingredient to the CMOs resilience from extreme stress? It was compassion for others! They found that for *91 percent* of CMOs, actively practicing compassion for others in their CMO roles reduced or counteracted their stress and also reduced their risk of burnout. They found that compassion was one of the CMOs' secrets for resilience.

> Physicians who had the most *dissatisfaction* with the quality of their relationships with patients had a *22-fold higher* risk of burnout.

There is more compelling data that the relationships physicians have with their patients matters for the well-being of physicians. In a cross-sectional study of 839 physicians across multiple specialties, researchers found that physicians who had the most *dissatisfaction* with the quality of their relationships with patients had a *22-fold higher* risk of burnout.[423]

Another study found that among primary care physicians, high emotional intelligence of the physician was associated with not only better patient experience, but also higher physician professional satisfaction and lower burnout.[424] These data support that connecting with patients in a meaningful way produces a better patient experience that can also transform the physician's experience in a meaningful way. And that leads to lower risk of burnout.

Similarly, other research—in primary care physicians, specifically—has identified that compassion for patients is a vital contributor to professional satisfaction.[425] Also notable: Research demonstrates that a *minimum level* of compassion is needed for a physician to benefit from the positive aspects of professional fulfillment and quality of life in the practice of medicine.[426]

> Compassionate physicians are more likely to be considered a "role model."

In case you were wondering, there is evidence that colleagues take notice when health care providers are especially compassionate. In fact, a study from Johns Hopkins University, published in *The New England Journal of Medicine*, found that compassionate physicians are more likely to be considered a "role model."[427]

The researchers asked Johns Hopkins resident physicians to name the supervising attending physicians that they believed to be the best role models. They then studied all attending physicians to determine which qualities were the most admirable.

They found that attending physicians who consistently stressed the importance of a compassionate doctor-patient relationship in their teaching had *2.6 times higher odds* of being perceived as a role model by the trainees. Certainly, being thought of as a role model can enhance professional fulfilment, well-being, and a sense of purpose in a physician's career.

Compassion for *Yourself*

Imagine you are a health care provider and one of your patients suffers a poor outcome. Now imagine what it feels like if you think that maybe you could have done something differently. Maybe things would have turned out differently.

Maybe, in retrospect, you are second-guessing what you did or the decisions you made. Even worse, maybe you clearly made a mistake. Now imagine the worst-case scenario of all: your patient has died. Imagine what all the second-guessing must feel like. Imagine the weight of that on your mind.

In intensive care medicine and emergency medicine—two of the fields with the highest physician burnout rates in all of medicine—health care providers feel this weight frequently. In these fields, health care providers often have to make split-second decisions based on limited information with someone's life hanging in the balance. And they see the worst patient outcomes imaginable.

Even the most knowledgeable and skilled clinicians find themselves with cases where, in retrospect, they wish they could turn back time and choose a different approach that just maybe could have saved a life. Imagine what that feels like to have tried and failed. Maybe there were forks in the road where if different decisions were made it could have changed things just enough to alter an outcome.

The guilt and the pain weigh on the mind…and the soul. In struggling with the weight of that, health care providers can go to dark places: depression, anxiety, insomnia, nightmares, and even flashbacks. They can't stop replaying these situations in their heads.

Repeatedly, they beat themselves up over what they could have or should have done differently. If one was already suffering from burnout, a bad patient outcome (with a sense of a missed opportunity to make a difference) could be the thing that sends a health care provider "over the edge."

What do we tell a health care provider in the midst of this struggle? What should they be telling *themselves?*

As Lama Yeshe, a Tibetan spiritual teacher advised, "*Be gentle first with yourself if you wish to be gentle with others.*" A similar approach is recommended by Dr. Kristin Neff, one of the world's leading researchers on the topic of "self-compassion."

With self-compassion, we offer ourselves the same kindness and care we would offer to a good friend going through the same circumstances.[428] A foundation of self-compassion is the recognition that failure and imperfection are part of the human condition.

Dr. Neff further explains self-compassion this way:

> "*Instead of mercilessly judging and criticizing yourself for various inadequacies or shortcomings, self-compassion means you are kind and understanding when confronted with personal failings—after all, who ever said you were supposed to be perfect?*"[429]

If you realize the importance of compassion for others in a time of personal failure, then when you are in need of that compassion yourself, you must make sure that your internal dialogue reflects the same encouragement and compassion you would show to others in your situation.

Of course, when a bad patient outcome occurs, thoughtful introspection and accountability are important. But the quality of this internal dialogue is key. For far too many health care providers, the internal dialogue that they hear repeatedly is not the voice of understanding and compassion, but rather a horrible, berating voice that can lead to an overwhelming depression they cannot escape.

In her book, *Self-Compassion: The Proven Power of Being Kind to Yourself*, Dr. Neff walks readers through the rigorous science behind self-compassion, and the evidence-based approaches to increase one's self-compassion. But one simple way to think about it is this: When you are struggling with failure, what would your best friend say to you (or about you)? Does your internal dialogue match what your best friend would say?

A poignant example of this comes from the work of psychology researcher Dr. James Kirby, who you were introduced to earlier in this chapter. Kirby relates a story of working with a 17-year-old male on self-compassion.[430] Kirby asked this young man to consider scenarios where serious failure was experienced and then write down five things he would say to a friend going through that failure.

Then, Kirby asked him to write down five things he would say to himself in that exact same failure. The results were startling:

To a friend, this teenager said: "There's always next time." "They don't deserve you." "You're only human." "I'm stupid too." "Don't listen to them."

But to *himself* he said: "I'm a failure." "No one likes me." "I'm an idiot." "I'm stupid." "He's right."

Kirby appropriately sums up the boy's internal dialogue to himself in just one word: "*Devastating.*"

Dr. Dennis Tirch, a renowned expert in compassion-focused therapy, describes self-compassion like this: *"It isn't about negating or rejecting undesirable thoughts like self-criticism or shame. It's about extending validation, warmth and caring to them, and recognizing where they're coming from. The same as we would do to a friend who was suffering."*[431]

In this chapter, you have seen the scientific evidence that compassion can be an antidote to burnout and a powerful promoter of resilience and one's own well-being. But that was compassion for *others*. It is also vital to realize that another powerful promoter of resilience is treating *yourself* with the same compassion that you already know makes a meaningful difference in the treatment of others.

Your internal dialogue must also be a voice of compassion—for yourself.

When it comes to health care providers who struggle with the reality of a poor patient outcome, they often mercilessly beat themselves up over what they could have or should have done differently. This is fuel to the fire of burnout.

If you find yourself in that moment…*stop*. *Stop* beating yourself up.

Instead, remember this question: *Is that what your best friend would say to you?*

Steve's Story: A Life-Changing (n=1) Experiment[432]

So this is where the science converges with the personal. A couple of years ago, after nearly twenty years of working in an ICU, and literally meeting people on the worst day of their lives, I came to a stark realization…I had almost every symptom of burnout.

Let me assure you, it's not a good place to be. It can be a dark place.

Currently, the recommended prescription for burnout in health care workers is "escapism." Get away. Pull back. Detach. Go on a nature hike. Meditate…or do yoga.

I get it. Sometimes you just need to get away, and I believe that things that help you relax (like nature hikes or yoga) have their place. But I was not buying that escapism was the answer.

My intuition, and my twenty years of experience, told me that the true antidote to burnout was not in escaping, but rather at the point of care. After a rigorous systematic review of the biomedical literature, and newly armed with all the scientific data that compassion can be a powerful therapy for the giver, too, I believed the solution was in more human connection, not less. That was my hypothesis.

So, in searching for recovery from burnout, I did the only thing I knew how to do…I took the "research nerd" approach. I decided to test my hypothesis. I decided to do an experiment—on myself. In this experiment, there was only one study subject: me. I was the "n of 1."

I tested the hypothesis that having more compassion for others would transform my experience. I gave patients my forty seconds of compassion. I connected more, not less. I cared more, not less. I leaned in, rather than pulling back.

And that was when the "fog" of burnout began to lift for me. Being intentional about compassion, and giving others my forty seconds of compassion, changed everything.

But let's be clear: You don't have to be a health care worker to feel burned out. If you are feeling this way, consider testing the compassion hypothesis…for yourself.

Try your "n of 1" experiment.

See those in need around you and give them your forty seconds of compassion, every opportunity that you have. See how it transforms your experience.

But don't do it because I say so; do it because science says so.

—Stephen Trzeciak, M.D., TEDxPenn, April 7, 2018

CONCLUSION:

"We live in a time when science is validating what humans have known throughout the ages: that compassion is not a luxury; it is a necessity for our well-being, resilience, and survival."

—Joan Halifax

When we started on this journey together, we set out to answer this question: Does compassion *really* matter?

In these pages, we have laid out all the evidence: the results of a systematic review of the biomedical literature in which we curated and synthesized the data from more than 1,000 scientific abstracts and more than 250 original science research papers.

You've seen the unmistakable difference that compassion can make.

> Compassion matters—for patients, for patient care, and for those who care for patients.

After analyzing all of the evidence, we conclude with confidence: compassion *matters*—for patients, for patient care, and for those who care for patients.

Compassion matters in not only meaningful ways, but also in measurable ways. Compassionate care is more effective than health care without compassion, by virtue of the fact that human connection confers distinct and measurable benefits.

Remember that these data are not what we *think*, nor are they what we *believe*. Rather, they are what we *found*. Compassionate care belongs in the domain of evidence-based medicine.

Compassionomics, therefore, is where the science and the art of medicine *converge*. There is science in the art of medicine, and the science is strong.

This journey represents a scientific awakening for us—an awakening to a truth that was right in front of us all along. We see it now. And now, after you have seen all the data, we hope that you, too, are awakened to the true power of compassion.

If you've read this far, it is likely that you already knew in your heart that compassion was powerful. But we never aimed to change your heart; your heart was already in the right place. Rather, in writing this book we aimed to change your *mind*...to help open your eyes to the scientific basis of what you already know to be the right thing to do.

And yet, a scientific justification for compassion was never *really* necessary. Compassion was, and always will be, the right thing to do. It's about treating patients the way they ought to be treated, the way they want to be treated, and the way we would want to be treated ourselves.

Still, after seeing all the science behind the power of compassion, we hope that you will be even more inspired to use your compassion at every opportunity you have.

You are *powerful*. Science shows that your compassion can be more powerful than you've ever dreamed. You don't have to be board-certified—or even go to medical school or nursing school—to make a critical difference in the lives of others. (Or even in your own life.)

Way back in Chapter 1, you saw a list of reasons (excuses, really) to justify why health care providers frequently fail to treat patients with compassion. Some people, for example, just don't see that there's a problem. But now you know that's just not true. There's a compassion crisis in health care.

Some people say they just don't have time to be compassionate. But now you know that's not true either—that it takes, on average, just forty seconds to confer all the benefits that compassion provides. You *do*, in fact, have time.

Others say they just don't know how to be compassionate. It's not in their nature. But now you understand that compassionate behaviors can be learned. You can learn, if you adopt a "growth mindset" and sincerely try.

Then there are the burned out health care providers who say they just don't care anymore; they don't care enough to show compassion. But you've learned that compassion can be so powerful for the *giver* that using compassion can actually help people begin to care again.

And finally, there are the health care providers who just don't believe compassion is that important. They think of compassion as just a "nice to have", not a science-backed intervention that must never be omitted.

But you have now reviewed a tidal wave of data on compassion's effects across a multitude of diseases and conditions. You've seen the physiological and psychological benefits, the improvement in patient self-care, and the effects on health care quality and financial sustainability that compassion delivers.

So any health care provider reading this book should be fresh out of excuses. No one that cares about delivering quality care today has a defensible reason to omit compassion from patient care. Rather, as Dr. Francis Peabody, a distinguished Harvard professor and physician, taught in a landmark *JAMA* article many decades ago, "The secret of the care of the patient is in *caring for the patient*."[433]

One last thing: and this is perhaps the most important lesson of the book. It's so important that we saved it for last.

> **Even when compassion can't "make a difference," it makes a difference.**

There are many times when compassion won't be able to change an outcome for patients and their families…when it just can't alter tragic circumstances. But always remember this: Even when compassion can't "make a difference," it makes a difference.

And that's why we—or rather, Anthony specifically— wanted to share a very personal experience with just how true this is in the most difficult of times.

Anthony's Story[434]

When I started medical school, compassion wasn't explicitly part of our curriculum. It wasn't the title of any lecture. It wasn't the answer on any test. And yet, I know that as a student I learned about compassion in the halls and patient rooms of our hospital.

For instance, in the triage area of our obstetrics (OB) department, I recall very clearly in my mind learning how to care for concerned mothers-to-be. I specifically remember one time that I watched as a concerned mother was waiting anxiously to be evaluated. Through the curtains, she could hear the heartbeat monitors for all the other patients.

I could see the worry on her face as the OB triage nurse started to do her evaluation. The nurse could tell the patient was concerned, but the nurse was clearly trying to stay upbeat.

The mother was worried because, even though she was full-term and the baby was due in a few days, she hadn't felt the baby move for hours. The nurse was moving the monitor pads around trying to find a heartbeat. It's not that unusual to have trouble finding a heartbeat, but it just added to the tension and the mother knew it.

It fed her panic. But the nurse remained calm; her voice soothing.

The patient looked up at me, but I wasn't going to go anywhere near those monitor pads. Nothing in my education was going to make me any better at understanding what was going on than the triage nurse. I remember the nurse finally said that she would get the physician, but she didn't leave before offering some more reassuring words to this mother who was now really starting to worry.

The physician rolled in the ultrasound machine, introduced herself, and offered the same calming tone. It was somewhere between, "I know this might be really bad," and, "Everything's gonna be okay." It seemed to strike the right balance which was, "You're in the right place, and you're going to get the right care, and the right thing's happening right now."

It only took a few seconds before the worst-case scenario was obvious even to me. There was no heartbeat in that fully formed baby. The mother knew the answer was clear to the physician.

"Is there a heartbeat?" asked the mother.

The physician gave it to her straight: "There is not a heartbeat."

I'll never forget the absolute sorrow at that moment. I relive that moment over and over again. Because while I had encountered this exact situation as a medical student, in this particular case, everything was alarmingly different.

In the very same room where I had experienced this situation as a medical student, I was actually now an attending physician.

And this baby was not just the patient's baby, but my son.

And this patient was not just the mother, but my wife.

And I was not just the person standing there observing, but I was the father and the husband.

While I had witnessed this scene before, I had never experienced such moments from that perspective. I have relived it hundreds, if not thousands, of times in my mind since, and I cannot tell you how much I still remember and appreciate every small aspect of compassion from everyone involved that day.

From every carefully chosen word, every supportive inflection and tone, every warm touch or moment of silence in support, the littlest things matter deeply in these situations.

And not just in the moments when patients first learn of a devastating loss or tragic diagnosis. No, the memories of those moments—and the compassion that was shared then—will be replayed again, and again, and again in all the years to come.

Their importance is magnified well beyond what caregivers realize. So I try to remember that, not only for the patients that I care for, but also for their families as well.

Patients and families may not remember your name or your face, but they will never forget the smallest comforts you offered in those moments because they will never forget the memory of what they were feeling.

—Anthony Mazzarelli, M.D., *Annals of Internal Medicine*, April 4, 2017

In such moments of unspeakable pain, let us always remember the enduring words of Kenneth B. Schwartz: Compassion "makes the unbearable *bearable*."

Compassion *always* matters.

ACKNOWLEDGMENTS:

Mutually, we want to express our deep gratitude for all of the people who made this project possible. First, we want to thank all of those that shared their personal stories with us, whether they were ultimately used in these pages or not. The willingness of so many to share heartfelt stories about themselves and their patients not only helped the data come alive but also it inspired us throughout the process of writing the book. Especially, we thank: Kacey Zorzi, Christine Fox, Meredith Johanson, Alann Solina, Mark Angelo, John Baxter, Alexandra Lane, and Jennifer Abraczinskas.

We also want to thank important pioneers in the field: the late Kenneth B. Schwartz and the Schwartz Center for Compassionate Healthcare, and the late Dr. Arnold P. Gold, Dr. Sandra Gold, and the Arnold P. Gold Foundation. For decades, they have been a guiding light toward more compassionate care in medicine.

We thank our colleagues at Cooper University Health Care. We are honored to work with such an impressive group of people. They have embraced this project and these concepts from the start, and we are continually impressed with their desire to increase compassionate care. Every day, they reinforce to us that caring makes a difference. In particular, we want to thank the physician and nursing leaders for their dedication to patients and to each other's success.

Dr. Ed Viner, mentioned multiple times in these pages, has been (and continues to be) a champion of all of the ideals contained in this book. Thank you Ed for your leadership, and for lighting the spark in us to "science this up."

We also thank the Board of Trustees at Cooper University Health Care, particularly our Chairman, George E. Norcross, III. His efforts to revitalize Camden, the city invincible, are a fantastic demonstration of compassion - for an entire community.

It is rare to find a medical school Dean that is as approachable and supportive as Annette Reboli, MD, the Dean of Cooper Medical School of Rowan University. Dean Reboli has not only been a supporter of this work from the beginning, but she has a deep understanding of these concepts from her own experience as a physician. We believe that the students, trainees, and faculty of CMSRU will be on the forefront of the research, education, and practice of compassionomics in the future, and it will be in large part because of her vision. We truly appreciate all she has done for us.

We would be remiss if we did not point out how much we appreciate the leadership of Cooper's CEO for the last six years, Adrienne Kirby, PhD, FACHE. Her influence and guidance has been felt through the entire institution and it has no doubt left a mark on this book.

We are incredibly grateful for the talents and commitment of Chris Roman, who was with us every step of the way in writing this book, and kept us moving forward and on track. Likewise, we are thankful for the tireless efforts of Jamie Stewart. Jamie not only brought the book to life, but she also had the extra patience needed to work with two science geeks who have never written a book before. We also thank Lindy Sikes, for her excellent work in proofreading and polishing. Many thanks also to Craig Deao, not only for nudging us at the very beginning and helping us believe that we could write a book, but also for keeping an eye on this project through to its completion.

We are especially grateful for Dr. Brian Roberts, who is the Science Director for our compassion research program at Cooper. In these pages, you read about Brian's ongoing research on the effects of compassionate care in the Emergency Department. He was an invaluable resource for us, helping us analyze much of the statistics in the studies included in this book. Brian is a brilliant scientist, and undoubtedly in the years to come he will leave an indelible mark on the field of compassion science. At the end of our careers, we predict that our main "claim to fame" will be that we once worked with the famous Dr. Roberts.

We are grateful for the mentorship and leadership of Dr. Michael Chansky, the Chief of Emergency Medicine at Cooper University Health Care and Chair of Emergency Medicine at Cooper Medical School of Rowan University. It is under Mike's leadership that such creative and cutting edge ideas and research happen. Much of our compassion science research is occurring in his department. Specifically in that regard, we thank Hope Kilgannon, Chris Jones, Valerie Braz, Lisa Shea, Jeena Moss, and the entire team, for embracing the hypotheses and believing that they must be tested rigorously in order for our work to have the greatest impact.

It is important to us to acknowledge our appreciation of Dr. Eric Kupersmith, the Chief Physician Executive at Cooper University Health Care. Without Eric's support and tireless efforts, there is no way we could have considered embarking on this project. Eric is a Jedi Knight when it comes to practicing compassion in physician leadership, and he is a role model for how to approach people with the utmost compassion and simultaneously holding them accountable. We suspect that the next book in this arena will likely have his name on it.

We also thank Dr. Jeffrey Brenner. Jeff's compassion for the most vulnerable citizens of Camden City led him to groundbreaking health care discoveries that have become a national model for bringing better health to the most at-risk populations. He has served as a resource, sounding board, and mentor to both us for many years. Jeff built the practice that generated some memorable stories contained in this book. He created an environment that was infused with a distinctive kind of caring, and that compassionate culture continues to this day.

We owe a special debt of gratitude to our colleague Anthony Welch. Anthony not only gave us feedback on an early draft of the book, but he was a tireless advocate in other ways as well. Before coming to Cooper, Anthony had not previously worked in the health care field, but we believe he has found a home in health care where his talents will help countless others in meaningful ways for years to come.

We also want to thank Stacey Burling of the Philadelphia Inquirer and John Kopp of Philly Voice, for their early "buy in" on compassionomics, and for helping us realize how the message resonates with people.

There are many others whose help was incredibly valuable to this project, and we are very grateful for their efforts: Tom Rubino, Jennifer Knorr, Maureen Miller, Dina Matthews, Rebecca Smith, Anthony Perno, Jennifer Perno, Jake Gordon, Jason Dravis, Lauren Westwood, Lynne Mahoney, Tasha Wells, Jared Hart, Ben Haney, Greg Stocker, and John McDonald.

For each person we have named here, there are many more that have helped in so many ways. We are grateful for all of you.

Lastly, we are grateful for the hundreds of researchers whose collective studies, some that date back half a century, comprise the message of this book. It is the works of these scholars that opened our eyes to the true power of compassion, and compelled us to tell this story.

Personal Acknowledgments from Stephen Trzeciak:

First, I thank my parents, Vi and Walt, for starting me on this journey, and encouraging me and supporting me unconditionally every step of the way.

I thank Dr. Ed Viner for being an inspiration for this book, and an exemplary role model for compassionate care. It is a tremendous honor to follow in his footsteps as the Chair of Medicine at Cooper, a role that was his for more than two decades. I am very grateful for all the support and encouragement he has given me, and continues to give me.

I am especially grateful for Dr. Phil Dellinger. He has been not only an amazing mentor and ardent supporter for me over the years, but also a very close friend. I am not sure where I would be today if not for him. Definitely not writing a book, that's for sure.

I am so thankful for Dr. Sergio Zanotti, the real Professor. I thank him for his friendship and constant encouragement over the years, and for helping me believe I could do this.

I also thank Dr. Nitin Puri, who is not only an amazing friend, but also the leader of our group of critical care physicians at Cooper (in which I still practice). Nitin is an inspirational leader who cares deeply about people, and I am very thankful to be one of those people. Nitin is already doing a way better job of leading our critical care team than the guy who did it before him, and I am thankful for that.

I thank all of the nurses that I have been so fortunate to work alongside in the intensive care unit at Cooper for the past 16 years. They put their hearts and souls into caring for the critically ill. They have been a wellspring of compassion for patients that continues to amaze me to this day. My medical training and textbooks taught me how to treat patients, but these nurses have helped me understand what it really means to *take care* of patients.

I owe a special debt of gratitude, one I could not possibly repay, to the patients and families I have had the privilege of caring for in the Cooper ICU over the past 16 years. The lessons they taught me were part of the genesis of this book, and a common thread through all of its pages.

I am so fortunate to be part of an incredible group of people in the Adult Health Institute (AHI) at Cooper, especially: Pam Ladu, Megan Avila,

Sunil Marwaha, Jim Haddock, Karen Kutner, Dan Hyman, Eddie Mahamitra, Mark Angelo, and so many others. Thank you for helping our health care providers give great care. I look forward to collaborating with you to infuse the lessons from compassionomics into everything that we do.

I am especially thankful for Rebecca Smith, my awesome assistant. I would love to say that Rebecca and I make a great team, but that would be giving me too much credit. She is responsible for so much of our success, and this book would never have come together without her support. In addition, Rebecca shows great kindness to everyone we collaborate with, and that sets a great example for me and the whole AHI team to follow.

Sometimes people can be instrumental in writing a book just by being early "believers". To that end, I want to thank Carson Marr and the entire team at TEDx Penn. I wasn't sure this message would resonate until they believed in it and invited me to share it on the TEDx stage. That experience inspired me to tell this story, and without it, this book may never have happened. Thank you.

I want to thank another great encourager, my colleague Dr. Dominic Vachon, and the team at the Ruth M. Hillebrand Center for Compassionate Care in Medicine at the University of Notre Dame. I am eternally grateful to my whole Notre Dame family, for always supporting me and encouraging me to dream big.

There are dozens of people in my church family that have encouraged and supported me through this project, but I especially want to thank: Lorenzo Eagles, Brian Catanella, Dan Wonneberger, Jonathan Miller, Dick Herman, Cal Knowlton, and Stuart Spencer. You guys live the principles of compassionomics every day, and you are amazing role models for me.

Above all, I am forever grateful for the support of my loving wife Tamara, who is the most compassionate person I have ever known, and who has taught me more about compassion than anyone ever could.

Lastly, I thank my wonderful children - Christian, Isabel, Bethany, and Jonathan - for inspiring me every day. People will say that this book is written for the health care industry, but the secret of this book is that the message contained in these pages is actually for *them*.

—Steve Trzeciak

Personal Acknowledgments from Anthony Mazzarelli:

Above all I would like to thank my wife Joanne. I am incredibly lucky to have such a supportive partner and friend. As a practicing cardiologist, she is not only clinically excellent but loved by her patients which made her perfect when I needed her during key moments when I would get stuck or needed advice during the writing process. She is always unbelievably supportive no matter the endeavor, but her particular support on this project, I believe, comes from the fact that she herself is a regular practitioner of the ideas expressed in this book. There were many nights where I'm sure that Joanne just wanted to go to sleep, but I kept her up to listen to an idea for a chapter or to get her opinion on the framing of a story. I sometimes wonder how she is so patient with me.

I would also like to thank my parents, Joe and Virginia, who have always supported everything I have done with such passion that I have always had no choice but to see things through to the end to make sure the value of their support was fully realized. As my children grow older I wonder how I could ever measure up to be even a fraction of the supportive and loving parent as each of them.

To my children - Sophia, JP, Leo, and forever in our hearts Joseph - you have all inspired me not only to write this book but to want people to read it. Don't tell our publisher, but we don't really care about how many books we sell. We do, however, care deeply about increasing the amount of compassionate care that exists in the world. That's the world in which I hope you can grow old.

My most heartfelt thanks goes to Michael Smerconish whose mentorship, guidance, and influence over the years is likely the reason I even participated in writing this book. "You need to write a book," has been his advice for probably a decade now. In Chapter 1 we postulate that the compassion crisis might be an extension of the decrease of compassion in our society in general as evidenced by the growing polarization among those that identify with political parties. For those that know Michael, you know this is one of his mantras and you may even recognize the data we quote. Michael is the SiriusXM and CNN host that is treating the disease of polarization with data-driven, thoughtful, independent discussion. Since compassion is the desire to take action in response to others pain, he is media's compassionate host.

I need to thank TC Scornavacchi since she was the first person I ever showed the book pitch. It was awful. However, she had the compassion to not only give me advice to make it better but to never, not for one second, take the position that it shouldn't happen. Her encouragement, support, and friendship is enduring and much appreciated. It should come as no surprise to those that know TC that she is the voice for the Audible version of the book. She has the perfect pipes and the perfect personality to convey this message.

I am very grateful to Rich Zeoli. Not only did Rich read early drafts of the book to offer guidance, but his continual counsel has been invaluable. Rich is a rising star and will soon be a national name. However, that never stops him from remembering his New Jersey roots and to spend whatever time I needed from him for help with this project.

I also want to thank Sacha Montas, MD, JD, MBE. If you are thinking, "What a nerd with all those degrees," I completely agree. Sacha is the person that first got me interested in the academic side of medicine many years ago in college when he introduced me to the world of bioethics. He continues to be the best sounding board a friend can have, and played that same role with respect to this book.

I would be remiss if I did not give a special thanks to Jennifer Knorr. In the world of executive assistants she has few, if any, equals. Her job would be exponentially easier if she did not choose to show compassion and kindness to others when dealing with them. She has never wavered from this practice, on good days and bad, which I appreciate almost as much as the fact that without her I would be completely lost. She also keeps the train running on time.

Thank you to the senior leadership team at Cooper. I know how hard you work to serve our patients and our employees, and your desire to have a culture of compassion within our organization. That dedication has also served as a muse for this book.

I especially want to thank my Co-President, Kevin O'Dowd, who I have the pleasure to work with closely every day. Health care is incredibly tumultuous and unpredictable, so having such a steady, calm, thoughtful, intelligent partner, especially one that excels more than me in all those traits, is incredibly valuable. His belief that the concepts in this book can help us serve patients, providers, and the entire health care system better is particularly inspiring.

Lastly, I would like to thank all of the past, present, and future patients I have ever been given the privilege to take care of in the Emergency Department. I hope I continue to grow in my journey to provide more compassionate care so that I can serve you better.

—Anthony Mazzarelli

REFERENCES:

1. Lown, B. A., J. Rosen, and J. Marttila. "An Agenda for Improving Compassionate Care: A Survey Shows About Half of Patients Say Such Care Is Missing." *Health Affairs* 30, no. 9 (September, 2011): 1772-8.
2. Burling, Stacey. "Cooper Doctors Study 'Compassion Crisis' in Health Care." *Philadelphia Inquirer.* March 15, 2018.
3. Darwin, Charles. *The Descent of Man, and Selection in Relation to Sex.* London: John Murray, 1871.
4. Spinrad, Tracy L., and Cynthia A. Stifter. "Toddlers' Empathy-Related Responding to Distress: Predictions from Negative Emotionality and Maternal Behavior in Infancy." *Infancy* 10, no. 2 (2006): 97-121.
5. Hepach, Robert, Amrisha Vaish, and Michael Tomasello. "Young Children Are Intrinsically Motivated to See Others Helped." *Psychological Science* 23, no. 9 (September 1, 2012): 967-72.
6. Warneken, Felix, and Michael Tomasello. "Helping and Cooperation at 14 Months of Age." *Infancy* 11, no. 3 (2007): 271-94.
7. Goetz, Jennifer L., Dacher Keltner, and Emiliana Simon-Thomas. "Compassion: An Evolutionary Analysis and Empirical Review." *Psychological Bulletin* 136, no. 3 (May, 2010): 351-74.
8. "AMA Principles of Medical Ethics." 2001, accessed November 12, 2018, https://www.ama-assn.org/about/publications-newsletters/ama-principles-medical-ethics.
9. "The NHS Consitution for England." 2015, accessed November 12, 2018, https://www.gov.uk/government/publications/the-nhs-constitution-for-england/the-nhs-constitution-for-england#nhs-values.
10. Lamm, Claus, Jean Decety, and Tania Singer. "Meta-Analytic Evidence for Common and Distinct Neural Networks Associated with Directly Experienced Pain and Empathy for Pain." *Neuroimage* 54, no. 3 (February 1, 2011): 2492-502.
11. Klimecki, Olga M., Susanne Leiberg, Matthieu Ricard, and Tania Singer. "Differential Pattern of Functional Brain Plasticity after Compassion and Empathy Training." *Social Cognitive and Affective Neuroscience* 9, no. 6 (June, 2014): 873-9.
12. Klimecki, Olga M., Susanne Leiberg, Claus Lamm, and Tania Singer. "Functional Neural Plasticity and Associated Changes in Positive Affect after Compassion Training." *Cerebral Cortex* 23, no. 7 (July, 2013): 1552-61.
13. McNeill, Donald P., Donald A. Morrison, and Henri J. Nouwen. *Compassion, a Reflection on the Christian Life.* Garden City: Doubleday, 1982.

14. Trzeciak, Stephen, Brian W. Roberts, and Anthony J. Mazzarelli. "Compassionomics: Hypothesis and Experimental Approach." *Medical Hypotheses* 107 (September, 2017): 92-97.
15. The Local. "Bus Driver Convicted for Deadly Crash." (2008). Published electronically April 28, 2008.
16. "Six Dead and Dozens Injured after Two Buses Collide." 2007, accessed November 10, 2018, https://sverigesradio.se/sida/artikel.aspx?programid=2054&artikel=1226195.
17. Lennquist, Sten (Ed.). *Medical Response to Major Incidents and Disasters: A Practical Guide for All Medical Staff.* Berlin: Springer, 2012.
18. Doohan, Isabelle, and Britt-Inger Saveman. "Need for Compassion in Prehospital and Emergency Care: A Qualitative Study on Bus Crash Survivors' Experiences." *International Emergency Nursing* 23, no. 2 (April, 2015): 115-9.
19. Graham, David A. "Really, Would You Let Your Daughter Marry a Democrat?" *The Atlantic*, September 27, 2012.
20. Davis, Lauren. "Dignity Health Survey Finds Majority of Americans Rate Kindness as Top Factor in Quality Health Care." news release, November 13, 2013.
21. Konrath, Sara H., Edward H. O'Brien, and Courtney Hsing. "Changes in Dispositional Empathy in American College Students over Time: A Meta-Analysis." *Personality and Social Psychology Review* 15, no. 2 (May, 2011): 180-98.
22. Making Caring Common Project, "The Children We Mean to Raise: The Real Messages Adults Are Sending About Values," (Cambridge: Harvard Graduate School of Education, 2014).
23. Doherty, Carroll, Jocelyn Kiley, and Bridget Johnson. "A Divided and Pessimistic Electorate." Pew Research Center, 2016.
24. Darley, John M., and C. Daniel Batson. ""From Jerusalem to Jericho": A Study of Situational and Dispositional Variables in Helping Behavior." *Journal of Personality and Social Psychology* 27, no. 1 (1973): 100-08.
25. The Schwartz Center for Compassionate Healthcare. "National Survey Data Presented at the Compassion in Action Conference Show Mixed Reactions on State of Compassion in U.S. Healthcare." news release, June 27, 2017, https://www.prnewswire.com/news-releases/national-survey-data-presented-at-the-compassion-in-action-conference-show-mixed-reactions-on-state-of-compassion-in-us-healthcare-300480125.html.
26. Bernstein, Lenny. "Once Again, U.S. Has Most Expensive, Least Effective Health Care System in Survey." *The Washington Post*, June 16, 2014.
27. Francis, Robert. "Report of the Mid Staffordshire NHS Foundation Trust Public Inquiry." London: Department of Health, 2013.
28. Campbell, Denis. "David Cameron's Prescription for NHS Failings: Target Pay for Nurses." *The Guardian*, February 6, 2013.
29. Lown, Beth A., Hilary Dunne, Steven J. Muncer, and Raymond Chadwick. "How Important Is Compassionate Healthcare to You? A Comparison of the Perceptions of People in the United States and Ireland." *Journal of Research in Nursing* 22, no. 1-2 (2017): 60-69.

30. Shanafelt, Tait D., Omar Hasan, Lotte N. Dyrbye, Christine Sinsky, Daniel Satele, Jeff Sloan, and Colin P. West. "Changes in Burnout and Satisfaction with Work-Life Balance in Physicians and the General Us Working Population between 2011 and 2014." *Mayo Clinic Proceedings* 90, no. 12 (December, 2015): 1600-13.
31. Soler, Jean Karl, Hakan Yaman, Magdalena Esteva, Frank Dobbs, Radost Spiridonova Asenova, Milica Katic, Zlata Ozvacic, *et al.* "Burnout in European Family Doctors: The EGPRN Study." *Family Practice* 25, no. 4 (August, 2008): 245-65.
32. Rosen, Ilene M., Phyllis A. Gimotty, Judy A. Shea, and Lisa M. Bellini. "Evolution of Sleep Quantity, Sleep Deprivation, Mood Disturbances, Empathy, and Burnout among Interns." *Academic Medicine* 81, no. 1 (January, 2006): 82-5.
33. Bellini, Lisa M., Michael Baime, and Judy A. Shea. "Variation of Mood and Empathy During Internship." *JAMA* 287, no. 23 (June 19, 2002): 3143-6.
34. Beckman, H. B., and R. M. Frankel. "The Effect of Physician Behavior on the Collection of Data." *Annals of Internal Medicine* 101, no. 5 (November, 1984): 692-6.
35. Marvel, M. K., R. M. Epstein, K. Flowers, and H. B. Beckman. "Soliciting the Patient's Agenda: Have We Improved?". *JAMA* 281, no. 3 (January 20, 1999): 283-7.
36. Singh Ospina, Naykky, Kari A. Phillips, Rene Rodriguez-Gutierrez, Ana Castaneda-Guarderas, Michael R. Gionfriddo, Megan E. Branda, and Victor M. Montori. "Eliciting the Patient's Agenda- Secondary Analysis of Recorded Clinical Encounters." *Journal of General Internal Medicine* 34, no. 1 (July 2, 2018): 36-40.
37. Levinson, W., and N. Chaumeton. "Communication between Surgeons and Patients in Routine Office Visits." *Surgery* 125, no. 2 (February, 1999): 127-34.
38. Mendes, Elizabeth. "Americans Down on Congress, OK with Own Representative." *Gallup*. Published electronically May 9, 2013.
39. Kenny, David A., Wernke Veldhuijzen, Trudy van der Weijden, Annie Leblanc, Jocelyn Lockyer, France Legare, and Craig Campbell. "Interpersonal Perception in the Context of Doctor-Patient Relationships: A Dyadic Analysis of Doctor-Patient Communication." *Social Science and Medicine* 70, no. 5 (March, 2010): 763-8.
40. Hall, J. A., T. S. Stein, D. L. Roter, and N. Rieser. "Inaccuracies in Physicians' Perceptions of Their Patients." *Medical Care* 37, no. 11 (November, 1999): 1164-8.
41. Block, Lauren, Lindsey Hutzler, Robert Habicht, Albert W. Wu, Sanjay V. Desai, Kathryn Novello Silva, Timothy Niessen, Nora Oliver, and Leonard Feldman. "Do Internal Medicine Interns Practice Etiquette-Based Communication? A Critical Look at the Inpatient Encounter." *Journal of Hospital Medicine* 8, no. 11 (November, 2013): 631-4.
42. Davis, David A., Paul E. Mazmanian, Michael Fordis, R. Van Harrison, Kevin E. Thorpe, and Laure Perrier. "Accuracy of Physician Self-Assessment Compared with Observed Measures of Competence: A Systematic Review." *JAMA* 296, no. 9 (September, 6 2006): 1094-102.

43. Weng, Hui-Ching, Hung-Chi Chen, Han-Jung Chen, Kang Lu, and Shin-Yuan Hung. "Doctors' Emotional Intelligence and the Patient-Doctor Relationship." *Medical Education* 42, no. 7 (July, 2008): 703-11.
44. Pollak, Kathryn I., Robert M. Arnold, Amy S. Jeffreys, Stewart C. Alexander, Maren K. Olsen, Amy P. Abernethy, Celette Sugg Skinner, Keri L. Rodriguez, and James A. Tulsky. "Oncologist Communication About Emotion During Visits with Patients with Advanced Cancer." *Journal of Clinical Oncology* 25, no. 36 (December 20, 2007): 5748-52.
45. Pollak, Kathryn I., Robert M. Arnold, Stewart C. Alexander, Amy S. Jeffreys, Maren K. Olsen, Amy P. Abernethy, Keri L. Rodriguez, and James A. Tulsky. "Do Patient Attributes Predict Oncologist Empathic Responses and Patient Perceptions of Empathy?" *Supportive Care in Cancer* 18, no. 11 (November, 2010): 1405-11.
46. Easter, David W., and Wayne Beach. "Competent Patient Care Is Dependent Upon Attending to Empathic Opportunities Presented During Interview Sessions." *Current Surgery* 61, no. 3 (May-June, 2004): 313-8.
47. Morse, Diane S., Elizabeth A. Edwardsen, and Howard S. Gordon. "Missed Opportunities for Interval Empathy in Lung Cancer Communication." *Archives of Internal Medicine* 168, no. 17 (September 22, 2008): 1853-8.
48. Weiss, Rachel, Eric Vittinghoff, Margaret C. Fang, Jenica E. W. Cimino, Kristen A. Chasteen, Robert M. Arnold, Andrew D. Auerbach, and Wendy G. Anderson. "Associations of Physician Empathy with Patient Anxiety and Ratings of Communication in Hospital Admission Encounters." *Journal of Hospital Medicine* 12, no. 10 (October, 2017): 805-10.
49. Levinson, W., R. Gorawara-Bhat, and J. Lamb. "A Study of Patient Clues and Physician Responses in Primary Care and Surgical Settings." *JAMA* 284, no. 8 (August 23-30, 2000): 1021-7.
50. Ahmedani, Brian K., Christine Stewart, Gregory E. Simon, Frances Lynch, Christine Y. Lu, Beth E. Waitzfelder, Leif I. Solberg, *et al.* "Racial/Ethnic Differences in Health Care Visits Made Before Suicide Attempt Across the United States." *Medical Care* 53, no. 5 (May, 2015): 430-5.
51. Posner, Kelly, Gregory K. Brown, Barbara Stanley, David A. Brent, Kseniya V. Yershova, Maria A. Oquendo, Glenn W. Currier, *et al.* "The Columbia–Suicide Severity Rating Scale: Initial Validity and Internal Consistency Findings from Three Multisite Studies with Adolescents and Adults." *American Journal of Psychiatry* 168, no. 12 (2011): 1266-77.
52. Joiner, Thomas. *Why People Die by Suicide.* Cambridge: Harvard University Press, 2007.
53. Carrese, Joseph A., Gail Geller, Emily D. Branyon, Lindsay K. Forbes, Rachel J. Topazian, Brian W. Weir, Omar Khatib, and Jeremy Sugarman. "A Direct Observation Checklist to Measure Respect and Dignity in the ICU." *Critical Care Medicine* 45, no. 2 (February, 2017): 263-70.
54. Selph, R. Brac, Julia Shiang, Ruth Engelberg, J. Randall Curtis, and Douglas B. White. "Empathy and Life Support Decisions in Intensive Care Units." *Journal of General Internal Medicine* 23, no. 9 (September, 2008): 1311-7.

55. Howick, J., L. Steinkopf, A. Ulyte, N. Roberts, and K. Meissner. "How Empathic Is Your Healthcare Practitioner? A Systematic Review and Meta-Analysis of Patient Surveys." *BMC Medical Education* 17, no. 1 (August 21, 2017): 136.
56. Larson, Eric B., and Xin Yao. "Clinical Empathy as Emotional Labor in the Patient-Physician Relationship." *JAMA* 293, no. 9 (March 2, 2005): 1100-6.
57. Neumann, Melanie, Friedrich Edelhauser, Diethard Tauschel, Martin R. Fischer, Markus Wirtz, Christiane Woopen, Aviad Haramati, and Christian Scheffer. "Empathy Decline and Its Reasons: A Systematic Review of Studies with Medical Students and Residents." *Academic Medicine* 86, no. 8 (August, 2011): 996-1009.
58. Cowell, Richard N. *The Hidden Curriculum: A Theoretical Framework and a Pilot Study.* Cambridge: Harvard Graduate School of Education, 1972.
59. Shem, Samuel. *House of God.* New York: Richard Marek, 1978.
60. Tai-Seale, Ming, Cliff W. Olson, Jinnan Li, Albert S. Chan, Criss Morikawa, Meg Durbin, Wei Wang, and Harold S. Luft. "Electronic Health Record Logs Indicate That Physicians Split Time Evenly Between Seeing Patients and Desktop Medicine." *Health Affairs* 36, no. 4 (April 1, 2017): 655-62.
61. Sinsky, Christine, Lacey Colligan, Ling Li, Mirela Prgomet, Sam Reynolds, Lindsey Goeders, Johanna Westbrook, Michael Tutty, and George Blike. "Allocation of Physician Time in Ambulatory Practice: A Time and Motion Study in 4 Specialties." *Annals of Internal Medicine* 165, no. 11 (December 6, 2016): 753-60.
62. Toll, Elizabeth "A Piece of My Mind. The Cost of Technology." *JAMA* 307, no. 23 (June 20, 2012): 2497-8.
63. "The Doctor." 2018, accessed May 15, 2018, https://www.tate.org.uk/art/artworks/fildes-the-doctor-n01522.
64. Block, Lauren, Robert Habicht, Albert W. Wu, Sanjay V. Desai, Kevin Wang, Kathryn N. Silva, Timothy Niessen, Nora Oliver, and Leonard Feldman. "In the Wake of the 2003 and 2011 Duty Hours Regulations, How Do Internal Medicine Interns Spend Their Time?" *Journal of General Internal Medicine* 28, no. 8 (August, 2013): 1042-7.
65. Wenger, Nathalie, Marie Mean, Julien Castioni, Pedro Marques-Vidal, Gerard Waeber, and Antoine Garnier. "Allocation of Internal Medicine Resident Time in a Swiss Hospital: A Time and Motion Study of Day and Evening Shifts." *Annals of Internal Medicine* 166, no. 8 (April 18, 2017): 579-86.
66. Markel, Howard. "In 1850, Ignaz Semmelweis Saved Lives with Three Words: Wash Your Hands." *PBS News Hour.* Published electronically May 15, 2015.
67. Smajdor, Anna. "Compassion Is Not the Answer to Failings in the NHS." *The Guardian.* Published electronically September 19, 2013.
68. The Cochrane Collaboration. "Cochrane Handbook for Systematic Reviews of Interventions." edited by Julian P.T. Higgins and Sally Green, updated March 2011.
69. Greenhalgh, Trisha, and Richard Peacock. "Effectiveness and Efficiency of Search Methods in Systematic Reviews of Complex Evidence: Audit of Primary Sources." *BMJ* 331, no. 7524 (November 5, 2005): 1064-5.

70. Sinclair, Shane, Jill M. Norris, Shelagh J. McConnell, Harvey Max Chochinov, Thomas F. Hack, Neil A. Hagen, Susan McClement, and Shelley R. Bouchal. "Compassion: A Scoping Review of the Healthcare Literature." *BMC Palliative Care* 15 (January 19, 2016): 6.
71. Boulton, Terynn. "'Blowing Smoke up Your Ass' Used to Be Literal." *Gizmodo.* Published electronically May 20, 2014.
72. Brummet, Jack "The Etymology of 'Blowing Smoke Up Your A**'," *All This is That.* Published electronically February 8, 2013.
73. Boulton, Terynn. "When Doctors Literally 'Blew Smoke Up Your Arse'." *Today I Found Out.* Published electronically May 19, 2014.
74. House, J. S., K. R. Landis, and D. Umberson. "Social Relationships and Health." *Science* 241, no. 4865 (July 29, 1988): 540-5.
75. Lewis, Thomas, Fari Amini, and Richard Lannon. *A General Theory of Love.* New York: Random House, 2000.
76. Holt-Lunstad, Julianne, and Timothy B. Smith. "Loneliness and Social Isolation as Risk Factors for CVD: Implications for Evidence-Based Patient Care and Scientific Inquiry." *Heart* 102, no. 13 (July 1, 2016): 987-9.
77. Holt-Lunstad, Julianne, Timothy B. Smith, and J. Bradley Layton. "Social Relationships and Mortality Risk: A Meta-Analytic Review." *PLOS Medicine* 7, no. 7 (July 27, 2010): e1000316.
78. Holt-Lunstad, Julianne, Timothy B. Smith, Mark Baker, Tyler Harris, and David Stephenson. "Loneliness and Social Isolation as Risk Factors for Mortality: A Meta-Analytic Review." *Perspectives on Psychological Science* 10, no. 2 (March, 2015): 227-37.
79. Rico-Uribe, Laura Alejandra, Francisco Felix Caballero, Natalia Martin-Maria, Maria Cabello, Jose Luis Ayuso-Mateos, and Marta Miret. "Association of Loneliness with All-Cause Mortality: A Meta-Analysis." *PLOS One* 13, no. 1 (2018): e0190033.
80. Perissinotto, Carla M., Irena Stijacic Cenzer, and Kenneth E. Covinsky. "Loneliness in Older Persons: A Predictor of Functional Decline and Death." *Archives of Internal Medicine* 172, no. 14 (July 23, 2012): 1078-83.
81. Donovan, Nancy J., Qiong Wu, Dorene M. Rentz, Reisa A. Sperling, Gad A. Marshall, and M. Maria Glymour. "Loneliness, Depression and Cognitive Function in Older U.S. Adults." *International Journal of Geriatric Psychiatry* 32, no. 5 (May, 2017): 564-73.
82. Berkman, L. F., L. Leo-Summers, and R. I. Horwitz. "Emotional Support and Survival after Myocardial Infarction. A Prospective, Population-Based Study of the Elderly." *Annals of Internal Medicine* 117, no. 12 (December 15, 1992): 1003-9.
83. "Health Impact Assessment, Determinants of Health." *World Health Organization*, accessed June 18, 2018, http://www.who.int/hia/evidence/doh/en/.
84. Brody, Jane E. "The Surprising Effects of Loneliness on Health." *New York Times*, December 11, 2017.
85. Yeginsu, Ceylan. "U.K. Appoints a Minister for Loneliness." *New York Times*, January 17, 2018.

86. TEDxBeaconStreet. "What Makes a Good Life? Lessons from the Longest Study on Happiness." https://www.ted.com/talks/robert_waldinger_what_makes_a_good_life_lessons_from_the_longest_study_on_happiness.
87. Eisenberger, Naomi I., and Steve W. Cole. "Social Neuroscience and Health: Neurophysiological Mechanisms Linking Social Ties with Physical Health." *Nature Neuroscience* 15, no. 5 (April 15, 2012): 669-74.
88. Hawkley, Louise C., Ronald A. Thisted, Christopher M. Masi, and John T. Cacioppo. "Loneliness Predicts Increased Blood Pressure: 5-Year Cross-Lagged Analyses in Middle-Aged and Older Adults." *Psychology and Aging* 25, no. 1 (March, 2010): 132-41.
89. Valtorta, Nicole K., Mona Kanaan, Simon Gilbody, Sara Ronzi, and Barbara Hanratty. "Loneliness and Social Isolation as Risk Factors for Coronary Heart Disease and Stroke: Systematic Review and Meta-Analysis of Longitudinal Observational Studies." *Heart* 102, no. 13 (July 1, 2016): 1009-16.
90. Pressman, Sarah D., Sheldon Cohen, Gregory E. Miller, Anita Barkin, Bruce S. Rabin, and John J. Treanor. "Loneliness, Social Network Size, and Immune Response to Influenza Vaccination in College Freshmen." *Health Psychology* 24, no. 3 (May, 2005): 297-306.
91. Cohen, S., W. J. Doyle, D. P. Skoner, B. S. Rabin, and J. M. Gwaltney, Jr. "Social Ties and Susceptibility to the Common Cold." *JAMA* 277, no. 24 (June 25, 1997): 1940-4.
92. Cole, Steve W., Louise C. Hawkley, Jesusa M. Arevalo, Caroline Y. Sung, Robert M. Rose, and John T. Cacioppo. "Social Regulation of Gene Expression in Human Leukocytes." *Genome Biology* 8, no. 9 (2007): R189.
93. Manczak, Erika M., Anita DeLongis, and Edith Chen. "Does Empathy Have a Cost? Diverging Psychological and Physiological Effects within Families." *Health Psychology* 35, no. 3 (March, 2016): 211-8.
94. Rozanski, A., J. A. Blumenthal, and J. Kaplan. "Impact of Psychological Factors on the Pathogenesis of Cardiovascular Disease and Implications for Therapy." *Circulation* 99, no. 16 (April 27, 1999): 2192-217.
95. Tawakol, Ahmen, Amorina Ishai, Richard A. Takx, Amparo L. Figueroa, Abdelrahman Ali, Yannick Kaiser, Quynh A. Truong, *et al.* "Relation between Resting Amygdalar Activity and Cardiovascular Events: A Longitudinal and Cohort Study." *Lancet* 389, no. 10071 (February 25, 2017): 834-45.
96. Maiti, Abhishek, and Abhijeet Dhoble. "Takotsubo Cardiomyopathy." *New England Journal of Medicine* 377, no. 16 (October 19, 2017): e24.
97. Fogarty, L. A., B. A. Curbow, J. R. Wingard, K. McDonnell, and M. R. Somerfield. "Can 40 Seconds of Compassion Reduce Patient Anxiety?" *Journal of Clinical Oncology* 17, no. 1 (January, 1999): 371-9.
98. Egbert, L. D., G. Battit, H. Turndorf, and H. K. Beecher. "The Value of the Preoperative Visit by an Anesthetist. A Study of Doctor-Patient Rapport." *JAMA* 185, no. 7 (August 17, 1963): 553-5.

99. Egbert, L. D., G. E. Battit, C. E. Welch, and M. K. Bartlett. "Reduction of Postoperative Pain by Encouragement and Instruction of Patients. A Study of Doctor-Patient Rapport." *New England Journal of Medicine* 270 (April 16, 1964): 825-7.
100. Pereira, Ligia, Margarida Figueiredo-Braga, and Irene P. Carvalho. "Preoperative Anxiety in Ambulatory Surgery: The Impact of an Empathic Patient-Centered Approach on Psychological and Clinical Outcomes." *Patient Education and Counseling* 99, no. 5 (May, 2016): 733-8.
101. Bergland, Christopher. "Face-to-Face Connectedness, Oxytocin, and Your Vagus Nerve." *Psychology Today*. Published electronically May 19, 2017.
102. Kok, Bethany E., Kimberly A. Coffey, Michael A. Cohn, Lahnna I. Catalino, Tanya Vacharkulksemsuk, Sara B. Algoe, Mary Brantley, and Barbara L. Fredrickson. "How Positive Emotions Build Physical Health: Perceived Positive Social Connections Account for the Upward Spiral between Positive Emotions and Vagal Tone." *Psychological Science* 24, no. 7 (July 1, 2013): 1123-32.
103. Kemper, Kathi J., and Hossam A. Shaltout. "Non-Verbal Communication of Compassion: Measuring Psychophysiologic Effects." *BMC Complementary and Alternative Medicine* 11 (December 20, 2011): 132.
104. Shaltout, Hossam A., Janet A. Tooze, Erica Rosenberger, and Kathi J. Kemper. "Time, Touch, and Compassion: Effects on Autonomic Nervous System and Well-Being." *Explore* 8, no. 3 (May-June, 2012): 177-84.
105. Shahrestani, Sara, Elizabeth M. Stewart, Daniel S. Quintana, Ian B. Hickie, and Adam J. Guastella. "Heart Rate Variability During Adolescent and Adult Social Interactions: A Meta-Analysis." *Biological Psychology* 105 (February, 2015): 43-50.
106. Holt-Lunstad, Julianne, Wendy A. Birmingham, and Kathleen C. Light. "Influence of a 'Warm Touch' Support Enhancement Intervention among Married Couples on Ambulatory Blood Pressure, Oxytocin, Alpha Amylase, and Cortisol." *Psychosomatic Medicine* 70, no. 9 (November, 2008): 976-85.
107. Christenfeld, N., and W. Gerin. "Social Support and Cardiovascular Reactivity." *Biomedicine & Pharmacotherapy* 54, no. 5 (June, 2000): 251-7.
108. Lepore, S. J., K. A. Allen, and G. W. Evans. "Social Support Lowers Cardiovascular Reactivity to an Acute Stressor." *Psychosomatic Medicine* 55, no. 6 (November-December, 1993): 518-24.
109. Mumford, E., H. J. Schlesinger, and G. V. Glass. "The Effect of Psychological Intervention on Recovery from Surgery and Heart Attacks: An Analysis of the Literature." *American Journal of Public Health* 72, no. 2 (February, 1982): 141-51.
110. Steinhausen, Simone, Oliver Ommen, Sunya-Lee Antoine, Thorsten Koehler, Holger Pfaff, and Edmund Neugebauer. "Short- and Long-Term Subjective Medical Treatment Outcome of Trauma Surgery Patients: The Importance of Physician Empathy." *Patient Preference and Adherence* 8 (2014): 1239-53.
111. National Institutes of Health. "The Science of Compassion: Future Directions in End-of-Life and Palliative Care." In *The Science of Compassion: Future Directions in End-of-Life and Palliative Care*. Bethesda, MD, 2011.

112. Temel, Jennifer S., Joseph A. Greer, Alona Muzikansky, Emily R. Gallagher, Sonal Admane, Vicki A. Jackson, Constance M. Dahlin, *et al.* "Early Palliative Care for Patients with Metastatic Non-Small-Cell Lung Cancer." *New England Journal of Medicine* 363, no. 8 (August 19, 2010): 733-42.
113. Goldstein, Pavel, Simone G. Shamay-Tsoory, Shahar Yellinek, and Irit Weissman-Fogel. "Empathy Predicts an Experimental Pain Reduction During Touch." *Journal of Pain* 17, no. 10 (October, 2016): 1049-57.
114. Goldstein, Pavel, Irit Weissman-Fogel, and Simone G. Shamay-Tsoory. "The Role of Touch in Regulating Inter-Partner Physiological Coupling During Empathy for Pain." *Scientific Reports* 7, no. 1 (June 12, 2017): 3252.
115. Goldstein, Pavel, Irit Weissman-Fogel, Guillaume Dumas, and Simone G. Shamay-Tsoory. "Brain-to-Brain Coupling During Handholding Is Associated with Pain Reduction." *Proceedings of the National Academy of Sciences of the United States of America* 115, no. 11 (March 13, 2018): E2528-E37.
116. Coan, James A., Hillary S. Schaefer, and Richard J. Davidson. "Lending a Hand: Social Regulation of the Neural Response to Threat." *Psychological Science* 17, no. 12 (December, 2006): 1032-9.
117. Coan, James A., Lane Beckes, Marlen Z. Gonzalez, Erin L. Maresh, Casey L. Brown, and Karen Hasselmo. "Relationship Status and Perceived Support in the Social Regulation of Neural Responses to Threat." *Social Cognitive and Affective Neuroscience* 12, no. 10 (October 1, 2017): 1574-83.
118. Hagerty, Barbara Bradley. *Midlife Friendships Key to a Longer, Healthier Life.* National Public Radio Podcast audio. Morning Edition 7:02. Accessed June 27, 2018. https://www.npr.org/2016/03/16/470635733/midlife-friendship-key-to-a-longer-healthier-life.
119. Goodwin, P. J., M. Leszcz, M. Ennis, J. Koopmans, L. Vincent, H. Guther, E. Drysdale, *et al.* "The Effect of Group Psychosocial Support on Survival in Metastatic Breast Cancer." *New England Journal of Medicine* 345, no. 24 (December 13, 2001): 1719-26.
120. Kim, Sung Soo, Stan Kaplowitz, and Mark V. Johnston. "The Effects of Physician Empathy on Patient Satisfaction and Compliance." *Evaluation & the Health of Professions* 27, no. 3 (September, 2004): 237-51.
121. Sarinopoulos, Issidoros, Ashley M. Hesson, Chelsea Gordon, Seungcheol A. Lee, Lu Wang, Francesca Dwamena, and Robert C. Smith. "Patient-Centered Interviewing Is Associated with Decreased Responses to Painful Stimuli: An Initial fMRI Study." *Patient Education and Counseling* 90, no. 2 (February, 2013): 220-5.
122. Manchikanti, L. "Epidemiology of Low Back Pain." *Pain Physician* 3, no. 2 (April, 2000): 167-92.
123. Fuentes, Jorge, Susan Armijo-Olivo, Martha Funabashi, Maxi Miciak, Bruce Dick, Sharon Warren, Saifee Rashiq, David J. Magee, and Douglas P. Gross. "Enhanced Therapeutic Alliance Modulates Pain Intensity and Muscle Pain Sensitivity in

Patients with Chronic Low Back Pain: An Experimental Controlled Study." *Physical Therapy* 94, no. 4 (April, 2014): 477-89.

124. Dibbelt, Susanne, Monika Schaidhammer, Christian Fleischer, and Bernhard Greitemann. "Patient-Doctor Interaction in Rehabilitation: The Relationship between Perceived Interaction Quality and Long-Term Treatment Results." *Patient Education and Counseling* 76, no. 3 (September, 2009): 328-35.
125. Attar, Hatim S., and Srinath Chandramani. "Impact of Physician Empathy on Migraine Disability and Migraineur Compliance." *Annals of Indian Academy of Neurology* 15, supplement 1 (August, 2012): S89-94.
126. Kaptchuk, Ted J., John M. Kelley, Lisa A. Conboy, Roger B. Davis, Catherine E. Kerr, Eric E. Jacobson, Iriving Kirsch, *et al.* "Components of Placebo Effect: Randomised Controlled Trial in Patients with Irritable Bowel Syndrome." *BMJ* 336, no. 7651 (May 3, 2008): 999-1003.
127. Katz, Josh. "Drug Deaths in America Are Rising Faster Than Ever." *New York Times*, June 5, 2017.
128. Hall, Amanda M., Paula H. Ferreira, Christopher G. Maher, Jane Latimer, and Manuela L. Ferreira. "The Influence of the Therapist-Patient Relationship on Treatment Outcome in Physical Rehabilitation: A Systematic Review." *Physical Therapy* 90, no. 8 (August, 2010): 1099-110.
129. Ambady, Nalini, Jasook Koo, Robert Rosenthal, and Carol H. Winograd. "Physical Therapists' Nonverbal Communication Predicts Geriatric Patients' Health Outcomes." *Psychology and Aging* 17, no. 3 (September, 2002): 443-52.
130. Dillingham, Timothy R., Liliana E. Pezzin, and Ellen J. MacKenzie. "Limb Amputation and Limb Deficiency: Epidemiology and Recent Trends in the United States." *Southern Medical Journal* 95, no. 8 (August, 2002): 875-83.
131. American Academy of Physical Medicine and Rehabilitation. "Lower Limb Amputations - Epidemiology and Assessment." Updated May 3, 2016, accessed November 12, 2018, https://now.aapmr.org/lower-limb-amputations-epidemiology-and-assessment.
132. Centers for Disease Control and Prevention. "National Diabetes Statistics Report." Atlanta: Centers for Disease Control and Prevention, U.S. Department of Health and Human Services; 2017.
133. American Diabetes Association. "Economic Costs of Diabetes in the U.S. In 2017." *Diabetes Care* 41, no. 5 (May, 2018): 917-28.
134. Centers for Desease Control. "About Underlying Cause of Death, 1999-2016." 2016, accessed July 1, 2018, https://wonder.cdc.gov/controller/datarequest/D76;jsessionid=AFF6080EF101C8E18774845C6AC5C055.
135. Hojat, Mohammadreza, Salvatore Mangione, Thomas J. Nasca, Mitchell J. M. Cohen, Joseph S. Gonnella, James B. Erdmann, Jon Veloski, and Mike Magee. "The Jefferson Scale of Physician Empathy: Development and Preliminary Psychometric Data." *Educational and Psychological Measurement* 61, no. 2 (2001): 349-65.
136. Hojat, Mohammadreza, Daniel Z. Louis, Fred W. Markham, Richard Wender, Carol Rabinowitz, and Joseph S. Gonnella. "Physicians' Empathy and Clinical

Outcomes for Diabetic Patients." *Academic Medicine* 86, no. 3 (March, 2011): 359-64.

137. Del Canale, Stefano, Daniel Z. Louis, Vittorino Maio, Xiaohong Wang, Giuseppina Rossi, Mohammadreza Hojat, and Joseph S. Gonnella. "The Relationship between Physician Empathy and Disease Complications: An Empirical Study of Primary Care Physicians and Their Diabetic Patients in Parma, Italy." *Academic Medicine* 87, no. 9 (September, 2012): 1243-9.
138. Lee, Yin-Yang, and Julia L. Lin. "The Effects of Trust in Physician on Self-Efficacy, Adherence and Diabetes Outcomes." *Social Science & Medicine* 68, no. 6 (March, 2009): 1060-8.
139. Ratanawongsa, Neda, Andrew J. Karter, Melissa M. Parker, Courtney R. Lyles, Michele Heisler, Howard H. Moffet, Nancy Adler, E. Margaret Warton, and Dean Schillinger. "Communication and Medication Refill Adherence: The Diabetes Study of Northern California." *JAMA Internal Medicine* 173, no. 3 (February 11, 2013): 210-8.
140. Kiecolt-Glaser, J. K., P. T. Marucha, W. B. Malarkey, A. M. Mercado, and R. Glaser. "Slowing of Wound Healing by Psychological Stress." *Lancet* 346, no. 8984 (November 4, 1995): 1194-6.
141. Kiecolt-Glaser, J. K., T. J. Loving, J. R. Stowell, W. B. Malarkey, S. Lemeshow, S. L. Dickinson, and R. Glaser. "Hostile Marital Interactions, Proinflammatory Cytokine Production, and Wound Healing." *Archives of General Psychiatry* 62, no. 12 (December, 2005): 1377-84.
142. Cohen, Sheldon, Denise Janicki-Deverts, Ronald B. Turner, and William J. Doyle. "Does Hugging Provide Stress-Buffering Social Support? A Study of Susceptibility to Upper Respiratory Infection and Illness." *Psychological Science* 26, no. 2 (February, 2015): 135-47.
143. Rakel, David P., Theresa J. Hoeft, Bruce P. Barrett, Betty A. Chewning, Benjamin M. Craig, and Min Niu. "Practitioner Empathy and the Duration of the Common Cold." *Family Medicine* 41, no. 7 (July-August, 2009): 494-501.
144. Viner, E. D. "Life at the Other End of the Endotracheal Tube: A Physician's Personal View of Critical Illness." *Progress in Critical Care* 2 (1985): 3-13.
145. Viner, E. D. Personal communication to Stephen Trzeciak. August 13, 2018.
146. TEDxMiddlebury. "The Power of Empathy." https://www.youtube.com/watch?v=baHrcC8B4WM: YouTube.
147. Marci, Carl, and Helen Riess. "The Clinical Relevance of Psychophysiology: Support for the Psychobiology of Empathy and Psychodynamic Process." *American Journal of Psychotherapy* 59, no. 3 (2005): 213-26.
148. Elliott, Robert, Arthur C. Bohart, Jeanne C. Watson, and Leslie S. Greenberg. "Empathy." *Psychotherapy* 48, no. 1 (March, 2011): 43-9.
149. Empathetics Homepage. 2018, accessed November 12, 2018, www.empathetics.com.

150. Kamal, Rabah, Cynthia Cox, David Rousseau, and Kaiser Family Foundation. "Costs and Outcomes of Mental Health and Substance Use Disorders in the US." *JAMA* 318, no. 5 (August 1, 2017): 415.
151. Graser, Johannes, and Ulrich Stangier. "Compassion and Loving-Kindness Meditation: An Overview and Prospects for the Application in Clinical Samples." *Harvard Review of Psychiatry* 26, no. 4 (July/August, 2018): 201-15.
152. Laithwaite, Heather, Martin O'Hanlon, Padraig Collins, Patrick Doyle, Lucy Abraham, Shauneen Porter, and Andrew Gumley. "Recovery after Psychosis (RAP): A Compassion Focused Programme for Individuals Residing in High Security Settings." *Behavioural and Cognitive Psychotherapy* 37, no. 5 (October, 2009): 511-26.
153. Braehler, Christine, Andrew Gumley, Janice Harper, Sonia Wallace, John Norrie, and Paul Gilbert. "Exploring Change Processes in Compassion Focused Therapy in Psychosis: Results of a Feasibility Randomized Controlled Trial." *British Journal of Clinical Psychology* 52, no. 2 (June, 2013): 199-214.
154. Kelly, Allison Catherine, Lucene Wisniewski, Caitlin Martin-Wagar, and Ellen Hoffman. "Group-Based Compassion-Focused Therapy as an Adjunct to Outpatient Treatment for Eating Disorders: A Pilot Randomized Controlled Trial." *Clinical Psychology & Psychotherapy* 24, no. 2 (March, 2017): 475-87.
155. Au, Teresa M., Shannon Sauer-Zavala, Matthew W. King, Nicola Petrocchi, David H. Barlow, and Brett T. Litz. "Compassion-Based Therapy for Trauma-Related Shame and Posttraumatic Stress: Initial Evaluation Using a Multiple Baseline Design." *Behavior Therapy* 48, no. 2 (March, 2017): 207-21.
156. Beaumont, Elaine, Mark Durkin, Sue McAndrew, and Colin R. Martin. "Using Compassion Focused Therapy as an Adjunct to Trauma-Focused CBT for Fire Service Personnel Suffering with Trauma-Related Symptoms." *The Cognitive Behavior Therapist* 9 (2016): e34.
157. Johnson, Suzanne B., Bradley L. Goodnight, Huaiyu Zhang, Irene Daboin, Bobbi Patterson, and Nadine J. Kaslow. "Compassion-Based Meditation in African Americans: Self-Criticism Mediates Changes in Depression." *Suicide & Life-Threatening Behavior* 48, no. 2 (April, 2018): 160-68.
158. Noorbala, Fatemeh, Ahmad Borjali, Mohammad Mahdi Ahmadian-Attari, and Ahmad Ali Noorbala. "Effectiveness of Compassionate Mind Training on Depression, Anxiety, and Self-Criticism in a Group of Iranian Depressed Patients." *Iranian Journal of Psychiatry* 8, no. 3 (August, 2013): 113-7.
159. Graser, Johannes, Volkmar Höfling, Charlotte Weßlau, Adriana Mendes, and Ulrich Stangier. "Effects of a 12-Week Mindfulness, Compassion, and Loving Kindness Program on Chronic Depression: A Pilot Within-Subjects Wait-List Controlled Trial." *Journal of Cognitive Psychotherapy* 30, no. 1 (2016): 35-49.
160. Gilbert, Paul, and Sue Procter. "Compassionate Mind Training for People with High Shame and Self-Criticism: Overview and Pilot Study of a Group Therapy Approach." *Clinical Psychology and Psychotherapy,* Issue 13, no. 6 (2006): 353-79.
161. Judge, Lorna, Ailish Cleghorn, Kirsten McEwan, and Paul Gilbert. "An Exploration of Group-Based Compassion Focused Therapy for a Heterogeneous

Range of Clients Presenting to a Community Mental Health Team." *International Journal of Cognitive Therapy* 5, no. 4 (December 1, 2012): 420-29.

162. Kirby, James N., Cassandra L. Tellegen, and Stanley R. Steindl. "A Meta-Analysis of Compassion-Based Interventions: Current State of Knowledge and Future Directions." *Behavior Therapy* 48, no. 6 (November 1, 2017): 778-92.
163. Elkin, I., M. B. Parloff, S. W. Hadley, and J. H. Autry. "NIMH Treatment of Depression Collaborative Research Program. Background and Research Plan." *Archives of General Psychiatry* 42, no. 3 (March, 1985): 305-16.
164. Elkin, I., M. T. Shea, J. T. Watkins, S. D. Imber, S. M. Sotsky, J. F. Collins, D. R. Glass, *et al.* "National Institute of Mental Health Treatment of Depression Collaborative Research Program. General Effectiveness of Treatments." *Archives of General Psychiatry* 46, no. 11 (November, 1989): 971-82; discussion 83.
165. McKay, Kevin M., Zac E. Imel, and Bruce E. Wampold. "Psychiatrist Effects in the Psychopharmacological Treatment of Depression." *Journal of Affective Disorders* 92, no. 2-3 (June, 2006): 287-90.
166. Blatt, S. J., D. M. Quinlan, D. C. Zuroff, and P. A. Pilkonis. "Interpersonal Factors in Brief Treatment of Depression: Further Analyses of the National Institute of Mental Health Treatment of Depression Collaborative Research Program." *Journal of Consulting and Clinical Psychology* 64, no. 1 (February, 1996): 162-71.
167. Burns, D. D., and S. Nolen-Hoeksema. "Therapeutic Empathy and Recovery from Depression in Cognitive-Behavioral Therapy: A Structural Equation Model." *Journal of Consulting and Clinical Psychology* 60, no. 3 (June, 1992): 441-9.
168. Ilardi, Stephen S., and W. Edward Craighead. "The Role of Nonspecific Factors in Cognitive-Behavior Therapy for Depression." *Clinical Psychology: Science and Practice* 1, no. 2 (1994): 138-56.
169. Neumann, Melanie, Markus Wirtz, Elfriede Bollschweiler, Stewart W. Mercer, Mathias Warm, Jurgen Wolf, and Holger Pfaff. "Determinants and Patient-Reported Long-Term Outcomes of Physician Empathy in Oncology: A Structural Equation Modelling Approach." *Patient Education and Counseling* 69, no. 1-3 (December, 2007): 63-75.
170. Zachariae, R., C. G. Pedersen, A. B. Jensen, E. Ehrnrooth, P. B. Rossen, and H. von der Maase. "Association of Perceived Physician Communication Style with Patient Satisfaction, Distress, Cancer-Related Self-Efficacy, and Perceived Control over the Disease." *British Journal of Cancer* 88, no. 5 (March 10, 2003): 658-65.
171. Kaplan, Jessica E., Robert D. Keeley, Matthew Engel, Caroline Emsermann, and David Brody. "Aspects of Patient and Clinician Language Predict Adherence to Antidepressant Medication." *Journal of the American Board of Family Medicine* 26, no. 4 (July-August, 2013): 409-20.
172. Hollinger-Samson, N., and J. L. Pearson. "The Relationship between Staff Empathy and Depressive Symptoms in Nursing Home Residents." *Aging & Mental Health* 4, no. 1 (February 1, 2000): 56-65.

173. Brandriet, Lois M. "Changing Nurse Aide Behavior to Decrease Learned Helplessness in Nursing Home Elders." *Gerontology & Geriatrics Education* 16, no. 2 (May 3, 1996): 3-19.
174. van Osch, Mara, Milou Sep, Liesbeth M. van Vliet, Sandra van Dulmen, and Jozien M. Bensing. "Reducing Patients' Anxiety and Uncertainty, and Improving Recall in Bad News Consultations." *Health Psychology* 33, no. 11 (November, 2014): 1382-90.
175. Sep, Milou S. C., Mara van Osch, Liesbeth M. van Vliet, Ellen M. A. Smets, and Jozien M. Bensing. "The Power of Clinicians' Affective Communication: How Reassurance About Non-Abandonment Can Reduce Patients' Physiological Arousal and Increase Information Recall in Bad News Consultations. An Experimental Study Using Analogue Patients." *Patient Education and Counseling* 95, no. 1 (April, 2014): 45-52.
176. Verheul, William, Ariette Sanders, and Jozien Bensing. "The Effects of Physicians' Affect-Oriented Communication Style and Raising Expectations on Analogue Patients' Anxiety, Affect and Expectancies." *Patient Education and Counseling* 80, no. 3 (September, 2010): 300-6.
177. Lelorain, Sophie, Anne Bredart, Sylvie Dolbeault, and Serge Sultan. "A Systematic Review of the Associations between Empathy Measures and Patient Outcomes in Cancer Care." *Psycho-oncology* 21, no. 12 (December, 2012): 1255-64.
178. Roberts, C. S., C. E. Cox, D. S. Reintgen, W. F. Baile, and M. Gibertini. "Influence of Physician Communication on Newly Diagnosed Breast Patients' Psychologic Adjustment and Decision-Making." *Cancer* 74, supplement 1 (July 1, 1994): 336-41.
179. Mager, Wendy M., and Michael A. Andrykowski. "Communication in the Cancer 'Bad News' Consultation: Patient Perceptions and Psychological Adjustment." *Psycho-oncology* 11, no. 1 (January-February, 2002): 35-46.
180. "Adjustment to Cancer: Anxiety and Distress." National Cancer Institute accessed July 17, 2018, https://www.cancer.gov/about-cancer/coping/feelings/anxiety-distress-hp-pdq#section/_6.
181. Shanafelt, Tait D., Deborah A. Bowen, Chaya Venkat, Susan L. Slager, Clive S. Zent, Neil E. Kay, Megan Reinalda, *et al.* "The Physician-Patient Relationship and Quality of Life: Lessons from Chronic Lymphocytic Leukemia." *Leukemia Research* 33, no. 2 (February, 2009): 263-70.
182. Ong, L. M., M. R. Visser, F. B. Lammes, and J. C. de Haes. "Doctor-Patient Communication and Cancer Patients' Quality of Life and Satisfaction." *Patient Education and Counseling* 41, no. 2 (September, 2000): 145-56.
183. Spiegel, D., J. R. Bloom, and I. Yalom. "Group Support for Patients with Metastatic Cancer. A Randomized Outcome Study." *Archives of General Psychiatry* 38, no. 5 (May, 1981): 527-33.
184. Little, Paul, Peter White, Joanne Kelly, Hazel Everitt, and Stewart Mercer. "Randomised Controlled Trial of a Brief Intervention Targeting Predominantly Non-Verbal Communication in General Practice Consultations." *British Journal of General Practice* 65, no. 635 (June, 2015): e351-6.

185. Roter, D. L., J. A. Hall, D. E. Kern, L. R. Barker, K. A. Cole, and R. P. Roca. "Improving Physicians' Interviewing Skills and Reducing Patients' Emotional Distress. A Randomized Clinical Trial." *Archives of Internal Medicine* 155, no. 17 (September, 25 1995): 1877-84.
186. Mercer, Stewart W., Melanie Neumann, Markus Wirtz, Bridie Fitzpatrick, and Gaby Vojt. "General Practitioner Empathy, Patient Enablement, and Patient-Reported Outcomes in Primary Care in an Area of High Socio-Economic Deprivation in Scotland--a Pilot Prospective Study Using Structural Equation Modeling." *Patient Education and Counseling* 73, no. 2 (November, 2008): 240-5.
187. Roberts, Michael B., Lindsey J. Glaspey, Anthony Mazzarelli, Christopher W. Jones, Hope J. Kilgannon, Stephen Trzeciak, and Brian W. Roberts. "Early Interventions for the Prevention of Posttraumatic Stress Symptoms in Survivors of Critical Illness: A Qualitative Systematic Review." *Critical Care Medicine* 46, no. 8 (August, 2018): 1328-33.
188. Edmondson, Donald, Safiya Richardson, Jennifer K. Fausett, Louise Falzon, Virginia J. Howard, and Ian M. Kronish. "Prevalence of PTSD in Survivors of Stroke and Transient Ischemic Attack: A Meta-Analytic Review." *PLOS One* 8, no. 6 (2013): e66435.
189. Edmondson, Donald, Nina Rieckmann, Jonathan A. Shaffer, Joseph E. Schwartz, Matthew M. Burg, Karina W. Davidson, Lynn Clemow, Daichi Shimbo, and Ian M. Kronish. "Posttraumatic Stress Due to an Acute Coronary Syndrome Increases Risk of 42-Month Major Adverse Cardiac Events and All-Cause Mortality." *Journal of Psychiatric Research* 45, no. 12 (December, 2011): 1621-6.
190. Griffiths, John, Gillian Fortune, Vicki Barber, and J. Duncan Young. "The Prevalence of Post Traumatic Stress Disorder in Survivors of ICU Treatment: A Systematic Review." *Intensive Care Medicine* 33, no. 9 (September, 2007): 1506-18.
191. Barefoot, John C., Beverly H. Brummett, Redford B. Williams, Ilene C. Siegler, Michael J. Helms, Stephen H. Boyle, Nancy E. Clapp-Channing, and Daniel B. Mark. "Recovery Expectations and Long-Term Prognosis of Patients with Coronary Heart Disease." *Archives of Internal Medicine* 171, no. 10 (May 23, 2011): 929-35.
192. Mondloch, M. V., D. C. Cole, and J. W. Frank. "Does How You Do Depend on How You Think You'll Do? A Systematic Review of the Evidence for a Relation between Patients' Recovery Expectations and Health Outcomes." *CMAJ* 165, no. 2 (July 24, 2001): 174-9.
193. Schwartz, Kenneth B. "A Patient's Story." *The Boston Globe Magazine*, July 16, 1995.
194. Brody, Jane E. "The Cost of Not Taking Your Medicine." *New York Times*, April 17, 2017.
195. Nieuwlaat, Robby, Nancy Wilczynski, Tamara Navarro, Nicholas Hobson, Rebecca Jeffery, Arun Keepanasseril, Thomas Agoritsas, *et al.* "Interventions for Enhancing Medication Adherence." *Cochrane Database of Systemic Reviews*, no. 11 (November 20, 2014): CD000011.

196. Viswanathan, Meera, Carol E. Golin, Christine D. Jones, Mahima Ashok, Susan J. Blalock, Roberta C. M. Wines, Emmanuel J. L. Coker-Schwimmer, *et al.* "Interventions to Improve Adherence to Self-Administered Medications for Chronic Diseases in the United States: A Systematic Review." *Annals of Internal Medicine* 157, no. 11 (December 4, 2012): 785-95.
197. luga, Aurel O, and Maura J McGuire. "Adherence and Health Care Costs." *Risk Management and Healthcare Policy* 7 (2014): 35-44.
198. Zullig, Leah L., and Hayden Bosworth. "Engaging Patients to Optimize Medication Adherence." *NEJM Catalyst*, March 29, 2017.
199. Miller, Tricia A., and M. Robin Dimatteo. "Importance of Family/Social Support and Impact on Adherence to Diabetic Therapy." *Diabetes, Metabolic Syndrome and Obesity* 6 (November 6, 2013): 421-6.
200. DiMatteo, M. Robin. "Social Support and Patient Adherence to Medical Treatment: A Meta-Analysis." *Health Psychology* 23, no. 2 (March, 2004): 207-18.
201. Beach, Mary Catherine, Jeanne Keruly, and Richard D. Moore. "Is the Quality of the Patient-Provider Relationship Associated with Better Adherence and Health Outcomes for Patients with HIV?". *Journal of General Internal Medicine* 21, no. 6 (June, 2006): 661-5.
202. Flickinger, Tabor E., Somnath Saha, Debra Roter, P. Todd Korthuis, Victoria Sharp, Jonathan Cohn, Susan Eggly, Richard D. Moore, and Mary Catherine Beach. "Clinician Empathy Is Associated with Differences in Patient-Clinician Communication Behaviors and Higher Medication Self-Efficacy in HIV Care." *Patient Education and Counseling* 99, no. 2 (February, 2016): 220-6.
203. Zolnierek, Kelly B. Haskard, and M. Robin Dimatteo. "Physician Communication and Patient Adherence to Treatment: A Meta-Analysis." *Medical Care* 47, no. 8 (August, 2009): 826-34.
204. Hall, J. A., D. L. Roter, and N. R. Katz. "Meta-Analysis of Correlates of Provider Behavior in Medical Encounters." *Medical Care* 26, no. 7 (July, 1988): 657-75.
205. Slepian, Michael L., and James N. Kirby. "To Whom Do We Confide Our Secrets?" *Personality & Social Psychology Bulletin* 44, no. 7 (July, 2018): 1008-23.
206. Hibbard, Judith H., Jean Stockard, Eldon R. Mahoney, and Martin Tusler. "Development of the Patient Activation Measure (PAM): Conceptualizing and Measuring Activation in Patients and Consumers." *Health Services Research* 39, no. 4 pt. 1 (August, 2004): 1005-26.
207. Hibbard, Judith H., and Jessica Greene. "What the Evidence Shows About Patient Activation: Better Health Outcomes and Care Experiences; Fewer Data on Costs." *Health Affairs* 32, no. 2 (February, 2013): 207-14.
208. Heszen-Klemens, I., and E. Lapinska. "Doctor-Patient Interaction, Patients' Health Behavior and Effects of Treatment." *Social Science & Medicine* 19, no. 1 (1984): 9-18.
209. Howie, J. G., D. J. Heaney, M. Maxwell, J. J. Walker, G. K. Freeman, and H. Rai. "Quality at General Practice Consultations: Cross Sectional Survey." *BMJ* 319, no. 7212 (September 18, 1999): 738-43.

210. Bikker, Annemieke P., Stewart W. Mercer, and David Reilly. "A Pilot Prospective Study on the Consultation and Relational Empathy, Patient Enablement, and Health Changes over 12 Months in Patients Going to the Glasgow Homoeopathic Hospital." *Journal of Alternative and Complementary Medicine* 11, no. 4 (August, 2005): 591-600.
211. Mercer, Stewart W., Bhautesh D. Jani, Margaret Maxwell, Samuel Y. S. Wong, and Graham C. M. Watt. "Patient Enablement Requires Physician Empathy: A Cross-Sectional Study of General Practice Consultations in Areas of High and Low Socioeconomic Deprivation in Scotland." *BMC Family Practice* 13 (February 8, 2012): 6.
212. Bordin, Edward S. *The Generalizability of the Psychoanalytic Concept of the Working Alliance.* Vol. 16, 1979.
213. Fuertes, Jairo N., Laura S. Boylan, and Jessie A. Fontanella. "Behavioral Indices in Medical Care Outcome: The Working Alliance, Adherence, and Related Factors." *Journal of General Internal Medicine* 24, no. 1 (January, 2009): 80-5.
214. Bennett, Jennifer K., Jairo N. Fuertes, Merle Keitel, and Robert Phillips. "The Role of Patient Attachment and Working Alliance on Patient Adherence, Satisfaction, and Health-Related Quality of Life in Lupus Treatment." *Patient Education and Counseling* 85, no. 1 (October, 2011): 53-9.
215. Francis, V., B. M. Korsch, and M. J. Morris. "Gaps in Doctor-Patient Communication. Patients' Response to Medical Advice." *New England Journal of Medicine* 280, no. 10 (March 6, 1969): 535-40.
216. Kerse, Ngaire, Stephen Buetow, Arch G. Mainous III, Gregory Young, Gregor Coster, and Bruce Arroll. "Physician-Patient Relationship and Medication Compliance: A Primary Care Investigation." *Annals of Family Medicine* 2, no. 5 (September-October, 2004): 455-61.
217. Mahmoudian, Ahmad, Ahmadreza Zamani, Neda Tavakoli, Ziba Farajzadegan, and Fariba Fathollahi-Dehkordi. "Medication Adherence in Patients with Hypertension: Does Satisfaction with Doctor-Patient Relationship Work?" *Journal of Research in Medical Sciences* 22 (2017): 48.
218. Kahn, Katherine L., Eric C. Schneider, Jennifer L. Malin, John L. Adams, and Arnold M. Epstein. "Patient Centered Experiences in Breast Cancer: Predicting Long-Term Adherence to Tamoxifen Use." *Medical Care* 45, no. 5 (May, 2007): 431-9.
219. O'Malley, Ann S., Christopher B. Forrest, and Jeanne Mandelblatt. "Adherence of Low-Income Women to Cancer Screening Recommendations." *Journal of General Internal Medicine* 17, no. 2 (February, 2002): 144-54.
220. Frankl, Viktor. *Man's Search for Meaning.* Boston: Beacon Press, 1959.
221. Cohen, Randy, Chirag Bavishi, and Alan Rozanski. "Purpose in Life and Its Relationship to All-Cause Mortality and Cardiovascular Events: A Meta-Analysis." *Psychosomatic Medicine* 78, no. 2 (February-March, 2016): 122-33.

222. McKnight, Patrick E., and Todd B. Kashdan. "Purpose in Life as a System That Creates and Sustains Health and Well-Being: An Integrative, Testable Theory." *Review of General Psychology* 13, no. 3 (2009): 242-51.
223. Hill, Patrick L., and Nicholas A. Turiano. "Purpose in Life as a Predictor of Mortality across Adulthood." *Psychological Science* 25, no. 7 (Jul 2014): 1482-6.
224. Kim, Eric S., Jennifer K. Sun, Nansook Park, and Christopher Peterson. "Purpose in Life and Reduced Incidence of Stroke in Older Adults: 'The Health and Retirement Study'." *Journal of Psychosomatic Research* 74, no. 5 (May, 2013): 427-32.
225. Kim, Eric S., Jennifer K. Sun, Nansook Park, Laura D. Kubzansky, and Christopher Peterson. "Purpose in Life and Reduced Risk of Myocardial Infarction among Older U.S. Adults with Coronary Heart Disease: A Two-Year Follow-Up." *Journal of Behavioral Medicine* 36, no. 2 (April, 2013): 124-33.
226. Kim, Eric S., Ichiro Kawachi, Ying Chen, and Laura D. Kubzansky. "Association between Purpose in Life and Objective Measures of Physical Function in Older Adults." *JAMA Psychiatry* 74, no. 10 (October 1, 2017): 1039-45.
227. Kim, Eric S., Shelley D. Hershner, and Victor J Strecher. "Purpose in Life and Incidence of Sleep Disturbances." *Journal of Behavioral Medicine* 38, no. 3 (June, 2015): 590-7.
228. Kim, Eric S., Victor J. Strecher, and Carol D. Ryff. "Purpose in Life and Use of Preventive Health Care Services." *Proceedings of the National Academy of Sciences of the United States of America* 111, no. 46 (November 18, 2014): 16331-6.
229. Long, P., M. Abrams, A. Milstein, G. Anderson, K. Lewis Apton, M. Lund Dahlberg, and D. Whicher. *Effective Care for High-Need Patients: Opportunities for Improving Outcomes, Value, and Health.* Washington, DC: National Academy of Medicine, 2017.
230. McCarthy, Douglas, Jamie Ryan, and Sarah Klein. "Models of Care for High-Need, High-Cost Patients: An Evidence Synthesis." *Commonwealth Fund* 31, no. 1843 (2015).
231. Gawande, Atul. "The Hot Spotters: Can We Lower Medical Costs by Giving the Neediest Patients Better Care?" *New Yorker*, January 24, 2011, 40-51.
232. National Institute for Health Care Management. "The Concentration of U.S. Health Care Spending." Published online 2017.
233. National Academy of Medicine. "Crossing the Quality Chasm: The IOM Health Care Quality Initiative." news release, 2018, http://www.nationalacademies.org/hmd/Global/News%20Announcements/Crossing-the-Quality-Chasm-The-IOM-Health-Care-Quality-Initiative.aspx.
234. Batson, C. Daniel, Bruce D. Duncan, Paula Ackerman, Terese Buckley, and Kimberly Birch. "Is Empathic Emotion a Source of Altruistic Motivation?" *Journal of Personality and Social Psychology* 40, no. 2 (1981): 290-302.
235. Toi, Miho, and C. Daniel Batson. "More Evidence That Empathy Is a Source of Altruistic Motivation." *Journal of Personality and Social Psychology* 43, no. 2 (1982): 281-92.

236. West, Colin P., Angelina D. Tan, Thomas M. Habermann, Jeff A. Sloan, and Tait D. Shanafelt. "Association of Resident Fatigue and Distress with Perceived Medical Errors." *JAMA* 302, no. 12 (September 23, 2009): 1294-300.
237. West, Colin P., Mashele M. Huschka, Paul J. Novotny, Jeff A. Sloan, Joseph C. Kolars, Thomas M Habermann, and Tait D. Shanafelt. "Association of Perceived Medical Errors with Resident Distress and Empathy: A Prospective Longitudinal Study." *JAMA* 296, no. 9 (September 6, 2006): 1071-8.
238. Shanafelt, Tait D., Katharine A. Bradley, Joyce E. Wipf, and Anthony L. Back. "Burnout and Self-Reported Patient Care in an Internal Medicine Residency Program." *Annals of Internal Medicine* 136, no. 5 (March 5, 2002): 358-67.
239. Shanafelt, Tait D., Charles M. Balch, Gerald Bechamps, Tom Russell, Lotte Dyrbye, Daniel Satele, Paul Collicott, *et al.* "Burnout and Medical Errors among American Surgeons." *Annals of Surgery* 251, no. 6 (June, 2010): 995-1000.
240. Welp, Annalena, Laurenz L. Meier, and Tanja Manser. "The Interplay between Teamwork, Clinicians' Emotional Exhaustion, and Clinician-Rated Patient Safety: A Longitudinal Study." *Critical Care* 20, no. 1 (April 19, 2016): 110.
241. Dasan, Sunil, Poonam Gohil, Victoria Cornelius, and Cath Taylor. "Prevalence, Causes and Consequences of Compassion Satisfaction and Compassion Fatigue in Emergency Care: A Mixed-Methods Study of UK NHS Consultants." *Emergency Medicine Journal* 32, no. 8 (August, 2015): 588-94.
242. Sokol-Hessner, Lauge, Patricia Folcarelli, and Kenneth E. Sands. "The Practice of Respect." *NEJM Catalyst*, June 23, 2016.
243. Sokol-Hessner, Lauge, Patricia Henry Folcarelli, and Kenneth E. F. Sands. "Emotional Harm from Disrespect: The Neglected Preventable Harm." *BMJ Quality & Safety* 24, no. 9 (September, 2015): 550-3.
244. Casalino, Lawrence P., David Gans, Rachel Weber, Meagan Cea, Amber Tuchovsky, Tara F. Bishop, Yesenia Miranda, *et al.* "US Physician Practices Spend More Than $15.4 Billion Annually to Report Quality Measures." *Health Affairs* 35, no. 3 (March, 2016): 401-6.
245. Masso Guijarro, P., J. M. Aranaz Andres, J. J. Mira, E. Perdiguero, and C. Aibar. "Adverse Events in Hospitals: The Patient's Point of View." *Quality & Safety in Health Care* 19, no. 2 (April, 2010): 144-7.
246. Kuzel, Anton J., Steven H. Woolf, Valerie J. Gilchrist, John D. Engel, Thomas A. LaVeist, Charles Vincent, and Richard M. Frankel. "Patient Reports of Preventable Problems and Harms in Primary Health Care." *Annals of Family Medicine* 2, no. 4 (July-August, 2004): 333-40.
247. Ruben, Brent D. "What Patients Remember: A Content Analysis of Critical Incidents in Health Care." *Health Communication* 5, no. 2 (1993): 99-112.
248. Jackman, Tom. "Anesthesiologist Trashes Sedated Patient - and It Ends up Costing Her." *Washington Post*, June 23, 2015.
249. Burack, J. H., D. M. Irby, J. D. Carline, R. K. Root, and E. B. Larson. "Teaching Compassion and Respect. Attending Physicians' Responses to Problematic Behaviors." *Journal of General Internal Medicine* 14, no. 1 (January, 1999): 49-55.

250. Ogle, Jessica, John A. Bushnell, and Peter Caputi. "Empathy Is Related to Clinical Competence in Medical Care." *Medical Education* 47, no. 8 (August, 2013): 824-31.
251. van Vliet, Liesbeth M., Elsken van der Wall, Akke Albada, Peter M. M. Spreeuwenberg, William Verheul, and Jozien M. Bensing. "The Validity of Using Analogue Patients in Practitioner-Patient Communication Research: Systematic Review and Meta-Analysis." *Journal of General Internal Medicine* 27, no. 11 (November, 2012): 1528-43.
252. Kraft-Todd, Gordon T., Diego A. Reinero, John M. Kelley, Andrea S. Heberlein, Lee Baer, and Helen Riess. "Empathic Nonverbal Behavior Increases Ratings of Both Warmth and Competence in a Medical Context." *PLOS One* 12, no. 5 (2017): e0177758.
253. Chau, V. M., J. T. Engeln, S. Axelrath, S. J. Khatter, R. Kwon, M. A. Melton, M. C. Reinsvold, *et al.* "Beyond the Chief Complaint: Our Patients' Worries." *Journal of Medical Humanities* 38, no. 4 (December, 2017): 541-47.
254. Chau, Mimi. Personal communication to Stephen Trzeciak, December 1, 2017.
255. "NHE Projections 2017-2026 - Forecast Summary." Centers for Medicare & Medicaid Services. Updated August 1, 2018, accessed November 14, 2018, https://www.cms.gov/Research-Statistics-Data-and-Systems/Statistics-Trends-and-Reports/NationalHealthExpendData/Downloads/ForecastSummary.pdf.
256. Walker, Joseph. "Why Americans Spend So Much on Health Care-in 12 Charts." *Wall Street Journal*, July 31, 2018.
257. Sakowski, Julie Ann, James G. Kahn, Richard G. Kronick, Jeffrey M. Newman, and Harold S. Luft. "Peering into the Black Box: Billing and Insurance Activities in a Medical Group." *Health Affairs* 28, no. 4 (July-August, 2009): w544-54.
258. Kahn, James G., Richard Kronick, Mary Kreger, and David N. Gans. "The Cost of Health Insurance Administration in California: Estimates for Insurers, Physicians, and Hospitals." *Health Affairs* 24, no. 6 (November-December, 2005): 1629-39.
259. "How Has U.S. Spending on Healthcare Changed over Time?" The Peterson Center on Healthcare and the Kaiser Family Foundation, Updated December 20, 2017, accessed November 14, 2018, https://www.healthsystemtracker.org/chart-collection/u-s-spending-healthcare-changed-time/#item-administrative-costs-risen-time-recently-moderated_2017.
260. "50 of the Most Powerful People in Healthcare." Becker's Hospital Review. Updated January 3, 2014, accessed November 14, 2018, https://www.beckershospitalreview.com/lists/50-of-the-most-powerful-people-in-healthcare-2013.html.
261. Brill, Stephen. "Bitter Pill: Why Medical Bills Are Killing Us." *Time*, March 4, 2013.
262. "NHE Fact Sheet." Centers for Medical & Medicaid Services. Updated December 6, 2018, accessed November 14, 2018, https://www.cms.gov/research-statistics-data-and-systems/statistics-trends-and-reports/nationalhealthexpenddata/nhe-fact-sheet.html.
263. Comlossy, Megan, and Jacob Walden. "Silver Tsunami." *State Legislatures*, Vol. 39. No. 10. December 2013. pg. 14-19.

264. Smith, Mark, Robert Saunders, Leigh Stuckhardt, and J. Michael McGinnis, eds. *Best Care at Lower Cost: The Path to Continuously Learning Health Care in America.* Washington, DC: National Academies Press, 2013.
265. "Federal Subsidies for Health Insurance Coverage for People Under Age 65: 2017 to 2027." Congressional Budget Office. September 14, 2017.
266. Barnett, Jessica C., and Marina S. Vornovitsky. "Health Insurance Coverage in the United States: 2015." Washington, DC: Census Bureau.
267. Pugh, Tony. "Family Health Costs Outpace Inflation and Wage Growth." *McClatchy.* Published electronically September 15, 2009.
268. Bannow, Tara. "Not-for-Profit Hospital Downgrades Surged in 2017." *Modern Healthcare.* Published electronically March 6, 2018.
269. Moody's Investors Service. "Moody's - US NFP & Public Hospitals' Annual Medians Show Expense Growth Topping Revenues for Second Year." news release, August 28, 2018, https://www.moodys.com/research/Moodys-US-NFP-public-hospitals-annual-medians-show-expense-growth--PBM_1139331.
270. "What Is Patient Experience?" Agency for Healthcare Research and Quality. Updated March 2017, accessed November 14, 2018, http://www.ahrq.gov/cahps/about-cahps/patient-experience/index.html.
271. "About Z." accessed November 14, 2018, https://zdoggmd.com/about-z/.
272. ZDoggMD. "Doc Vader Vs. Patient Satisfaction Scores." https://www.youtube.com/watch?v=jjCu4nxOHlQ: YouTube, 2016.
273. Betts, David, Andreea Balan-Cohen, Maulesh Shukla, and Navneet Kumar. "The Value of Patient Experience: Hospitals with Better Patient-Reported Experience Perform Better Financially." Washington, DC: Deloitte Center for Health Solutions, 2016.
274. McClelland, Laura E., and Timothy J. Vogus. "Compassion Practices and HCAHPS: Does Rewarding and Supporting Workplace Compassion Influence Patient Perceptions?" *Health Services Research* 49, no. 5 (October, 2014): 1670-83.
275. Gregoire, Carolyn. "The Amazing Way This Hospital Is Fighting Physician Burnout." *Huffington Post.* Published electronically December 12, 2013.
276. Stone, Susan B. "Code Lavender: A Tool for Staff Support." *Nursing* 48, no. 4 (April, 2018): 15-17.
277. Centers for Medicare & Medicaid Services. "Hospital Value-Based Purchasing Fact Sheet." edited by Medicare Learning Network, 2017. https://www.cms.gov/Outreach-and-Education/Medicare-Learning-Network-MLN/MLNProducts/downloads/Hospital_VBPurchasing_Fact_Sheet_ICN907664.pdf.
278. Trzeciak, Stephen, John P. Gaughan, Joshua Bosire, Mark Angelo, Adam S. Holzberg, and Anthony J. Mazzarelli. "Association between Medicare Star Ratings for Patient Experience and Medicare Spending Per Beneficiary for US Hospitals." *Journal of Patient Experience* 4, no. 1 (March, 2017): 17-21.
279. "Doctors' Interpersonal Skills Are Valued More Than Training." *Wall Street Journal*, September 28, 2004.

280. Wen, Leana S., and Suhavi Tucker. "What Do People Want from Their Health Care? A Qualitative Study." *Journal for Participatory Medicine* 7, no. 10 (June 18, 2015).
281. Healthgrades. "Patient Sentiment Report: An Analysis of 7 Million Physician Reviews." 2018. https://www.healthgrades.com/content/patient-sentiment-report.
282. Menendez, Mariano E., Neal C. Chen, Chaitanya S. Mudgal, Jesse B. Jupiter, and David Ring. "Physician Empathy as a Driver of Hand Surgery Patient Satisfaction." *Journal of Hand Surgery* 40, no. 9 (September, 2015): 1860-5 e2.
283. Hojat, Mohammadreza, Daniel Z. Louis, Kaye Maxwell, Fred W. Markham, Richard C. Wender, and Joseph S. Gonnella. "A Brief Instrument to Measure Patients' Overall Satisfaction with Primary Care Physicians." *Family Medicine* 43, no. 6 (June, 2011): 412-7.
284. Comstock, L. M., E. M. Hooper, J. M. Goodwin, and J. S. Goodwin. "Physician Behaviors That Correlate with Patient Satisfaction." *Journal of Medical Education* 57, no. 2 (February, 1982): 105-12.
285. HealthTap. "Survey Reveals 85 Percent of Patients Choose Compassion over Pricing When Choosing a Doctor." news release, February 6, 2018, https://www.businesswire.com/news/home/20180206005704/en/Survey-Reveals-85-Percent-Patients-Choose-Compassion.
286. Van Den Bos, Jill, Karan Rustagi, Travis Gray, Michael Halford, Eva Ziemkiewicz, and Jonathan Shreve. "The $17.1 Billion Problem: The Annual Cost of Measurable Medical Errors." *Health Affairs* 30, no. 4 (April, 2011): 596-603.
287. Shreve, Jon, Jill Van Den Bos, Travis Gray, Michael Halford, Karan Rustagi, and Eva Ziemkiewicz. "The Economic Measurement of Medical Errors." Society of Actuaries, 2012.
288. Andel, Charles, Stephen L. Davidow, Mark Hollander, and David A. Moreno. "The Economics of Health Care Quality and Medical Errors." *Journal of Health Care Finance* 39, no. 1 (Fall 2012): 39-50.
289. Stewart, M., J. B. Brown, A. Donner, I. R. McWhinney, J. Oates, W. W. Weston, and J. Jordan. "The Impact of Patient-Centered Care on Outcomes." *Journal of Family Practice* 49, no. 9 (September, 2000): 796-804.
290. Bertakis, Klea D., and Rahman Azari. "Patient-Centered Care Is Associated with Decreased Health Care Utilization." *Journal of the American Board of Family Medicine* 24, no. 3 (May-June, 2011): 229-39.
291. Epstein, Ronald M., Peter Franks, Cleveland G. Shields, Sean C. Meldrum, Katherine N. Miller, Thomas L. Campbell, and Kevin Fiscella. "Patient-Centered Communication and Diagnostic Testing." *Annals of Family Medicine* 3, no. 5 (September-October, 2005): 415-21.
292. Little, P., H. Everitt, I. Williamson, G. Warner, M. Moore, C. Gould, K. Ferrier, and S. Payne. "Observational Study of Effect of Patient Centredness and Positive Approach on Outcomes of General Practice Consultations." *BMJ* 323, no. 7318 (October 20, 2001): 908-11.

293. Barsade, Sigal G., and Olivia A. O'Neill. "What's Love Got to Do with It? A Longitudinal Study of the Culture of Companionate Love and Employee and Client Outcomes in a Long-Term Care Setting." 59, no. 4 (2014): 551-98.
294. Gleichgerrcht, Ezequiel, and Jean Decety. "Empathy in Clinical Practice: How Individual Dispositions, Gender, and Experience Moderate Empathic Concern, Burnout, and Emotional Distress in Physicians." *PLOS One* 8, no. 4 (2013): e61526.
295. American Psychological Association. "Psychologically Healthy Workplace Program Fact Sheet: By the Numbers." 2008. http://www.phwa.org/dl/phwp_fact_sheet.pdf.
296. American Psychological Association. "Stress in America." 2007. http://apahelpcenter.mediaroom.com/file.php/138/Stress+in+America+REPORT+FINAL.doc.
297. Bureau of Labor Statistics. "Number and Percent Distribution of Nonfatal Occupational Injuries and Illnesses Involving Days Away from Work by Nature of Injury or Illness and Number of Days Away from Work." 2001. http://www.bls.gov/iif/oshwc/osh/case/ostb1222.pdf.
298. Rosch, P. J. *The Quandary of Job Stress Compensation.*Health & Stress. Vol. 3, 2001.
299. Seppälä, Emma. *The Happiness Track.* San Francisco: HarperOne, 2016.
300. Seppälä, Emma. "Why Compassion in Business Makes Sense." *Greater Good Science Center.* Published online April 15, 2013.
301. Peckham, Carol. "Medscape National Physician Burnout & Depression Report." Medscape (2018).
302. Young, Aaron, Humayun J. Chaudhry, Xiaomei Pei, Katie Arnhart, Michael Dugan, and Gregory B. Snyder. "A Census of Actively Licensed Physicians in the United States, 2016." *Journal of Medical Regulation* 103, no. 2 (2017): 7-21.
303. American Medical Association. "Creating the Organizational Foundation for Joy in Medicine." https://edhub.ama-assn.org/steps-forward/module/2702510.
304. Richter, Ruthann. "In a First for U.S. Academic Medical Center, Stanford Medicine Hires Chief Physician Wellness Officer." news release, June 22, 2017, https://med.stanford.edu/news/all-news/2017/06/stanford-medicine-hires-chief-physician-wellness-officer.html.
305. Shanafelt, Tait D., Joel Goh, and Christine A. Sinsky. "The Business Case for Investing in Physician Well-Being." *JAMA Internal Medicine* 177, no. 12 (December 1, 2017): 1826-32.
306. Shanafelt, Tait D., Michelle Mungo, Jaime Schmitgen, Kristin A. Storz, David Reeves, Sharonne N. Hayes, Jeff A. Sloan, Stephen J. Swensen, and Steven J. Buskirk. "Longitudinal Study Evaluating the Association between Physician Burnout and Changes in Professional Work Effort." *Mayo Clinic Proceedings* 91, no. 4 (2016): 422-31.
307. Mello, Michelle M., Amitabh Chandra, Atul A. Gawande, and David M. Studdert. "National Costs of the Medical Liability System." *Health Affairs* 29, no. 9 (September, 2010): 1569-77.
308. Bal, B. Sonny. "An Introduction to Medical Malpractice in the United States." *Clinical Orthopaedics and Related Research* 467, no. 2 (February, 2009): 339-47.

309. Harvard Medical Practice Study. "Patients, Doctors, and Lawyers: Medical Injury, Malpractice Litigation, and Patient Compensation in New York: The Report of the Harvard Medical Practice Study to the State of New York." Cambridge, 1990.
310. Studdert, D. M., E. J. Thomas, H. R. Burstin, B. I. Zbar, E. J. Orav, and T. A. Brennan. "Negligent Care and Malpractice Claiming Behavior in Utah and Colorado." *Medical Care* 38, no. 3 (March, 2000): 250-60.
311. Weiler, Paul C., Howard Hiatt, Joseph P. Newhouse, Troyen Brennan, and Lucian Leape. *A Measure of Malpractice: Medical Injury, Malpractice Litigation, and Patient Compensation.* Cambridge: Harvard University Press, 1993.
312. Beckman, H. B., K. M. Markakis, A. L. Suchman, and R. M. Frankel. "The Doctor-Patient Relationship and Malpractice. Lessons from Plaintiff Depositions." *Archives of Internal Medicine* 154, no. 12 (June 27, 1994): 1365-70.
313. Hickson, G. B., E. W. Clayton, S. S. Entman, C. S. Miller, P. B. Githens, K. Whetten-Goldstein, and F. A. Sloan. "Obstetricians' Prior Malpractice Experience and Patients' Satisfaction with Care." *JAMA* 272, no. 20 (November 23-30, 1994): 1583-7.
314. Slawson, P. F. "Psychiatric Malpractice: Some Aspects of Cause." *Psychiatric Hospital* 15, no. 3 (Summer 1984): 141-4.
315. Lieberman, J.A. *The Litigious Society.* New York: Basic Books, 1985.
316. Friedman, L. *Total Justice.* New York: Russel Sage, 1985.
317. Eisenberg, H. "New Light on the Costliest Malpractice Mistakes." *Journal of Medical Economics* 16 (1973): 146-50.
318. Hicks, R. G. "Ounces of Prevention. I." *New York State Journal of Medicine* 73, no. 18 (September 15, 1973): 2268-9.
319. Vincent, C., M. Young, and A. Phillips. "Why Do People Sue Doctors? A Study of Patients and Relatives Taking Legal Action." *Lancet* 343, no. 8913 (June 25, 1994): 1609-13.
320. Moore, P. J., N. E. Adler, and P. A. Robertson. "Medical Malpractice: The Effect of Doctor-Patient Relations on Medical Patient Perceptions and Malpractice Intentions." *Western Journal of Medicine* 173, no. 4 (October, 2000): 244-50.
321. "Emergency Medical Treatment & Labor Act (EMTALA)." Updated March 26, 2012, accessed November 14, 2018, https://www.cms.gov/Regulations-and-Guidance/Legislation/EMTALA/.
322. Redelmeier, D. A., J. P. Molin, and R. J. Tibshirani. "A Randomised Trial of Compassionate Care for the Homeless in an Emergency Department." *Lancet* 345, no. 8958 (May 6, 1995): 1131-4.
323. Riess, Helen, John M. Kelley, Robert W. Bailey, Emily J. Dunn, and Margot Phillips. "Empathy Training for Resident Physicians: A Randomized Controlled Trial of a Neuroscience-Informed Curriculum." *Journal of General Internal Medicine* 27, no. 10 (October, 2012): 1280-6.
324. Bylund, Carma L., and Gregory Makoul. "Examining Empathy in Medical Encounters: An Observational Study Using the Empathic Communication Coding System." *Health Communication* 18, no. 2 (2005): 123-40.

325. Dempsey, Christina. *The Antidote to Suffering: How Compassionate Connected Care Can Improve Safety, Quality, and Experience.* New York: McGraw-Hill Education, 2017.
326. Mogilner, Cassie, Zoe Chance, and Michael I. Norton. "Giving Time Gives You Time." *Psychological Science* 23, no. 10 (October 1, 2012): 1233-8.
327. Youngson, Robin. *Time to Care: How to Love Your Patients and Your Job.* Scotts Valley: CreateSpace, 2012.
328. Youngson, Robin. "Practising Compassion in an Uncompassionate Health System." *Hearts in Healthcare.* Published electronically September 1, 2017.
329. Sturtevant, A. H. "A New Inherited Character in Man." *Proceedings of the National Academy of Sciences of the United States of America* 26, no. 2 (February 15, 1940): 100-2.
330. Hullinger, Jessica. "Tongue Rolling and 5 Other Oversimplified Genetic Traits." *Mental Floss.* Published electronically March 18, 2015.
331. Brown, Brené. *I Thought It Was Just Me: Women Reclaiming Power and Courage in a Culture of Shame.* New York: Gotham, 2007.
332. Maguire, E. A., D. G. Gadian, I. S. Johnsrude, C. D. Good, J. Ashburner, R. S. Frackowiak, and C. D. Frith. "Navigation-Related Structural Change in the Hippocampi of Taxi Drivers." *Proceedings of the National Academy of Sciences of the United States of America* 97, no. 8 (April 11, 2000): 4398-403.
333. Gladwell, Malcolm. *Outliers: The Story of Success.* New York: Little, Brown and Company, 2008.
334. TED. "The Habits of Happiness." https://www.ted.com/talks/matthieu_ricard_on_the_habits_of_happiness?language=en, 2004.
335. Goleman, Daniel, and Richard J. Davidson. *Altered Traits: Science Reveals How Meditation Changes Your Mind, Brain, and Body.* New York: Avery, 2017.
336. Lutz, Antoine, Lawrence L. Greischar, Nancy B. Rawlings, Matthieu Ricard, and Richard J. Davidson. "Long-Term Meditators Self-Induce High-Amplitude Gamma Synchrony During Mental Practice." *Proceedings of the National Academy of Sciences of the United States of America* 101, no. 46 (November 16, 2004): 16369-73.
337. Engen, Haakon G., Boris C. Bernhardt, Leon Skottnik, Matthieu Ricard, and Tania Singer. "Structural Changes in Socio-Affective Networks: Multi-Modal MRI Findings in Long-Term Meditation Practitioners." *Neuropsychologia* 116, pt. A (July 31, 2018): 26-33.
338. Leung, Mei-Kei, Chetwyn C. H. Chan, Jing Yin, Chack-Fan Lee, Kwok-Fai So, and Tatia M. C. Lee. "Increased Gray Matter Volume in the Right Angular and Posterior Parahippocampal Gyri in Loving-Kindness Meditators." *Social Cognitive and Affective Neuroscience* 8, no. 1 (January, 2013): 34-9.
339. Weng, Helen Y., Andrew S. Fox, Alexander J. Shackman, Diane E. Stodola, Jessica Z. K. Caldwell, Matthew C. Olson, Gregory M. Rogers, and Richard J. Davidson. "Compassion Training Alters Altruism and Neural Responses to Suffering." *Psychological Science* 24, no. 7 (July 1, 2013): 1171-80.

340. Rodrigues, Sarina M., Laura R. Saslow, Natalia Garcia, Oliver P. John, and Dacher Keltner. "Oxytocin Receptor Genetic Variation Relates to Empathy and Stress Reactivity in Humans." *Proceedings of the National Academy of Sciences of the United States of America* 106, no. 50 (December 15, 2009): 21437-41.
341. Huetter, Franz Korbinian, Hagen Sjard Bachmann, Anette Reinders, Doris Siffert, Patrick Stelmach, Dietmar Knop, Peter Alexander Horn, and Winfried Siffert. "Association of a Common Oxytocin Receptor Gene Polymorphism with Self-Reported 'Empathic Concern' in a Large Population of Healthy Volunteers." *PLOS One* 11, no. 7 (2016): e0160059.
342. Gong, Pingyuan, Huiyong Fan, Jinting Liu, Xing Yang, Kejin Zhang, and Xiaolin Zhou. "Revisiting the Impact of Oxtr Rs53576 on Empathy: A Population-Based Study and a Meta-Analysis." *Psychoneuroendocrinology* 80 (2017): 131-36.
343. Smith, R. C., J. S. Lyles, J. A. Mettler, A. A. Marshall, L. F. Van Egeren, B. E. Stoffelmayr, G. G. Osborn, and V. Shebroe. "A Strategy for Improving Patient Satisfaction by the Intensive Training of Residents in Psychosocial Medicine: A Controlled, Randomized Study." *Academic Medicine* 70, no. 8 (August, 1995): 729-32.
344. Ekman, Paul, and Eve Ekman. "Is Global Compassion Achieveable?" In *Oxford Handbook of Compassion Science*, edited by Emma M. Seppälä, Emiliana Simon-Thomas, Stephanie L. Brown, Monica C. Worline, C. Daryl Cameron and James R. Doty. Oxford: Oxford University Press, 2017.
345. English, Bella. "At MGH, Schooling Doctors in the Power of Empathy." *Boston Globe*, August 15, 2015.
346. Teding van Berkhout, Emily, and John M Malouff. "The Efficacy of Empathy Training: A Meta-Analysis of Randomized Controlled Trials." *Journal of Counseling Psychology* 63, no. 1 (January, 2016): 32-41.
347. Kelm, Zak, James Womer, Jennifer K. Walter, and Chris Feudtner. "Interventions to Cultivate Physician Empathy: A Systematic Review." *BMC Medical Education* 14 (October 14, 2014): 219.
348. Satterfield, Jason M., and Ellen Hughes. "Emotion Skills Training for Medical Students: A Systematic Review." *Medical Education* 41, no. 10 (October, 2007): 935-41.
349. Batt-Rawden, Samantha A., Margaret S. Chisolm, Blair Anton, and Tabor E. Flickinger. "Teaching Empathy to Medical Students: An Updated, Systematic Review." *Academic Medicine* 88, no. 8 (August, 2013): 1171-7.
350. Razavi, D., N. Delvaux, S. Marchal, J. F. Durieux, C. Farvacques, L. Dubus, and R. Hogenraad. "Does Training Increase the Use of More Emotionally Laden Words by Nurses When Talking with Cancer Patients? A Randomised Study." *British Journal of Cancer* 87, no. 1 (July 1, 2002): 1-7.
351. Gholamzadeh, Sakineh, Maryam Khastavaneh, Zahra Khademian, and Soraya Ghadakpour. "The Effects of Empathy Skills Training on Nursing Students' Empathy and Attitudes toward Elderly People." *BMC Medical Education* 18, no. 1 (August 15 ,2018): 198.

352. Wu, Li-Min, Chi-Chun Chin, and Chung-Hey Chen. "Evaluation of a Caring Education Program for Taiwanese Nursing Students: A Quasi-Experiment with Before and After Comparison." *Nurse Education Today* 29, no. 8 (November, 2009): 873-8.

353. Bas-Sarmiento, Pilar, Martina Fernandez-Gutierrez, Maria Baena-Banos, and Jose Manuel Romero-Sanchez. "Efficacy of Empathy Training in Nursing Students: A Quasi-Experimental Study." *Nurse Education Today* 59 (December, 2017): 59-65.

354. Kelley, John M., Gordon Kraft-Todd, Lidia Schapira, Joe Kossowsky, and Helen Riess. "The Influence of the Patient-Clinician Relationship on Healthcare Outcomes: A Systematic Review and Meta-Analysis of Randomized Controlled Trials." *PLOS One* 9, no. 4 (2014): e94207.

355. Chadwick, Kristen. "Study Confirms Impact of Clinician-Patient Relationship on Health Outcomes." news release, April 9, 2014, https://www.massgeneral.org/News/pressrelease.aspx?id=1691.

356. Dweck, Carol S. *Mindset: The New Psychology of Success.* New York: Ballantine Books, 2008.

357. Schumann, Karina, Jamil Zaki, and Carol S. Dweck. "Addressing the Empathy Deficit: Beliefs About the Malleability of Empathy Predict Effortful Responses When Empathy Is Challenging." *Journal of Personality and Social Psychology* 107, no. 3 (September, 2014): 475-93.

358. Weinstein, Netta, and Richard M. Ryan. "When Helping Helps: Autonomous Motivation for Prosocial Behavior and Its Influence on Well-Being for the Helper and Recipient." *Journal of Personality and Social Psychology* 98, no. 2 (February, 2010): 222-44.

359. American Psychiatric Association. *Diagnostic and Statistical Manual of Mental Disorders, 5th Edition.* Philadelphia: American Psychiatric Association, 2013.

360. Liu, T. T., and T. C. Hsu. "Tongue-Folding and Tongue-Rolling in a Sample of the Chinese Population." *Journal of Heredity* 40, no. 1 (January, 1949): 19-21.

361. Martin, N. G. "No Evidence for a Genetic Basis of Tongue Rolling or Hand Clasping." *Journal of Heredity* 66, no. 3 (1975): 179-80.

362. Matlock, P. "Identical Twins Discordant in Tongue-Rolling." *Journal of Heredity* 43, no. 24 (1952).

363. Komai, T. "Notes on Lingual Gymnastics: Frequency of Tongue Rollers and Pedigrees of Tied Tongues in Japan." *Journal of Heredity* 42 (1951): 293-97.

364. Woods, Catherine. "Debunking the Biggest Genetic Myth of the Human Tongue." *PBS News Hour.* Published electronically August 5, 2015.

365. Salyers, Michelle P., Kelsey A. Bonfils, Lauren Luther, Ruth L. Firmin, Dominique A. White, Erin L. Adams, and Angela L. Rollins. "The Relationship between Professional Burnout and Quality and Safety in Healthcare: A Meta-Analysis." *Journal of General Internal Medicine* 32, no. 4 (April, 2017): 475-82.

366. Tawfik, Daniel S., Jochen Profit, Timothy I. Morgenthaler, Daniel V. Satele, Christine A. Sinsky, Liselotte N. Dyrbye, Michael A. Tutty, Colin P. West, and Tait D. Shanafelt. "Physician Burnout, Well-Being, and Work Unit Safety Grades

in Relationship to Reported Medical Errors." *Mayo Clinic Proceedings* 93, no. 11 (November, 2018): 1571-80.

367. Makary, Martin A., and Michael Daniel. "Medical Error-the Third Leading Cause of Death in the US." *BMJ* 353 (May 3, 2016): i2139.
368. Dyrbye, Lotte N., Tait D. Shanafelt, Christine A. Sinsky, Pamela F. Cipriano, Jay Bhatt, Alexander Ommaya, Colin West, and David Meyers. *Burnout Among Health Care Professionals: A Call to Explore and Address This Underrecognized Threat to Safe, High-Quality Care.* Vol. 7, 2017.
369. Xu, Rena. "The Burnout Crisis in American Medicine." *The Atlantic*, May 11, 2018.
370. Mukherjee, Siddhartha "For Doctors, Delving Deeper as a Way to Avoid Burnout." *New York Times Magazine*, October 10, 2018.
371. Lagnado, Lucette. "Hospitals Address Widespread Doctor Burnout." *Wall Street Journal*, June 9, 2018.
372. Schernhammer, Eva S., and Graham A. Colditz. "Suicide Rates among Physicians: A Quantitative and Gender Assessment (Meta-Analysis)." *American Journal of Psychiatry* 161, no. 12 (December, 2004): 2295-302.
373. Anderson, Pauline. "Physicians Experience Highest Suicide Rate of Any Profession." *Medscape Medical News*. Published electronically May 7, 2018.
374. Davidson, Judy, Janet Mendis, Amy R. Stuck, Gianni DeMichele, and Sidney Zisook. *Nurse Suicide: Breaking the Silence.* Vol. 8, 2018.
375. Goodman, Michael and Michele Berlinerblau. "Discussion: Treating Burnout by Addressing Its Causes." *American Association for Physician Leadership*. Published electronically January 5, 2018.
376. Gawande, Atul. "Why Doctors Hate Their Computers." *The New Yorker*, November 12, 2018.
377. Seppälä, Emma, and Marissa King. "Burnout at Work Isn't Just About Exhaustion. It's Also About Loneliness." *Harvard Business Review*, June 29, 2017.
378. West, Colin P., Liselotte N. Dyrbye, Patricia J. Erwin, and Tait D. Shanafelt. "Interventions to Prevent and Reduce Physician Burnout: A Systematic Review and Meta-Analysis." *Lancet* 388, no. 10,057 (November 5, 2016): 2272-81.
379. Panagioti, Maria, Efharis Panagopoulou, Peter Bower, George Lewith, Evangelos Kontopantelis, Carolyn Chew-Graham, Shoba Dawson, *et al.* "Controlled Interventions to Reduce Burnout in Physicians: A Systematic Review and Meta-Analysis." *JAMA Internal Medicine* 177, no. 2 (February 1, 2017): 195-205.
380. Wilkinson, Helen, Richard Whittington, Lorraine Perry, and Catrin Eames. "Examining the Relationship between Burnout and Empathy in Healthcare Professionals: A Systematic Review." *Burnout Research* 6 (September, 2017): 18-29.
381. TEDWomen. "Compassion and the True Meaning of Empathy." https://www.ted.com/talks/joan_halifax: TED.com, 2010.
382. Vigen, Tyler. *Spurious Correlations.* New York: Hachette, 2015.
383. Vigen, Tyler. "Divorce Rate in Maine Correlates with Per Capita Consumption of Margarine." 2018, http://tylervigen.com/spurious-correlations.
384. Kim, Kristen. "To Feel or Not to Feel: Empathy and Physician Burnout." *Academic Psychiatry* 42, no. 1 (February, 2018): 157-58.

385. Thirioux, Berangere, Francois Birault, and Nematollah Jaafari. "Empathy Is a Protective Factor of Burnout in Physicians: New Neuro-Phenomenological Hypotheses Regarding Empathy and Sympathy in Care Relationship." *Frontiers in Psychology* 7 (2016): 763.
386. Atkins, P. W. B. "Empathy, Self-Other Differentiation and Mindfulness." In *Organizing through Empathy* edited by K. Pavlovich and K. Krahnke, 49-70. New York: Routledge, 2013.
387. Decety, Jean, and Claus Lamm. "Human Empathy through the Lens of Social Neuroscience." *Scientific World Journal* 6 (September 20, 2006): 1146-63.
388. Singer, Tania, and Olga M. Klimecki. "Empathy and Compassion." *Current Biology* 24, no. 18 (September 22, 2014): R875-R78.
389. Gillihan, Seth J., "Why Does Compassion Feel So Good? Here Are Five Reasons," *Think, Act, Be*, February 1, 2018, https://www.psychologytoday.com/us/blog/think-act-be/201802/why-does-compassion-feel-so-good-here-are-five-reasons.
390. Luks, Allen. "Doing Good: Helper's High." *Psychology Today* 22, no. 10 (1998): 39-42.
391. Raposa, Elizabeth B., Holly B. Laws, and Emily B. Ansell. "Prosocial Behavior Mitigates the Negative Effects of Stress in Everyday Life." *Clinical Psychological Science* 4, no. 4 (July, 2016): 691-98.
392. Schacter, Hannah L. "Teens Who Feel Down May Benefit from Picking Others Up." *The Conversation*. Published electronically August 24, 2018.
393. Mor, Nilly, and Jennifer Winquist. "Self-Focused Attention and Negative Affect: A Meta-Analysis." *Psychological Bulletin* 128, no. 4 (July, 2002): 638-62.
394. Shamay-Tsoory, Simone, and Claus Lamm. "The Neuroscience of Empathy - from Past to Present and Future." *Neuropsychologia* 116, pt. A (July 31, 2018): 1-4.
395. Stellar, Jennifer E., Adam Cohen, Christopher Oveis, and Dacher Keltner. "Affective and Physiological Responses to the Suffering of Others: Compassion and Vagal Activity." *Journal of Personality and Social Psychology* 108, no. 4 (April, 2015): 572-85.
396. Brown, Stephanie L., and R. Michael Brown. "Connecting Prosocial Behavior to Improved Physical Health: Contributions from the Neurobiology of Parenting." *Neuroscience and Biobehavioral Reviews* 55 (August, 2015): 1-17.
397. Cosley, Brandon J., Shannon K. McCoy, Laura R. Saslow, and Elissa S. Epel. "Is Compassion for Others Stress Buffering? Consequences of Compassion and Social Support for Physiological Reactivity to Stress." *Journal of Experimental Social Psychology* 46, no. 5 (2010): 816-23.
398. Pace, Thaddeus W. W., Lobsang Tenzin Negi, Daniel D. Adame, Steven P. Cole, Teresa I. Sivilli, Timothy D. Brown, Michael J. Issa, and Charles L. Raison. "Effect of Compassion Meditation on Neuroendocrine, Innate Immune and Behavioral Responses to Psychosocial Stress." *Psychoneuroendocrinology* 34, no. 1 (January, 2009): 87-98.
399. Weng, Helen Y., Regina C. Lapate, Diane E. Stodola, Gregory M. Rogers, and Richard J. Davidson. "Visual Attention to Suffering after Compassion Training Is

Associated with Decreased Amygdala Responses." *Frontiers in Psychology* 9 (2018): 771.
400. Engen, Haakon G., and Tania Singer. "Compassion-Based Emotion Regulation up-Regulates Experienced Positive Affect and Associated Neural Networks." *Social Cognitive and Affective Neuroscience* 10, no. 9 (September, 2015): 1291-301.
401. Hutcherson, Cendri A., Emma M. Seppala, and James J. Gross. "Loving-Kindness Meditation Increases Social Connectedness." *Emotion* 8, no. 5 (October, 2008): 720-4.
402. Seppälä, Emma M., Cendri A. Hutcherson, Dong T. H. Nguyen, James R. Doty, and James J. Gross. "Loving-Kindness Meditation: A Tool to Improve Healthcare Provider Compassion, Resilience, and Patient Care." *Journal of Compassionate Health Care* 1, no. 1 (December 19, 2014): 5.
403. Jazaieri, Hooria, Kelly McGonigal, Ihno A. Lee, Thupten Jinpa, James R. Doty, James J. Gross, and Philippe R. Goldin. "Altering the Trajectory of Affect and Affect Regulation: The Impact of Compassion Training." *Mindfulness* 9, no. 1 (February 1, 2018): 283-93.
404. Jazaieri, Hooria, Kelly McGonigal, Thupten Jinpa, James R. Doty, James J. Gross, and Philippe R. Goldin. "A Randomized Controlled Trial of Compassion Cultivation Training: Effects on Mindfulness, Affect, and Emotion Regulation." *Motivation and Emotion* 38, no. 1 (February 1, 2014): 23-35.
405. Mongrain, Myriam, Jacqueline M. Chin, and Leah B. Shapira. "Practicing Compassion Increases Happiness and Self-Esteem." *Journal of Happiness Studies* 12, no. 6 (December 1, 2011): 963-81.
406. Fredrickson, Barbara L., Michael A. Cohn, Kimberly A. Coffey, Jolynn Pek, and Sandra M. Finkel. "Open Hearts Build Lives: Positive Emotions, Induced through Loving-Kindness Meditation, Build Consequential Personal Resources." *Journal of Personality and Social Psychology* 95, no. 5 (November, 2008): 1045-62.
407. James Kirby Homepage. http://jameskirby.com.au/.
408. Tei, S., C. Becker, R. Kawada, J. Fujino, K. F. Jankowski, G. Sugihara, T. Murai, and H. Takahashi. "Can We Predict Burnout Severity from Empathy-Related Brain Activity?". *Translational Psychiatry* 4 (June 3, 2014): e393.
409. Shanafelt, Tait D., Colin West, Xinghua Zhao, Paul Novotny, Joseph Kolars, and Thomas Habermann. "Relationship between Increased Personal Well-Being and Enhanced Empathy among Internal Medicine Residents." *Journal of General Internal Medicine* 20, no. 7 (July, 2005): 559-64.
410. Thomas, Matthew R., Liselotte N. Dyrbye, Jefrey L. Huntington, Karen L. Lawson, Paul J. Novotny, Jeff A. Sloan, and Tait D. Shanafelt. "How Do Distress and Well-Being Relate to Medical Student Empathy? A Multicenter Study." *Journal of General Internal Medicine* 22, no. 2 (February, 2007): 177-83.
411. Lamothe, Martin, Emilie Boujut, Franck Zenasni, and Serge Sultan. "To Be or Not to Be Empathic: The Combined Role of Empathic Concern and Perspective Taking in Understanding Burnout in General Practice." *BMC Family Practice* 15 (January 23, 2014): 15.

412. Bourgault, Patricia, Stephan Lavoie, Emilie Paul-Savoie, Maryse Gregoire, Cecile Michaud, Emilie Gosselin, and Celeste C. Johnston. "Relationship between Empathy and Well-Being among Emergency Nurses." *Journal of Emergency Nursing* 41, no. 4 (July, 2015): 323-8.
413. Krasner, Michael S., Ronald M. Epstein, Howard Beckman, Anthony L. Suchman, Benjamin Chapman, Christopher J. Mooney, and Timothy E. Quill. "Association of an Educational Program in Mindful Communication with Burnout, Empathy, and Attitudes among Primary Care Physicians." *JAMA* 302, no. 12 (September 23, 2009): 1284-93.
414. Mascaro, Jennifer S., Sean Kelley, Alana Darcher, Lobsang Tenzin Negi, Carol Worthman, Andrew Miller, and Charles Raison. "Meditation Buffers Medical Student Compassion from the Deleterious Effects of Depression." *The Journal of Positive Psychology* 13, no. 2 (March 4, 2018): 133-42.
415. McClelland, Laura E., Allison S. Gabriel, and Matthew J. DePuccio. "Compassion Practices, Nurse Well-Being, and Ambulatory Patient Experience Ratings." *Medical Care* 56, no. 1 (January, 2018): 4-10.
416. Mineo, Liz. "Good Genes Are Nice, but Joy Is Better." *Harvard Gazette*, April 11, 2017.
417. Hojat, Mohammadreza, Michael Vergare, Gerald Isenberg, Mitchell Cohen, and John Spandorfer. "Underlying Construct of Empathy, Optimism, and Burnout in Medical Students." *International Journal of Medical Education* 6 (January 29, 2015): 12-6.
418. Brazeau, Chantal M. L. R., Robin Schroeder, Sue Rovi, and Linda Boyd. "Relationships between Medical Student Burnout, Empathy, and Professionalism Climate." *Academic Medicine* 85, no. 10 (October, 2010): S33-6.
419. Zenasni, Franck, E. Boujut, Bluffel du Vaure, A. Catu-Pinault, J.L. Tavani, L. Rigal, P. Jaury, *et al.* "Development of a French-Language Version of the Jefferson Scale of Physician Empathy and Association with Practice Characteristics and Burnout in a Sample of General Practitioners." *International Journal of Person Centered Medicine* 2, no. 4 (June 12, 2012): 8.
420. Wiens, Kandi, and Annie McKee. "Why Some People Get Burned out and Others Don't." *Harvard Business Review*, November 23, 2016.
421. McKee, Annie, and Kandi Wiens. "Prevent Burnout by Making Compassion a Habit." *Harvard Business Review*, May 11, 2017.
422. Wiens, Kandi. "Leading through Burnout: The Influence of Emotional Intelligence on the Ability of Executive Level Physician Leaders to Cope With Occupational Stress and Burnout." Doctoral dissertation, 2016.
423. Chen, Kuan-Yu, Che-Ming Yang, Che-Hui Lien, Hung-Yi Chiou, Mau-Roung Lin, Hui-Ru Chang, and Wen-Ta Chiu. "Burnout, Job Satisfaction, and Medical Malpractice among Physicians." *International Journal of Medical Sciences* 10, no. 11 (2013): 1471-8.
424. Weng, Hui-Ching, Chao-Ming Hung, Yi-Tien Liu, Yu-Jen Cheng, Cheng-Yo Yen, Chi-Chang Chang, and Chih-Kun Huang. "Associations between Emotional

Intelligence and Doctor Burnout, Job Satisfaction and Patient Satisfaction." *Medical Education* 45, no. 8 (August, 2011): 835-42.
425. Derksen, Frans, Jozien Bensing, Sascha Kuiper, Milou van Meerendonk, and Antoine Lagro-Janssen. "Empathy: What Does It Mean for GPs? A Qualitative Study." *Family Practice* 32, no. 1 (February, 2015): 94-100.
426. Gleichgerrcht, Ezequiel, and Jean Decety. "The Relationship between Different Facets of Empathy, Pain Perception and Compassion Fatigue among Physicians." *Frontiers in Behavioral Neuroscience* 8 (2014): 243.
427. Wright, S. M., D. E. Kern, K. Kolodner, D. M. Howard, and F. L. Brancati. "Attributes of Excellent Attending-Physician Role Models." *New England Journal of Medicine* 339, no. 27 (December 31, 1998): 1986-93.
428. Neff, Kristin. *Self-Compassion.* New York: William Morrow, 2011.
429. Neff, Kristin. "Definition of Self-Compassion." 2018, accessed November 3, 2018, https://self-compassion.org/the-three-elements-of-self-compassion-2/.
430. Kirby, James N. "I Was Working with a 17 Year Old Male on Compassion. Asked Him to Consider 5 Different Scenarios Where Failure Was Experienced. On Left Is What What He Would Say to a Friend. On Right What He'd Say to Himself. Devastating. #365daysofcompassion." Twitter, August 1, 2018. https://twitter.com/JamesNKirby/status/1024641468705595393.
431. Tirch, Dennis. "Compassion Isn't About Negating or Rejecting Undesirable Thought or Feelings Like Self-Criticism or Shame. It's About Extending Validation, Warmth and Caring to Them, Witnessing Them, & Recognizing Where They're Coming From. The Same as We Would to a Friend Who Was Suffering." Twitter, November 16, 2018. https://twitter.com/DennisTirchPhD/status/1063538458549985280.
432. TEDxPenn. "How 40 Seconds of Compassion Could Save a Life." https://youtu.be/elW69hyPUuI: YouTube.
433. Peabody, Francis W. "The Care of the Patient." *JAMA* 88 (March 19, 1927): 877-82.
434. Mazzarelli, Anthony. "Annals Story Slam - Humanism in Medical Education." *Annals of Internal Medicine* 166, no. 7 (2017): SS1.

ADDITIONAL RESOURCES:

About Huron:

Huron is a global consultancy that helps our clients drive growth, enhance performance, and sustain leadership in the markets they serve. We partner with them to develop strategies and implement solutions that enable the transformative change our clients need to own their future.

Learn more at www.huronconsultinggroup.com

About Studer Group, a Huron solution:

A recipient of the 2010 Malcolm Baldrige National Quality Award, Studer Group is an outcomes-based healthcare performance improvement firm that partners with healthcare organizations in the United States, Canada, and beyond, teaching them how to achieve, sustain, and accelerate exceptional clinical, operational, and financial results.

Working with Huron, we help to get the foundation right so organizations can build a sustainable culture that promotes accountability, fosters innovation, and consistently delivers a great patient experience and the best quality outcomes over time.

To learn more about Studer Group, visit www.studergroup.com or call 850-439-5839.

Coaching:

Studer Group coaches work with healthcare leaders to create an aligned culture accountable to achieving outcomes together. Working side-by-side, we help to establish, accelerate, and hardwire the necessary changes to create a culture of excellence. This leads to better transparency, higher accountability, and the ability to target and execute specific, objective results that organizations want to achieve.

Studer Group offers coaching based on organizational needs: Evidence-Based Leadership^{SM}, Health System, Emergency Department, Medical Group, and Rural Healthcare.

Learn more about Studer Group coaching by visiting www.studergroup.com/coaching.

Conferences:

Huron and Studer Group offer interactive learning events throughout the year that provide a fresh perspective from industry-leading keynote speakers and focused sessions that share evidence-based methods to improve consistency, reduce variance, increase engagement, and create highly profitable organizations. They also provide networking opportunities with colleagues and experts and help participants learn new competencies needed to continuously improve the quality and experience of patient-centered care.

Most learning events offer continuing education credits. Find out more about upcoming conferences and register at www.studergroup.com/conferences.

Speaking:

From large association events to exclusive executive training, Studer Group speakers deliver the perfect balance of inspiration and education for every audience. As experienced clinicians and administrators, each speaker has a unique journey to share filled with expertise on a variety of healthcare topics.

This personal touch along with hard-hitting healthcare improvement tactics empower your team to take action.

Learn more about Studer Group speakers by visiting www.studergroup.com/speaking.

Publishing:

Studer Group offers practical, purpose-driven books that help healthcare professionals develop the skills they need to improve and sustain results across their organizations. For over 15 years, our resources have addressed industry challenges, elevate care delivery, and provide solutions for quality patient experience.

With more than two million publications in circulation across the United States, Canada, Australia, New Zealand, China, and Japan, we are a trusted source for proven tactics and tools to help improve employee engagement, build leadership skills, and improve channels of communication.

Explore our catalog of resources by visiting www.publishing.studergroup.com.

ABOUT THE AUTHORS:

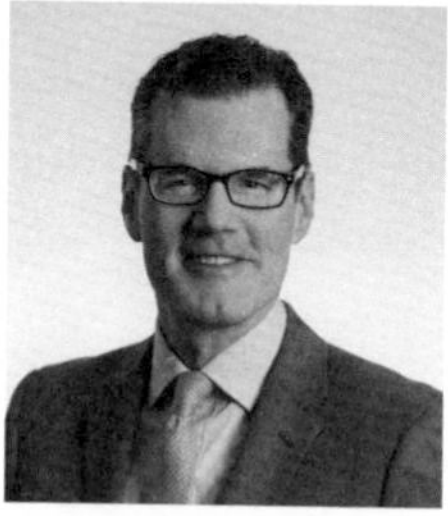

Stephen Trzeciak, MD, MPH is a physician scientist, professor and chair of medicine at Cooper Medical School of Rowan University, and the chief of medicine at Cooper University Health Care. Dr. Trzeciak is a practicing intensivist (specialist in intensive care medicine), and a National Institutes of Health (NIH)-funded clinical researcher with more than 100 publications in the scientific literature, primarily in the field of resuscitation science. Dr. Trzeciak's publications have been featured in some of the most prestigious medical journals, such as: Journal of the American Medical Association (JAMA), Circulation, and The New England Journal of Medicine. His scientific program has been supported by research grants from the American Heart Association and the NIH (National Institute of General Medical Sciences and the National Heart, Lung, and Blood Institute), with Dr. Trzeciak serving in the role of Principal Investigator.

Dr. Trzeciak is a graduate of the University of Notre Dame. He earned his medical degree at the University of Wisconsin-Madison, and his Masters in Public Health at the University of Illinois at Chicago. He completed his residency training at the University of Illinois at Chicago Medical Center, and his fellowship training in critical care medicine at Rush University Medical Center in Chicago. He is board-certified in internal medicine, emergency medicine, critical care medicine, and neurocritical care.

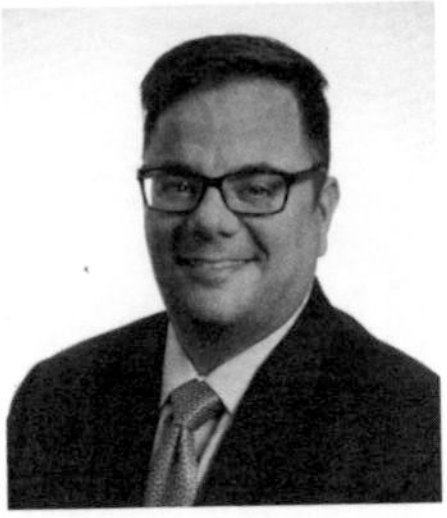

Anthony Mazzarelli, MD, JD, MBE is co-president of Cooper University Health Care and the associate dean of clinical affairs for Cooper Medical School of Rowan University. Prior to his current role, Dr. Mazzarelli served as Cooper's chief physician executive where he oversaw the physician practice, as well as quality/ patient safety and continuous process improvement efforts for the health system, the same topics for which he teaches within the medical school and residency programs. Dr. Mazzarelli has been named one of the 50 most powerful people in New Jersey health care by NJ Biz and was awarded the Halo Award for leading a team of health care providers from Cooper into Haiti in the days immediately following the 2010 earthquake. Dr. Mazzarelli has also received numerous commendations for his leadership and he speaks regularly on several local and national media outlets.

Dr. Mazzarelli received his medical degree from Robert Wood Johnson Medical School, his law degree from University of Pennsylvania Law School, and his master's degree in bioethics from the Perelman School of Medicine at the University of Pennsylvania. He trained in emergency medicine at Cooper University Hospital, where he also served as chief resident. He is board-certified in emergency medicine, and is actively practicing in the emergency department at Cooper.

About Cooper University Health Care and Cooper Medical School of Rowan University

Cooper University Health Care is the leading academic health system in southern New Jersey, and one of the most trusted health systems in the region. Located on the Health Sciences Campus in Camden, New Jersey, Cooper University Hospital is an academic, tertiary care medical center that is the academic affiliate for Cooper Medical School of Rowan University. Cooper is southern New Jersey's only Level I trauma center, and has one of the region's leading cancer centers, MD Anderson Cancer Center at Cooper. Cooper has over 100 ambulatory care locations throughout southern

New Jersey and Pennsylvania, with more than 1.4 million outpatient visits annually, and a 650-physician multi-specialty employed faculty practice plan.

Since Cooper is the only tertiary care academic health system in southern New Jersey and a regional referral center, Drs. Trzeciak, Mazzarelli, and their colleagues are fortunate to be able to take care of an incredible array of fascinating and complex patients.